Diagnosis and Treatment of Fungal Chest Infections

Editors

EVA M. CARMONA
ANDREW H. LIMPER

CLINICS IN
CHEST MEDICINE

www.chestmed.theclinics.com

September 2017 • Volume 38 • Number 3

ELSEVIER

1600 John F. Kennedy Boulevard • Suite 1800 • Philadelphia, Pennsylvania, 19103-2899

http://www.theclinics.com

CLINICS IN CHEST MEDICINE Volume 38, Number 3
September 2017 ISSN 0272-5231, ISBN-13: 978-0-323-54546-4

Editor: Katie Pfaff
Developmental Editor: Casey Potter

Clinics in Chest Medicine (ISSN 0272-5231) is published quarterly by Elsevier Inc., 360 Park Avenue South, New York, NY 10010-1710. Months of issue are March, June, September, and December. Periodicals postage paid at New York, NY and additional mailing offices. Subscription prices are $352.00 per year (domestic individuals), $652.00 per year (domestic institutions), $100.00 per year (domestic students/residents), $388.00 per year (Canadian individuals), $810.00 per year (Canadian institutions), $479.00 per year (international individuals), $810.00 per year (international institutions), and $230.00 per year (international and Canadian students/residents). International air speed delivery is included in all Clinics subscription prices. All prices are subject to change without notice. **POSTMASTER:** Send address changes to Clinics in Chest Medicine, Elsevier Health Sciences Division, Subscription Customer Service, 3251 Riverport Lane, Maryland Heights, MO 63043. **Customer Service: Telephone: 1-800-654-2452** (U.S. and Canada); **1-314-447-8871** (outside U.S. and Canada). **Fax: 1-314-447-8029. E-mail: journalscustomerservice-usa@elsevier.com (for print support); journalsonlinesupport-usa@elsevier.com (for online support).**

Reprints. For copies of 100 or more of articles in this publication, please contact the Commercial Reprints Department, Elsevier Inc., 360 Park Avenue South, New York, NY 10010-1710. Tel.: 212-633-3874; Fax: 212-633-3820; E-mail: reprints@elsevier.com.

Clinics in Chest Medicine is covered in *MEDLINE/PubMed (Index Medicus), Current Contents/Clinical Medicine, EMBASE/ Excerpta Medica, Science Citation Index*, and *ISI/BIOMED*.

Contributors

EDITORS

EVA M. CARMONA, MD, PhD
Thoracic Diseases Research Unit, Division of
Pulmonary Critical Care and Internal Medicine,
Assistant Professor, Department of Medicine,
Mayo Clinic, Rochester, Minnesota, USA

ANDREW H. LIMPER, MD
Thoracic Diseases Research Unit, Division of
Pulmonary Critical Care and Internal Medicine,
Professor, Department of Medicine, Mayo
Clinic College of Medicine & Science, Mayo
Clinic, Rochester, Minnesota, USA

AUTHORS

SANA ARIF, MB,BS
Instructor of Medicine, Division of Infectious
Diseases, Duke University Medical Center,
Durham, North Carolina, USA

MARWAN M. AZAR, MD
Fellow in Microbiology, Pathology Department,
Massachusetts General Hospital, Harvard
School of Medicine, Boston, Massachusetts,
USA

CASSANDRA M. BATZLAFF, MD
Instructor in Medicine, Thoracic Diseases
Research Unit, Division of Pulmonary Critical
Care and Internal Medicine, Mayo Clinic
College of Medicine, Mayo Clinic, Rochester,
Minnesota, USA

EVA M. CARMONA, MD, PhD
Thoracic Diseases Research Unit, Division of
Pulmonary Critical Care and Internal Medicine,
Assistant Professor, Department of Medicine,
Mayo Clinic, Rochester, Minnesota, USA

RACHEL CHASAN, MD, MPH
Division of Infectious Diseases, Icahn School of
Medicine at Mount Sinai, Mount Sinai Hospital,
New York, New York, USA

OLEG EPELBAUM, MD, FACP
Division of Pulmonary, Critical Care, and
Sleep Medicine, Westchester Medical
Center, New York Medical College, Valhalla,
New York, USA

SCOTT E. EVANS, MD, FCCP
Associate Professor, Division of Internal
Medicine, Department of Pulmonary Medicine,
The University of Texas MD Anderson Cancer
Center, Houston, Texas, USA

LUKE M. GABE, MD
Division of Pulmonary, Allergy, Critical
Care and Sleep Medicine, University of
Arizona College of Medicine – Tucson, Tucson,
Arizona, USA

GREGORY M. GAUTHIER, MD
Associate Professor, Division of Infectious
Disease, Department of Medicine, University of
Wisconsin School of Medicine and Public
Health, Madison, Wisconsin, USA

CHADI A. HAGE, MD, FCCP
Associate Professor of Clinical Medicine,
Indiana University, Thoracic Transplantation
Program, Indiana University Health,
Indianapolis, Indiana, USA

LAURENCE HUANG, MD
Department of Medicine, University of
California, San Francisco San Francisco,
California, USA

SHAUNNA HUSTON, PhD
Department of Physiology and Pharmacology,
Health Research Innovation Centre, University
of Calgary, Calgary, Alberta, Canada

CASSIE C. KENNEDY, MD
Assistant Professor of Medicine, Division of Pulmonary and Critical Care Medicine, William J. von Liebig Center for Transplantation and Clinical Regeneration, Robert D. and Patricia E. Kern Center for the Science of Health Care Delivery, Mayo Clinic, Rochester, Minnesota, USA

BRUCE S. KLEIN, MD
Professor, Division of Infectious Disease, Departments of Medicine, Pediatrics, and Medical Microbiology and Immunology, University of Wisconsin School of Medicine and Public Health, Madison, Wisconsin, USA

KENNETH S. KNOX, MD
Division of Pulmonary, Allergy, Critical Care and Sleep Medicine, University of Arizona College of Medicine – Tucson, Tucson, Arizona, USA

MIGUEL M. LEIVA JUAREZ, MD
Postdoctoral Fellow, Division of Internal Medicine, Department of Pulmonary Medicine, The University of Texas MD Anderson Cancer Center, Houston, Texas, USA

ANDREW H. LIMPER, MD
Thoracic Diseases Research Unit, Division of Pulmonary Critical Care and Internal Medicine, Professor, Department of Medicine, Mayo Clinic College of Medicine, Mayo Clinic, Rochester, Minnesota, USA

JOSHUA MALO, MD
Division of Pulmonary, Allergy, Critical Care and Sleep Medicine, University of Arizona College of Medicine – Tucson, Tucson, Arizona, USA

JOSEPH A. McBRIDE, MD
Fellow, Division of Infectious Disease, Departments of Medicine and Pediatrics, University of Wisconsin School of Medicine and Public Health, Madison, Wisconsin, USA

ROBERT F. MILLER, MBBS, CBiol, FRSB, FRCP
Research Department of Infection and Population Health, Institute of Global Health, University College London, Faculty of Infectious and Tropical Diseases, Department of Clinical Research, London School of Hygiene and Tropical Medicine, London, United Kingdom

CHRISTOPHER H. MODY, MD
Departments of Microbiology and Infectious Diseases and Internal Medicine, Health Research Innovation Centre, University of Calgary, Calgary, Alberta, Canada

EAVAN G. MULDOON, MD, MPH
National Aspergillosis Centre, University Hospital of South Manchester, Division of Infection, Immunity and Respiratory Medicine, University of Manchester, Manchester, United Kingdom

KAREN C. PATTERSON, MD
Assistant Professor, Division of Pulmonary, Allergy and Critical Care, University of Pennsylvania, Philadelphia, Pennsylvania, USA

JOHN R. PERFECT, MD
Professor of Medicine, Chair, Division of Infectious Diseases, Duke University Medical Center, Durham, North Carolina, USA

POORNIMA RAMANAN, MD
Clinical Microbiology Fellow, Division of Clinical Microbiology, Department of Laboratory Medicine and Pathology, Mayo Clinic, Rochester, Minnesota, USA

RAYMUND R. RAZONABLE, MD
Professor of Medicine, Division of Infectious Diseases, William J. von Liebig Center for Transplantation and Clinical Regeneration, Mayo Clinic, Rochester, Minnesota, USA

KATE SKOLNIK, MD
Division of Respirology, Department of Internal Medicine, Rockyview General Hospital, University of Calgary, Calgary, Alberta, Canada

MARY E. STREK, MD
Section of Pulmonary and Critical Care, Department of Medicine, The University of Chicago, Chicago, Illinois, USA

ELITZA S. THEEL, PhD
Laboratory Director, Infectious Diseases Serology, Division of Clinical Microbiology, Assistant Professor, Department of Laboratory Medicine and Pathology, Mayo Clinic, Rochester, Minnesota, USA

RICHARD J. WANG, MD
Department of Medicine, University of California San Francisco, San Francisco, California, USA

NANCY L. WENGENACK, PhD
Laboratory Director, Mycology and
Mycobacteriology, Division of Clinical
Microbiology, Professor, Department of
Laboratory Medicine and Pathology, Mayo
Clinic, Rochester, Minnesota, USA

ALISHA Y. YOUNG, MD
Clinical Fellow, Division of Pulmonary,
Critical Care and Sleep Medicine,
Department of Internal Medicine, The
University of Texas Health Sciences Center at
Houston, Houston, Texas, USA

Contents

Fungal infections are an important and increasingly prevalent cause of disease in certain patient populations. These infections can occur both in immune-compromised and immune-competent individuals. Because the number of patients who are immunocompromised is steadily growing, it is vital for clinicians to consider fungal disease in the differential diagnosis of these patients. This article reviews the epidemiology and approach to diagnosis of a variety of fungal infections.

Invasive fungal diseases cause high morbidity and mortality in an immunocompromised host. Antifungals are the drugs of choice and can be divided into 4 main groups: polyenes, azoles, echinocandins, and pyrimidine analogues. Each class has its specific mechanism of action, spectrum of activity, and pharmacokinetic and side effects. It is important to understand the precise use of the established and new antifungal agents to successfully manage these complex infections in an already tenuous and frail host. This article discusses the main characteristics, clinical uses, and secondary effects of the main antifungals used in clinical practice.

With increasing numbers of travelers and immunocompromised patients, histoplasmosis, caused by the dimorphic fungus *Histoplasma capsulatum*, has become a disease of national extent. The clinical spectrum of histoplasmosis is very wide, in terms of disease cadence, onset, distribution, and severity. A multipronged approach is recommended for diagnosis. Manifestations that are always treated include moderate to severe acute pulmonary histoplasmosis, disseminated disease, and histoplasmosis in immunocompromised individuals. Amphotericin B is the drug of choice for moderate to severe and disseminated presentations, whereas itraconazole is appropriate for mild disease and as step-down therapy.

Coccidioidomycosis is a leading cause of community-acquired pneumonia within its traditional endemic zone in the Southwestern United States and portions of Mexico and Central and South America. Its incidence has increased dramatically within the endemic region; its presence outside of the region, facilitated by a mobile society, is also now substantial. Although only a fraction of the incident disease progresses beyond subclinical illness, this proportion is large in absolute terms and causes substantial disease burden. Diagnosis often depends on serologic interpretation. Treatment has been revolutionized by azole therapy. Controversy remains regarding the decision to treat in less severe disease.

The causal agents of blastomycosis, *Blastomyces dermatitidis* and *Blastomyces gilchristii*, belong to a group of thermally dimorphic fungi that can infect healthy and immunocompromised individuals. Following inhalation of mycelial fragments and spores into the lungs, *Blastomyces* spp convert into pathogenic yeast and evade host immune defenses to cause pneumonia and disseminated disease. The clinical spectrum of pulmonary blastomycosis is diverse. The diagnosis of blastomycosis requires a high degree of clinical suspicion and involves culture-based and non–culture-based fungal diagnostic tests. The site and severity of infection, and the presence of underlying immunosuppression or pregnancy, influence the selection of antifungal therapy.

Cryptococcus is among the most common invasive fungal pathogens globally and is one of the leading causes of acquired immunodeficiency virus-related deaths. *Cryptococcus neoformans* and *Cryptococcus gattii* are the most clinically relevant species and account for most cryptococcal disease. Pulmonary manifestations can range from mild symptoms to life-threatening infection. Treatment is tailored based on the severity of pulmonary infection, the presence of disseminated or central nervous system disease, and patient immune status. Amphotericin B and flucytosine followed by fluconazole remain the standard agents for the treatment of severe cryptococcal infection.

Many fungi cause pulmonary disease in patients with human immunodeficiency virus (HIV) infection. Pathogens include *Pneumocystis jirovecii*, *Cryptococcus neoformans*, *Aspergillus* spp, *Histoplasma capsulatum*, *Coccidioides* spp, *Blastomyces dermatitidis*, *Paracoccidioides brasiliensis*, *Talaromyces marneffei*, and *Emmonsia* spp. Because symptoms are frequently nonspecific, a high index of suspicion for fungal infection is required for diagnosis. Clinical manifestations of fungal infection in HIV-infected patients frequently depend on the degree of immunosuppression and the CD4$^+$ helper T cell count. Establishing definitive diagnosis is important because treatments differ. Primary and secondary prophylaxes depend on CD4$^+$ helper T cell counts, geographic location, and local prevalence of disease.

Fungal pneumonias cause unacceptable morbidity among patients with hematologic malignancies (HM) and recipients of hematopoietic stem cell transplantation (HSCT). The high incidence of fungal pneumonias in HM/HSCT populations arises from their frequently severe, complex, and persistent immune dysfunction caused by the underlying disease and its treatment. The cytopenias, treatment toxicities, and other immune derangements that make patients susceptible to fungal pneumonia frequently complicate its diagnosis and increase the intensity and duration of antifungal therapy. This article addresses the host factors that contribute to susceptibility, summarizes diagnostic recommendations, and reviews current guidelines for management of fungal pneumonia in patients with HM/HSCT.

Candidemia presents several challenges to the intensive care unit (ICU) community. Recognition and treatment of this infection is frequently delayed, with dramatic clinical deterioration and death often preceding the detection of Candida in blood cultures. Identification of individual patients at the highest risk for developing candidemia remains an imperfect science; the role of antifungal therapy before culture diagnosis is yet to be fully defined in the ICU. The absence of well-established molecular techniques for early detection of candidemia hinders efforts to reduce the heavy clinical and economic impact of this infection. Echinocandins are the recommended antifungal drug class for the treatment of ICU candidemia.

Infection remains a significant source of morbidity and mortality after lung transplant, including fungal infection. Various antifungal prophylactic agents are administered for a variable duration after transplant with the goal of preventing invasive fungal infections. Alternatively, some programs target the use of antifungal agents only in those colonized with Aspergillus spp. Despite prophylaxis or preemptive therapy, a significant number of invasive fungal infections occur after lung transplant. Risk factors for fungal infections include single lung transplant, pretransplant Aspergillus colonization, environmental risks, structural lung disease such as cystic fibrosis, augmented immunosuppression, sinus disease, and use of indwelling airway stents.

Aspergillus spp are ubiquitous in the environment, and inhalation of Aspergillus spores is unavoidable. An intact immune system, with normal airway function, protects most people from disease. Globally, however, the toll from aspergillosis is high. The literature has largely focused on invasive aspergillosis, yet the burden in terms of chronicity and prevalence is higher for noninvasive Aspergillus conditions. This article discusses allergic aspergilloses and provides an update on the diagnosis and management of allergic bronchopulmonary aspergillosis, including in patients with cystic fibrosis, and an update on severe asthma with fungal sensitization. In addition, the presentation, investigation, and management of noninvasive infectious aspergilloses are reviewed.

This article reviews the current diagnostic approaches, both serologic and molecular, for the detection of fungi associated with pulmonary disease. Classic serologic techniques, including immunodiffusion and complement fixation, both of which remain a cornerstone for fungal diagnostic testing, are reviewed and their performance characteristics presented. More recent advances in this field, including novel lateral-flow assays for fungal antigen detection, are also described. Molecular techniques for fungal identification both from culture and directly from patient specimens, including nucleic acid probes, mass spectrometry–based methods, nucleic acid amplification testing, and traditional and broad-range sequencing, are discussed and their performance evaluated.

Emergence of the Molds Other than *Aspergillus* in Immunocompromised Patients 555

Sana Arif and John R. Perfect

Immunocompromised patients are at high risk for invasive fungal infections (IFIs); although *Aspergillus* remains the most common IFI caused by molds, other fungi, such as Mucorales, dematiaceous molds, and *Fusarium* spp, are being seen with increasing frequency. Presentations can vary, but sinopulmonary and disseminated infections are common. Our understanding of the pathogenesis of these infections is rudimentary. Fungal cultures and histopathology remain the backbone of diagnostics, as no good serologic markers are available. Polymerase chain reaction tests are being developed but currently remain investigational. Management of these infections is usually multidisciplinary, requiring surgical debridement along with antifungal therapy.

PROGRAM OBJECTIVE

The goal of the *Clinics in Chest Medicine* is to provide provide practitioners with state-of-the-art information that is clinically useful, concise, well referenced, and comprehensive.

TARGET AUDIENCE

All practicing physicians and healthcare professionals who provide patient care utilizing findings from *Chest Medicine Clinics of North America*.

LEARNING OBJECTIVES

Upon completion of this activity, participants will be able to:
1. Review the diagnosis and management of fungal chest infections.
2. Discuss fungal infections of the chest in special populations.
3. Recognize trends in the diagnosis and management of fungal chest infections.

ACCREDITATION

The Elsevier Office of Continuing Medical Education (EOCME) is accredited by the Accreditation Council for Continuing Medical Education (ACCME) to provide continuing medical education for physicians.

The EOCME designates this enduring material for a maximum of 15 *AMA PRA Category 1 Credit*(s)™. Physicians should claim only the credit commensurate with the extent of their participation in the activity.

All other healthcare professionals requesting continuing education credit for this enduring material will be issued a certificate of participation.

DISCLOSURE OF CONFLICTS OF INTEREST

The EOCME assesses conflict of interest with its instructors, faculty, planners, and other individuals who are in a position to control the content of CME activities. All relevant conflicts of interest that are identified are thoroughly vetted by EOCME for fair balance, scientific objectivity, and patient care recommendations. EOCME is committed to providing its learners with CME activities that promote improvements or quality in healthcare and not a specific proprietary business or a commercial interest.

The planning committee, staff, authors and editors listed below have identified no financial relationships or relationships to products or devices they or their spouse/life partner have with commercial interest related to the content of this CME activity:
Sana Arif, MB,BS; Marwan M. Azar, MD; Casandra M. Batzlaff, MD; Eva M. Carmona, MD, PhD; Rachel Chasan, MD, MPH; Oleg Epelbaum, MD, FACP; Anjali Fortna; Luke M. Gabe, MD; Gregory M. Gauthier, MD; Chadi A. Hage, MD, FCCP; Laurence Huang, MD; Shaunna Huston, PhD; Cassie C. Kennedy, MD; Bruce S. Klein, MD; Kenneth S. Knox, MD; Miguel M. Leiva Juarez, MD; Andrew H. Limper, MD; Joshua Malo, MD; Joseph A. McBride, MD; Christopher H. Mody, MD; Eavan G. Muldoon, MD, MPH; Karen C. Patterson, MD; Katie Pfaff; Poornima Ramanan, MD; Raymund R. Razonable, MD; Kate Skolnik, MD; Mary E. Strek, MD; Elitza S. Theel, PhD; Richard J. Wang, MD; Nancy L. Wengenack, PhD; Katie Widmeier; Amy Williams; Alisha Y. Young, MD.

The planning committee, staff, authors and editors listed below have identified financial relationships or relationships to products or devices they or their spouse/life partner have with commercial interest related to the content of this CME activity:
Scott E. Evans, MD, FCCP has stock ownership in Pulmotect, Inc.
Robert F. Miller, MBBS, CBiol, FRSB, FRCP is on the speakers' bureau for Gilead; Merck & Co., Inc.; Jannssen Pharmaceutical Companies of Johnson & Johnson; and ViiV Healthcare group of companies.
John R. Perfect, MD is a consultant/advisor for Astellas Pharma Inc.; Merck & Co., Inc.; Viamet Pharmaceuticals, Inc; Vical Inc.; Cidara Therapeutics, Inc.; and Synexis, LLC, and had research support from Pfizer Inc.

UNAPPROVED/OFF-LABEL USE DISCLOSURE

The EOCME requires CME faculty to disclose to the participants:
1. When products or procedures being discussed are off-label, unlabelled, experimental, and/or investigational (not US Food and Drug Administration [FDA] approved); and
2. Any limitations on the information presented, such as data that are preliminary or that represent ongoing research, interim analyses, and/or unsupported opinions. Faculty may discuss information about pharmaceutical agents that is outside of FDA-approved labelling. This information is intended solely for CME and is not intended to promote off-label use of these medications. If you have any questions, contact the medical affairs department of the manufacturer for the most recent prescribing information.

TO ENROLL

To enroll in the *Chest Medicine Clinics* Continuing Medical Education program, call customer service at 1-800-654-2452 or sign up online at http://www.theclinics.com/home/cme. The CME program is available to subscribers for an additional annual fee of USD $225.

METHOD OF PARTICIPATION

In order to claim credit, participants must complete the following:

1. Complete enrolment as indicated above.
2. Read the activity.
3. Complete the CME Test and Evaluation. Participants must achieve a score of 70% on the test. All CME Tests and Evaluations must be completed online.

CME INQUIRIES/SPECIAL NEEDS

For all CME inquiries or special needs, please contact elsevierCME@elsevier.com

CLINICS IN CHEST MEDICINE

THE CLINICS ARE AVAILABLE ONLINE!
Access your subscription at:
www.theclinics.com

Preface

Diagnosis and Treatment of Fungal Chest Infections

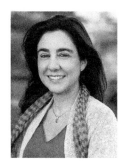   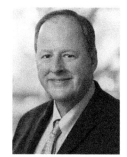

Eva M. Carmona, MD, PhD   Andrew H. Limper, MD

Editors

In an era where travel is increasing and even encouraged as a way to pursue one's dreams, as a way to enrich one's knowledge, and as a source of personal satisfaction, exposure to endemic fungi is not just limited to those living in at-risk areas, but also exposure occurs in the vast numbers of individuals traveling the world as well. In addition, when being older represents not just living longer, but also living with more chronic conditions where some degree of immunosuppression is part of the "new" aging process, fungal diseases become an ever-increasing threat.

Once rare entities with very limited diagnostic tools and even more limited treatment options, fungal infections are now part of the differential diagnosis of many patients with respiratory symptoms, fever, and pulmonary nodules and infiltrates. These are not occasional patients any longer, but patients that visit our practice on a regular basis, whether we are generalists, pulmonologists, infectious diseases specialists, intensivists, or hematologists, among other practitioners. Familiarity with the new diagnostic tools, clinical manifestations, and treatment of the most common and new

emerging fungal diseases has therefore become very important for our everyday practice.

In this issue of *Clinics in Chest Medicine*, expert clinicians and scientists in the field of fungal diseases have reviewed and summarized the latest knowledge of the most prevalent endemic fungi as well as the most common and new emerging molds and yeast infections. This issue also discusses when to consider the possibility of fungal infections, the contemporary diagnostic tools, and the latest treatments, with an article that specifically reviews the classic and new antifungal agents. Individual articles are also dedicated to reviewing fungal diseases in the most vulnerable populations, such as HIV-infected individuals, patients with malignancies, lung transplantation patients, and critically ill patients.

As we recognize the complexity of these patients, we should acknowledge that these are also exciting times when we are witnessing the emergence of a variety of less-invasive and more precise diagnostic tools, as well as new therapeutic drugs with potential for less toxicity and secondary effects, and greater effectiveness against these fungal infections. We believe that you will

Clin Chest Med 38 (2017) xv–xvi
http://dx.doi.org/10.1016/j.ccm.2017.06.002
0272-5231/17/© 2017 Published by Elsevier Inc.

chestmed.theclinics.com

find these reviews informative and a useful resource for your practice as you deal with fungal infections in a variety of patients.

Eva M. Carmona, MD, PhD
Thoracic Diseases Research Unit
Division of Pulmonary Critical Care
and Internal Medicine
Department of Medicine
Mayo Clinic and Foundation
200, 1st Street Southwest
Rochester, MN 55905, USA

Andrew H. Limper, MD
Thoracic Diseases Research Unit
Division of Pulmonary Critical Care
and Internal Medicine
Department of Medicine
Mayo Clinic and Foundation
200, 1st Street Southwest
Rochester, MN 55905, USA

E-mail addresses:
carmona.eva@mayo.edu (E.M. Carmona)
limper.andrew@mayo.edu (A.H. Limper)

When to Consider the Possibility of a Fungal Infection

An Overview of Clinical Diagnosis and Laboratory Approaches

Cassandra M. Batzlaff, MD, Andrew H. Limper, MD*

KEYWORDS

- Fungi • Pneumonia • Epidemiology • Diagnosis

KEY POINTS

- Fungal infections of the lung can occur both in immune-competent and immune-compromised individuals.
- Rising numbers of immune-compromised patients with human immunodeficiency virus, organ transplantation, and cancer chemotherapy, as well as patients receiving immunosuppressive agents, including corticosteroids and tumor necrosis factor (TNF)-α antagonists, has resulted in increased incidence of fungal infections.
- The clinician needs to consider both geographic endemic factors and the nature of the immune compromise in considering the most likely fungal organisms that may infect a given patient.
- Clinical features, including unresolving pulmonary infiltrates despite usual antibacterial antibiotics and the possible presence of skin, bone, genitourinary, and central nervous system manifestations, should raise the possibility of a fungal infection.

EPIDEMIOLOGY AND APPROACH TO THE DIAGNOSIS OF FUNGAL LUNG INFECTION

Fungal lung infections are increasingly prevalent and commonly encountered and managed by pulmonary and critical care physicians. The increasing incidence is likely multifactorial and related to an ever-growing population of susceptible patients, including immunocompromised individuals and transplantation patients, as well as heightened clinical awareness of these infections and advances in laboratory medicine used to confirm their diagnosis.[1,2]

Accordingly, the clinician must remain vigilant and consider fungal infections in the differential diagnosis especially in certain circumstances, such as when a patient presents with persistent lung infiltrates, with or without mediastinal lymphadenopathy, which does not respond to typical antibacterial antimicrobials. Frequently, the diagnosis of a fungal lung infection can be delayed because it is not strongly considered early in the clinical course. Other important clues for the clinician include the presence of a profound neutropenia (absolute neutrophil count <500/μL for >21 days), hematologic malignancy, a hematologic cell or solid organ transplant, or active chemotherapy. These should trigger enhanced suspicion for the potential of a fungal infection.[2] Candida bloodstream infections and invasive

Thoracic Diseases Research Unit, Division of Pulmonary Critical Care and Internal Medicine, Department of Medicine, Mayo Clinic College of Medicine, 200 First Street SW, Rochester, MN 55905, USA
* Corresponding author. Gonda 18-South, Mayo Clinic College of Medicine, 200 First Street SW, Rochester, MN 55905.
E-mail address: limper.andrew@mayo.edu

Clin Chest Med 38 (2017) 385–391
http://dx.doi.org/10.1016/j.ccm.2017.04.002
0272-5231/17/© 2017 Elsevier Inc. All rights reserved.

Aspergillus infections are still the most common infections among immunocompromised individuals in the United States and Europe.[3] However, worldwide, other fungal infections including *Cryptococcus* and *Pneumocystis* infections have significantly greater prevalence, particularly in resource poor settings and regions with high incidence of human immunodeficiency virus (HIV) infections.[4] Other patient populations considered of intermediate risk include those on chronic corticosteroids or novel immune suppressants, and those with HIV, chronic renal insufficiency, or chronic obstructive pulmonary disease (COPD). Furthermore, individuals with liver cirrhosis or diabetes mellitus are at increased risk due to impaired neutrophil function. Significantly, the endemic mycoses are often encountered among completely immunocompetent patients as well.[3] In that case, it is imperative to obtain a good travel history to review potential relevant exposures for those patients who have recently traveled to an endemic geographic region.

Radiographically, they can present as lung consolidation, hilar or mediastinal adenopathy alone, or nodules (**Fig. 1**). Pleural effusions are generally uncommon but may on occasion occur during certain fungal lung infections, particularly coccidioidomycosis, when a pleural-based nodule may erode into the pleural space. Skin lesions can also alert the clinician to a possibility of a fungal infection (**Box 1**). This includes erythema nodosum, which are red firm nodules, or erythema multiforme, which can range from papules to target-like lesions, which may occur with any of the endemic mycoses. In addition, ulcerative lesions

---

Box 1
Factors suggesting the possibility of a fungal lung infection

- Recent travel or exposure to endemic geographic regions
- Unresolving pulmonary infiltrates and fever despite usual antibiotics
- Associated adenopathy
- Associated skin, CNS, genitourinary, or bone abnormalities
- Significant neutropenia, blood malignancy, chemotherapy, or transplantation
- Emerging immune-compromising disease states (novel immune suppression, corticosteroid use, liver cirrhosis, renal failure, COPD, or diabetes mellitus)

---

can occur in disseminated fungal disease and may be a good source to identify the organisms.

Today, a wide range of advanced diagnostic tests are available to the clinician, including microscopic examination of respiratory secretions; fungal smear and culture; specific antigen testing of the serum, urine, or bronchoalveolar lavage (BAL) specimens; serologic testing for antibodies directed against certain fungal components; bronchoscopy with lavage or transbronchial biopsy; and polymerase chain reaction (PCR) assays. To ensure the greatest chance of successful diagnosis, multiple tests are often used simultaneously.

Aspergillus

Aspergillus is a common mold found in both indoor and outdoor environments. Recently, the incidence of *Aspergillus* infection seems to be increasing based on an analysis of 11,000 autopsies, which showed a rise in invasive fungal infections over the years of 1978 to 1992.[5] The traditional risk factors for invasive *Aspergillus* pulmonary infections were long thought to be profound and prolonged neutropenia, hematologic malignancy, and bone marrow transplantation.[6] However, more recently, additional risk factors have been identified including prolonged corticosteroid administration, cirrhosis, solid organ malignancy, HIV, acquired immune deficiency syndrome (AIDS), structural lung disease such as COPD, solid organ transplantation, novel biologic immune suppressants, and chemotherapy.[6] These features have now been clearly associated with enhanced risk for *Aspergillus* infection and demonstrate that the clinician must remain

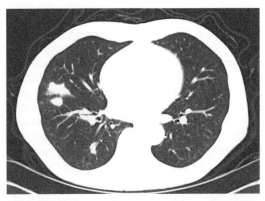

Fig. 1. Computerized tomography image from a 68-year-old white man with history of pancreatic carcinoma treated with chemotherapy. He reported 2 weeks of cough, fever, and dyspnea on exertion. The nodular lesions in the right lung proved to be due to *Cryptococcus neoformans*.

attentive for fungal infection even in those patients who would be considered only moderately immune compromised by traditional standards. *Aspergillosis* can present in the form of allergic bronchopulmonary aspergillosis, allergic *Aspergillus* sinusitis, aspergilloma (or fungus ball), chronic pulmonary aspergillosis, cutaneous aspergillosis, or invasive aspergillosis.

In addition to fungal smear and culture, 2 assays are primarily used for diagnosis of *Aspergillus* infection, namely galactomannan and beta-D-glucan. The galactomannan assays have good sensitivity and excellent specificity.[7] Of note, historically, the galactomannan assay has had cross-reactivity with antibiotic preparations containing beta-lactam, such as piperacillin-tazobactam, resulting in false positives, although in recent years improvements in manufacturing has resulted in a decline in this issue.[8] Galactomannan assays are generally applied to serum but may have enhanced utility when applied to BAL samples.[9] In contrast, beta-D-glucan assays exhibit good negative predictive value for excluding invasive fungal infection.[10] Although not specific, beta-D-glucan is present in many fungal species, including *Candida*, *Aspergillus*, and *Pneumocystis*. Hence, they lack specificity for identifying particular fungal organisms causing a particular fungal infection.[11]

Cryptococcus

Cryptococcus is a genus of encapsulated budding yeast with the species *C neoformans* being the most common cause of human disease. *C gattii* is an emerging cause of infection in tropical and subtropical regions, as well as in the US Pacific Northwest and in British Columbia.[12] Infection of the central nervous system (CNS) and pneumonitis are the most common presentations and those with HIV are at greatest risk. Worldwide, *Cryptococcosis* represents the most common and serious fungal infection, resulting in greater than 1,000,000 clinical cases being estimated annually.[4] Lung manifestations include nodular and mass-like lesions with or without adenopathy, as well as more diffuse infiltration and consolidation. The meningitis can be indolent or fulminate but insidiously progressive and lethal if untreated. Screening with antigen-detection methods in patients with HIV indicates that subclinical meningitis can occur and should be aggressively diagnosed in patients who are profoundly immune suppressed.[13] Diagnosis can be established via direct visualization of the organism, culture, or *Cryptococcus* antigen detection. Antigen testing can be done on blood, urine, or cerebrospinal fluid (CSF)

samples. The development of the highly sensitive and specific lateral flow assay has broadened the availability of effective testing throughout the world, including in those geographic regions with limited health care resources.[14]

Candida

There are more than 20 species of *Candida* that can cause infection in humans. The most common and, therefore, clinically relevant of the *Candida* species is *C albicans*.[15] Presentations can range from mild local mucous membrane infections to candidemia, disseminated disease, and multiorgan failure. Those with profound neutropenia, in intensive care or other immune-compromised states, are at highest risk for developing candidemia or invasive candidiasis.[15] The prevalence of *Candida* infections seems to be relatively stable, likely related to the routine use of antifungal prophylaxis in the immune-compromised patient population. Traditionally, the diagnostic approach for *Candida* bloodstream infection relied on culture identification of the fungus. Indeed, isolation of candidal species represents the most common fungal isolates from the bloodstream, though the cultures may take several days to ultimately verify the diagnosis. In addition, studies suggest that identification of circulating beta-D-glucan can be a useful diagnostic adjunct in documenting potential *Candida* bloodstream infections.[16]

Pneumocystis jirovecii

Pneumocystis jirovecii pneumonia remains the chief fungal pulmonary infection in HIV-infected patients who have a peripheral blood CD4 count of less than 200 cells. The worldwide incidence of *Pneumocystis* pneumonia has been estimated to be in excess of 400,000 cases annually.[4] Unfortunately, most cases are either undiagnosed or diagnosed late in the course of disease, particularly in regions of the world with limited health care resources. Strikingly, the mortality from *Pneumocystis* infection ranges from 10% to 30%, or higher, in various patient populations with comorbid factors or if the diagnosis is delayed, preventing the implementation of effective treatment.[17,18] In cases in which the infection is not diagnosed premortem, the infection is nearly universally fatal.[19] Although the incidence of *Pneumocystis* infections has been effectively suppressed by the use of highly active antiretroviral therapy, this important pneumonia continues to be a common occurrence in individuals who are unaware that they are infected with HIV, and in those who either fail or are intolerant of antiretroviral therapy.[20] Those patients with hematologic malignancy; on immunosuppressive medications; following organ transplantation; with inflammatory conditions, such as granulomatosis with polyangiitis; and with solid tumors are also at increased risk of contracting *Pneumocystis*. As such, prophylaxis may be warranted, most commonly with trimethoprim-sulfamethoxazole. In those patients without HIV who contract *Pneumocystis*, the disease often manifests as fulminant respiratory failure with cough, exertional dyspnea, and fever, as opposed to those with HIV who often have a more indolent clinical presentation. Diffuse, bilateral infiltrates are seen on radiographic imaging. Diagnosis is made by identification of the organism by microscopy with the use of Wright-Giemsa, Gram-Weigert, modified Papanicolaou, or monoclonal antibody immunofluorescence staining to visualize the trophic form of the organism. The cystic form can be appreciated with use of calcofluor white, methenamine silver, or toluidine blue. Notably, *Pneumocystis* cannot be readily cultured. The respiratory specimens studied often include induced sputum or specimens obtained via BAL. Typically, the organism burden is larger in HIV-infected patients despite their milder disease manifestation.[21] Additionally, PCR assays can be applied to nasopharyngeal aspirates, sputum, or BAL samples, and may be more sensitive for making the diagnosis than microscopy in non-HIV patients for the aforementioned reasons.

Scedosporium, Fusarium, and Mucormycosis Infections

Although these species of fungi are less common compared with those previously discussed, they are an emerging concern, particularly in light of the widening use of azole antifungal prophylaxis, which has rendered the host susceptible to resistant molds and other fungal species.[12] In particular, poorly controlled diabetics are at higher risk for invasive mucormycosis, which often manifests as a fungal sinusitis. Diagnosis of these fungal infections traditionally has relied on identifying the typical organisms in tissue or secretion using histopathology or culture.[22] More recently, assays using PCR and mass spectroscopy have been developed and are available through some reference laboratories.

Endemic Mycoses: Histoplasmosis capsulatum, Blastomyces dermatitidis, Coccidioides Species

These fungal organisms can infect both immunocompetent and immunocompromised persons.

Each of the previously discussed fungi has a particular geographic predilection and unique clinical features. Diagnosis can be made via PCR assays, relevant serologic and urinary antigen tests, fungal smear and culture, biopsy of involved sites, bronchoscopy, and lumbar puncture if warranted.[3] Of note, although skin manifestations, such as erythema nodosum or erythema multiforme, are common in those with endemic mycoses infections, the skin biopsies of those skin conditions do not contain detectable organisms and are of limited diagnostic value because these are an immune mediated reaction. In contrast, mucosal or cutaneous ulcerations, such as with histoplasmosis or blastomycosis, should be biopsied with demonstration of the relevant organisms on tissue histology and culture. The severity and presentation of these infections varies widely (see later discussion) and depends on the host's overall immune status, keeping in mind that many endemic mycoses exposures and low-grade infections remain subclinical and minimally asymptomatic in individuals with normal host defense.

Histoplasmosis

Histoplasmosis is endemic to the Ohio and Mississippi river valleys in the Midwest portions of the United States, where the fungus thrives in soils that have been enriched with bird and bat excrement. Histoplasmosis also occurs in regions of Central and South America, Asia, Africa, and in Australia.[23] The clinical presentation of histoplasmosis can range from mild transient fever and chills, to cough and pulmonary nodules, mediastinal lymphadenopathy, or broncholithiasis. More severe consequences of this infection include fibrosing mediastinitis, progressive and disseminated pulmonary histoplasmosis with associated acute respiratory distress syndrome (ARDS), and chronic pulmonary histoplasmosis.[24] Many cases with mild disease may not require treatment and can be simply managed with close observation and follow-up. Those with more significant active and symptomatic disease are treated with azole antifungal therapy. Life-threatening infections should be treated promptly with liposomal amphotericin B until signs of clinical improvement is established, followed by oral azole therapy.[12] The diagnostic approach for histoplasmosis includes several useful approaches, many of which may be used concurrently to increase the diagnostic yield. Typical organisms can be observed in tissues and respiratory secretions but the sensitivity of this approach is rather low. Culture can be useful in severe cases, though this approach may require several weeks before revealing the organisms. Enzyme-based immuno-assay detection of *Histoplasma* antigen can be applied to urine, blood, CSF, and BAL with good sensitivity and excellent specificity.[23,24] PCR assays for detecting histoplasmosis are available in some laboratories and exhibit good sensitivity and excellent specificity.

Blastomycosis

Blastomycosis is caused by inhalation of *Blastomyces dermatitidis*, which is endemic to damp soil and rotting wood in the central and south-eastern United States. As such, it tends to be isolated most commonly from river and creek beds and shores, and from wooded areas with rotted trees and beaver dam activity[25–27] Clinical presentation can range from acute to subacute to chronic respiratory infections. The most common pulmonary presentations include pulmonary nodules, lobar pneumonia, mass-like consolidations, and (at times) chronic fibrocavitary disease. Blastomycosis has the ability to disseminate from the lungs.[12] Hence, skin disease is the second most common manifestation of blastomycosis with the development of verrucous lesions with irregular borders. Biopsy of such lesions can prove useful in demonstrating the thick wall, broad-based, budding yeast. This fungus can additionally lead to ARDS, fulminant diffuse pneumonia, or dissemination to the bone, urogenital tract, and CNS infection. More severe pulmonary infections can follow large inoculum exposures, even in individuals with normal host defense. Diagnosis relies on identifying the typical organisms morphologically in respiratory secretions or in tissues. These organisms can be visualized using potassium hydroxide (KOH) preparations or following silver staining. Blastomyces serologic assays are available with moderate sensitivity but with some cross-reactivity to histoplasmosis. Blastomyces urinary antigen testing and PCR assays are also available.

Coccidioidomycosis

Coccidioidomycosis related to either *Coccidioides immitis* or *Coccidioides posadasii* is an endemic fungal infection that results from inhaling the spores from these species. These fungal organisms grow in the soil of the southwestern United States, regions of Mexico, and in parts of Central America and South America.[28] More recently, these organisms have been detected in south-central Washington.[29] Enhanced environmental fungal growth follows periods of rain, with disruption of the soil and dispersion of the spores during construction and other activities the following dry season, leading to environmental exposures for individual exposed to these inhalants. The organism has high infectivity, with laboratory exposures and infections being well-documented. A pneumonia-like presentation is the most common manifestation and can be accompanied by fatigue, night sweats, fever, peripheral blood eosinophilia, and erythema multiforme or erythema nodosum. This usual presentation is known as Valley Fever in endemic regions. With large inoculum exposures, severe pulmonary disease involvement can become fulminant. In addition, coccidioidomycosis can spread to the bone, joints, skin, and the CNS. A fraction of individuals go on to develop persistent pulmonary disease or dissemination. Patients receiving organ transplantation and patients with HIV infection with low CD4 cell counts are at significant risk for dissemination of coccidioidomycosis. Men of African and Filipino descent are also at higher risk for developing dissemination, as are pregnant women.[30] Furthermore, COPD and structural lung disease, congestive heart failure, chronic renal failure, diabetes mellitus, and those individuals receiving tumor necrosis factor (TNF)-α antagonists are also at enhanced risk for dissemination.[12] The diagnosis usually relies on documentation of anticoccidioidal antibodies circulating in the serum, which can be verified by enzyme-linked immunosorbent assay (ELISA) and immunodiffusion assays, or through the use of complement fixation or tube precipitin testing. In addition, laboratory identification of coccidioidal giant spherules of silver staining of tissue or by isolating the organisms by culture from a clinical specimen can be used to confirm the diagnosis.

SUMMARY

Fungal infections are being appreciated with increased frequency, both in individuals with impaired immunity as well as in immune-compromised hosts. Timely diagnosis first requires a heightened suspicion for the presence of a fungal infection using the clinical clues described in this article. Fortunately, a wide variety of both traditional and contemporary laboratory diagnostic tools are available. These include histopathology and cytopathology visualization of the organisms, and culture techniques. In addition, antigen detection and serologic demonstration of antibodies recognizing these organisms are useful tools for diagnosis. In recent years, modern techniques including PCR detection of the fungal nucleic acids, have enhanced the ability to diagnose these challenging infections. The concurrent application of multiple laboratory approaches increases the diagnostic yield and may be required in appropriate clinical settings.

REFERENCES

1. Limper AH. The changing spectrum of fungal infections in pulmonary and critical care practice: clinical approach to diagnosis. Proc Am Thorac Soc 2010; 7(3):163–8.

2. Limper AH, Hoyte JS, Standing JE. The role of alveolar macrophages in *Pneumocystis carinii* degradation and clearance from the lung. J Clin Invest 1997; 99(9):2110–7.

3. Limper AH. Clinical approach and management for selected fungal infections in pulmonary and critical care patients. Chest 2014;146(6):1658–66.

4. Brown GD, Denning DW, Gow NA, et al. Hidden killers: human fungal infections. Sci Transl Med 2012;4(165):165rv113.

5. Groll AH, Shah PM, Mentzel C, et al. Trends in the postmortem epidemiology of invasive fungal infections at a university hospital. J Infect 1996;33(1): 23–32.

6. Kousha M, Tadi R, Soubani AO. Pulmonary aspergillosis: a clinical review. Eur Respir Rev 2011;20(121): 156–74.

7. Heng SC, Morrissey O, Chen SC, et al. Utility of bronchoalveolar lavage fluid galactomannan alone or in combination with PCR for the diagnosis of invasive aspergillosis in adult hematology patients: a systematic review and meta-analysis. Crit Rev Microbiol 2015;41(1):124–34.

8. Mikulska M, Furfaro E, Del Bono V, et al. Piperacillin/tazobactam (Tazocin) seems to be no longer responsible for false-positive results of the galactomannan assay. J Antimicrob Chemother 2012; 67(7):1746–8.

9. Lehrnbecher T, Robinson PD, Fisher BT, et al. Galactomannan, Beta-D-Glucan and PCR-Based assays for the diagnosis of invasive fungal disease in pediatric cancer and hematopoietic stem cell transplantation: a systematic review and meta-analysis. Clin Infect Dis 2016;63(10):1340–8.

10. Theel ES, Jespersen DJ, Iqbal S, et al. Detection of (1, 3)-beta-D-glucan in bronchoalveolar lavage and serum samples collected from immunocompromised hosts. Mycopathologia 2013;175(1–2):33–41.

11. Skalski JH, Limper AH. Fungal, viral, and parasitic pneumonias associated with human immunodeficiency virus. Semin Respir Crit Care Med 2016; 37(2):257–66.

12. Limper AH, Knox KS, Sarosi GA, et al. An official American Thoracic Society statement: treatment of fungal infections in adult pulmonary and critical care patients. Am J Respir Crit Care Med 2011; 183(1):96–128.

13. Meya DB, Manabe YC, Castelnuovo B, et al. Cost-effectiveness of serum cryptococcal antigen screening to prevent deaths among HIV-infected persons with a CD4+ cell count ≤100 cells/microL who start HIV therapy in resource-limited settings. Clin Infect Dis 2010;51(4):448–55.

14. Kozel TR, Bauman SK. CrAg lateral flow assay for cryptococcosis. Expert Opin Med Diagn 2012;6(3): 245–51.

15. Montagna MT, Lovero G, Borghi E, et al. Candidemia in intensive care unit: a nationwide prospective observational survey (GISIA-3 study) and review of the European literature from 2000 through 2013. Eur Rev Med Pharmacol Sci 2014; 18(5):661–74.

16. Kohno S, Mitsutake K, Maesaki S, et al. An evaluation of serodiagnostic tests in patients with candidemia: beta-glucan, mannan, candida antigen by Cand-Tec and D-arabinitol. Microbiol Immunol 1993;37(3):207–12.

17. Thomas CF Jr, Limper AH. Current insights into the biology and pathogenesis of Pneumocystis pneumonia. Nat Rev Microbiol 2007;5(4):298–308.

18. Thomas CF Jr, Limper AH. Pneumocystis pneumonia. N Engl J Med 2004;350(24):2487–98.

19. Hui AN, Koss MN, Meyer PR. Necropsy findings in acquired immunodeficiency syndrome: a comparison of premortem diagnoses with postmortem findings. Hum Pathol 1984;15(7):670–6.

20. Lopez-Sanchez C, Falco V, Burgos J, et al. Epidemiology and long-term survival in HIV-infected patients with Pneumocystis jirovecii pneumonia in the HAART era: experience in a university hospital and review of the literature. Medicine 2015;94(12): e681.

21. Limper AH, Offord KP, Smith TF, et al. *Pneumocystis carinii* pneumonia. Differences in lung parasite number and inflammation in patients with and without AIDS. Am Rev Respir Dis 1989;140(5):1204–9.

22. Riley TT, Muzny CA, Swiatlo E, et al. Breaking the mold: a review of mucormycosis and current pharmacological treatment options. Ann Pharmacother 2016;50(9):747–57.

23. Hage CA, Azar MM, Bahr N, et al. Histoplasmosis: up-to-date evidence-based approach to diagnosis and management. Semin Respir Crit Care Med 2015;36(5):729–45.

24. Knox KS, Hage CA. Histoplasmosis. Proc Am Thorac Soc 2010;7(3):169–72.

25. Klein BS, Vergeront JM, Davis JP. Epidemiologic aspects of blastomycosis, the enigmatic systemic mycosis. Semin Respir Infect 1986;1(1):29–39.

26. Klein BS, Vergeront JM, DiSalvo AF, et al. Two outbreaks of blastomycosis along rivers in Wisconsin. Isolation of blastomyces dermatitidis from riverbank soil and evidence of its transmission along waterways. Am Rev Respir Dis 1987;136(6):1333–8.

27. Roy M, Benedict K, Deak E, et al. A large community outbreak of blastomycosis in Wisconsin with geographic and ethnic clustering. Clin Infect Dis 2013;57(5):655–62.

28. Ampel NM. Coccidioidomycosis: a review of recent advances. Clin Chest Med 2009;30(2):241 51, v.

29. Marsden-Haug N, Goldoft M, Ralston C, et al. Coccidioidomycosis acquired in Washington state. Clin Infect Dis 2013;56(6):847–50.

30. Ampel NM, Wieden MA, Galgiani JN. Coccidioidomycosis: clinical update. Rev Infect Dis 1989; 11(6).897–911.

Overview of Treatment Approaches for Fungal Infections

Eva M. Carmona, MD, PhD*, Andrew H. Limper, MD

KEYWORDS

- Antifungal • Fungal infections • Invasive mycoses • Amphotericin • Triazoles • Echinocandins
- Flucytosine

KEY POINTS

There are 4 main groups of antifungals and each one has a specific mechanism of action: polyenes and azoles disrupt the cell membrane, echinocandins affect the cell wall synthesis, and pyrimidine analogues block the DNA synthesis.

- Amphotericin B is still the drug of choice to treat empiric severe and invasive fungal infections due to its broad spectrum of activity.
- Triazoles are the preferred agents for the treatment and prevention of invasive aspergillosis in most patients, and for many endemic mycoses.
- Echinocandins are usually preferred among other antifungals for their activity against *Candida* spp.
- Fluocytosine is generally used in combination of amphotericin B to treat refractory *Candida* infections and cryptococcal meningitis.

INTRODUCTION

Fungi are eukaryotic organisms that cause both endemic and severe infections, predominantly in the immunocompromised and debilitated host. Yeasts (eg, *Candida* spp), molds (eg, *Aspergillus* spp), and dimorphic fungi (eg, *Histoplasma capsulatum*) are the 3 groups in which fungi are generally classified.

Structurally, fungi are usually formed by a cell membrane surrounded by a fungal cell wall. The cell membrane is mostly formed from ergosterol and zymosterol (fungi equivalents of cholesterol), whereas mannoproteins, chitin, and beta-glucans are the main components of the fungal wall. These elements not only confer rigidity to the fungus but can also alter the host immunity, causing some patients' exuberant inflammatory reactions responsible for tissue injury and other systemic manifestations, such as respiratory failure and even death.[1–3]

Antifungals are commonly used drugs for the treatment and prophylaxis of most fungal infections and can be divided into 4 main groups: polyenes, azoles (triazoles and imidazoles), echinocandins, and pyrimidine analogues. They have different mechanisms of action, which result in different spectrums of activity. Polyenes and azoles disrupt the cell membrane, echinocandins affect the synthesis of the cell wall, and pyrimidine

Disclosure Statement: E.M. Carmona: Co-I in ReSAPH study (registry for patients with sarcoidosis associated pulmonary hypertension). Sponsor by Gilead. A.H. Limper: Dr Limper has no conflicts of interest relevant to the contents of this article.
Thoracic Diseases Research Unit, Division of Pulmonary Critical Care and Internal Medicine, Department of Medicine, Mayo Clinic, Mayo Foundation, 200, 1st Street Southwest, Rochester, MN 55905, USA
* Corresponding author.
E-mail address: carmona.eva@mayo.edu

Clin Chest Med 38 (2017) 393–402
http://dx.doi.org/10.1016/j.ccm.2017.04.003
0272-5231/17/© 2017 Elsevier Inc. All rights reserved.

analogues block the DNA synthesis. This is important because additive effect may be achieved by combining different antifungal classes, particularly in very severe or invasive disease.

Understanding the precise use of the established and new antifungal agents is critical because fungal infections are on the rise. The increased mobility of patients to endemic fungal regions, together with an aging population with more chronic conditions, malignancies, transplants, and autoimmune diseases that require the use of potent immunosuppressant agents, represent the main contributors to this increase. This article reviews the main characteristics, clinical uses, and secondary effects of the main antifungals used in clinical practice to treat systemic and chest fungal infections.

Amphotericin B

Developed in the 1950s, amphotericin B (AmB) is a natural product of *Streptomyces nodosus*. Despite being among oldest drugs available to treat fungal diseases, it is still the drug of choice for severe and invasive fungal infections due to its broad spectrum of activity. It is effective for most clinical isolates of *Candida* spp and *Aspergillus* spp, *Cryptococcus neoformans*, endemic mycosis, *Zygomycetes*, and brown-black molds. However, there are well known AmB-resistant organisms, including chromoblastomycosis, *Aspergillus terreus*, *Candida lusitaniae*, *Scedosporium* spp, *Trichosporon* spp, and some *Fusarium* spp.[4]

AmB belongs to the polyenes group and it has been classically accepted that it exerts action by binding to ergosterol. AmB-ergosterol binding was thought to disrupt the fungal cell membrane by creating pores that allow the efflux of electrolytes and other molecules, causing the death of the organism. Recent evidence suggests that AmB also forms large, extramembranous aggregates that kill yeast by extracting ergosterol from lipid bilayers.[5] The AmB effect is not specific to ergosterol and in mammalian cells may also exhibit altered cholesterol content, causing cell damage, which is responsible for some of its known toxicity. Resistance to AmB is rare and has been attributed to a decreased content of ergosterol or other sterols in the fungal membrane.

AmB is poorly absorbed and, therefore, is commonly administered intravenously (IV). Deoxycholate is used to solubilize AmB and is responsible for some of the well-known drug-toxicities, particularly the nephrotoxicity. To avoid that, lipid formulations have been developed (liposomal AmB, AmB lipid complex, and AmB colloidal dispersion) and are generally preferred because they are more potent and have lower incidence of nephrotoxicity and other infusion-related reactions. Direct or local instillation (intraperitoneal, intrathecal, intravitreal, and bladder irrigation), as well as inhaled administration, are also available. Inhaled lipid formulations are favored over the deoxycholate preparation because the former has been shown to affect surfactant proteins.[6–8]

If nephrotoxicity develops, it usually improves after discontinuation of therapy. However, permanent effects may occur, particularly in patients receiving doses greater than 5 gm of AmB or when AmB is used in conjunction with other nephrotoxic drugs. Hydration and sodium repletion before initiation of AmB may decrease the risk of nephrotoxicity; frequent monitoring of renal function and avoidance of concomitant administration of other nephrotoxic agents is recommended. However, alternative safer options are generally preferred when available. Recommended monitoring includes regular cell blood count (CBC), serum electrolytes (magnesium and potassium), and renal and liver function tests.[9]

Infusion-related toxicities are also common, consisting mostly of fever, chills, hypotension, nausea, vomiting, and bronchospasm. Life-threating hyperkalemia and arrhythmias has been described after rapid infusion and, therefore, infusion over 2 to 6 hours is recommended.[10] Pulmonary toxicity is a concern with concomitant infusion of leukocytes and should be avoided.[11]

Despite the aforementioned secondary effects, IV liposomal formulation of AmB is a primary indication for empiric treatment of neutropenic fever, cryptococcal meningitis, *Zygomycetes*, and severe infections caused by endemic mycosis (*Histoplasma*, *Blastomyces*, *Coccidioides*, and *Sporothrix*).[9,12] It is an alternative to voriconazole for initial and salvage therapy for invasive aspergillosis. The inhaled formulation has been shown to be protective against the development of invasive aspergillosis in neutropenic patients with cancer and current guidelines recommend it use for prophylaxis in patients with prolonged neutropenia and lung transplant.[13] Inhaled AmB is also recommended as adjunctive therapy in the setting of tracheobronchial aspergillosis associated with anastomotic endobronchial ischemia or ischemic reperfusion injury due to airway ischemia associated with lung transplant.[13]

AmB is usually the preferred antifungal for severe fungal infections during pregnancy and is considered by the US Food and Drug Administration (FDA) as a class B agent. Infant risk cannot be ruled out and breast feeding is not recommended while receiving AmB.[9,14,15]

Triazoles

Triazoles are synthetic agents composed by a 5-membered ring of 2 carbon and 3 nitrogen atoms. Five members of this family are currently available in the United States: fluconazole, itraconazole, posaconazole, voriconazole, and the newer member isavuconazole.

Triazoles, unlike AmB, affect the synthesis of the fungal cell membrane by inhibiting the cytochrome (CYP)-450-dependent enzyme, lanosterol 14-alpha-demethylase, important for the conversion of lanosterol to ergosterol. This alters the biosynthesis of ergosterol, causing increased permeability of the cell membrane and fungal death. The affinity for this enzyme varies among the different triazoles and is largely responsible for their different potency and spectrum of activity. However, most triazoles are considered fungistatic, with the exception of voriconazole that can be fungicidal for *Aspergillus* spp.

Drug interactions and toxicities within the triazole family are mostly due to their interaction with the human CYP-dependent enzymes, causing inhibition of 3A4, 2C9, and 2C19 subtypes.[16] Triazoles can also cause QTc prolongation, so administration with other agents known to affect QTc should be avoided. They are associated with increased risk for birth defects and the FDA considers them class C (itraconazole, posaconazole, isavuconazole, and single-dose fluconazole for vaginal candidiasis) or class D (fluconazole and voriconazole); therefore, they are not recommended during pregnancy.[13] They are also secreted in breast milk; therefore, breast feeding is not advisable while taking these medications.[13,14,17]

The spectrum of activity varies among the different members, although all of them have similar activity against *Candida* isolates. The individual characteristics follow.

Fluconazole

Fluconazole is among the preferred triazoles because it has an excellent bioavailability, tolerability, and safety profile. Its activity is very good against *Candida* spp, except *Candida glabrata* (limited activity), and *Candida krusei* (no activity), and *Cryptococcus* spp. It has also some activity against endemic fungi, including *Histoplasma*, *Blastomyces*, *Coccidioides*, and *Paracoccidioides* spp (**Table 1**).

Fluconazole is available in oral and IV formulation. It is almost completely absorbed following oral administration and its absorption is not affected by gastric pH or food. Only 10% is protein bound and it has excellent penetration in cerebral spinal fluid (CSF). Its half-life is 27 to 34 hours and, therefore, it can be administered once a day. It is renally excreted and dosage adjustments are necessary in individuals with renal dysfunction. For patients undergoing hemodialysis, dosage replacement is needed after each dialysis session.[17]

Unlike other triazoles, fluconazole is a weak substrate of CYP450 and, therefore, causes less toxicity. However, caution is needed when administered with phenytoin, glipizide, glyburide, warfarin, rifabutin, or cyclosporine because levels of these drugs can increase in the presence of fluconazole. In contrast, concomitant use with rifampicin causes fluconazole levels to decrease.[18] Careful review of patient's medication interaction is, therefore, recommended.

Fluconazole is mainly indicated for the treatment of *Candida* esophagitis, the urogenital tract, and *Candida* vulvovaginitis. For candidemia, IV or oral fluconazole, 800 mg (12 mg/kg) loading dose followed by 400 mg (6 mg/kg) daily, is considered an acceptable alternative to an echinocandin as initial therapy in patients who are not critically ill and who are considered unlikely to have a fluconazole-resistant *Candida* spp.[19] The same regimen is an alternative choice for empiric treatment of suspected invasive candidiasis in nonneutropenic patients in the intensive care unit who have had no recent azole exposure and are not colonized with azole-resistant *Candida* spp.[19] Fluconazole is also a considered a step-down therapy, generally from echinocandins, in clinically stable patients who have susceptible isolates and documented bloodstream clearance. It is also indicated in the prophylaxis of candidiasis in bone marrow transplant patients. In addition to *Candida* infections, fluconazole can be used in cryptococcal meningitis and coccidiodomycosis.[12,20] Doses vary depending on the indication and serum drug monitoring is rarely needed.[19]

Itraconazole

Itraconazole has broader spectrum of activity than fluconazole, particularly for endemic fungi like *Histoplasma* and *Blastomyces*. It is also active against *Aspergillus* spp, *Candida* spp (except *Candida krusei*), *Sporothrix schenckii*, and brown-black molds (see **Table 1**).

It is only available for oral administration in either capsule form or as an oral solution. Their bioavailability differs substantially and the oral solution is preferred over the capsule because it is up to 30% more bioavailable. Furthermore, the capsule form is affected by gastric pH, requiring an acid environment or the presence of food for better absorption. Therefore, proton pump inhibitors, antihistamine 2 receptor blockers, and antacids

Table 1
Spectrum of activity to selected fungal organisms

Medication	Aspergillus spp	Candida albicans / Candida tropicalis / Candida parapsilosis	Candida glabrata	Candida krusei	Candida lusitaniae / Candida guilliermondii	Histoplasma spp	Blastomyces dermatitidis	Coccidioides spp	C spp	Fusarium spp	Zygomycetes
AmB	2	2	1–2	1–2	R	2	2	2	2	1	2
Fluconazole	0	2	1	0	1–2	1	1	1–2	2	0	0
Itraconazole	1–2	2	1	0	1	1–2	1–2	1–2	1	0	1–0
Isavuconazole	2	2	2	2	2	2a	2a	2a	2	2	2
Posaconazole	2	2	1–2	2	1–2	1–2	1–2	1–2	1–2	1	1–2
Voriconazole	2	2	1–2	2	1–2	1	1	1–2	1–2	1	0
Caspofungin	1–2	2	1–2	2	1–2	1	0–1	0	0	0	0
Micafungin	1–2	2	1–2	2	1–2	1	0–1	0	0	0	0
Anidulafungin	1–2	2	1–2	2	1–2	1	0–1	0	0	0	0
Flucytosineb	0	2	2	0	1	0	0	1	1–2	0	0

Abbreviations: 0, little or no activity; 1, moderate activity; 2, good activity; R, increase rates of resistance, do not use without susceptibility data.
a Limited clinical data.
b Usually not used alone.

should be avoided. Itraconazole has a long half-life (25–64 hours), allowing once a day administration. However, when doses of 400 mg a day are used, divided dosage is recommended for better absorption.[16]

Itraconazole and its active metabolite (hydroxyitraconazole) are bound to protein up to 99%. The unbound drug is very lipophilic and reaches high concentration in the lungs, kidneys, and skin. In contrast to fluconazole, itraconazole penetrates poorly into the CSF and eye; therefore, it is not optimal for central nervous system (CNS) or eye infections. Itraconazole is metabolized in the liver via CYP3A4 and inactive metabolites are excreted in the urine and feces. It cannot, therefore, be used to treat urinary tract infections. Dosage adjustments are not required in renal insufficiency but caution is needed in those with liver diseases.[21,22]

Itraconazole is FDA approved for salvage therapy for invasive aspergillosis, and is the antifungal of choice in mild and chronic histoplasmosis and mild-to-moderate blastomycosis (including skin and bone disease).[23] Itraconazole can also be used to treat coccidioidomycosis, cryptococcosis, oropharyngeal and esophageal candidiasis and allergic bronchopulmonary aspergillosis. The dosages vary depending on the indication and severity of infection.

Due to the unpredictable absorption of itraconazole, the Infectious Diseases Society of America recommends monitoring drug levels.[13,24,25] Random levels should be measured after steady state levels have been achieved, which is usually after 2 weeks of therapy. Two different methods are available: bioassay and high-pressure liquid chromatography. The former measures itraconazole and hydroxyitraconazole. The sum of both should be considered when calculating the drug levels, which are generally recommended between 1 to 10 μg/mL.[13,24,25] Higher levels associate with higher rates of complications and should be avoided. Monitoring of liver function test is also recommended.

Side effects with itraconazole are rare and may include pruritus or rash, nausea, vomiting, diarrhea, dizziness, headache, and edema. More serious, but very rare, are congestive heart failure or pulmonary edema, Stevens-Johnson syndrome, toxic epidermal necrolysis, and pancreatitis[13,23] Like most of the azoles, interactions may occur with medications that use CYP450 enzymes; therefore, medication interactions must be reviewed before institution of treatment.

Posaconazole

Among all the azoles, posaconazole has one of the broadest spectrums of activity. It is effective against most Candida spp, Aspergillus fumigatus, Cryptococcus, Zygomycetes, and endemic fungi (Histoplasma, Blastomyces, and Coccidioides) (see **Table 1**).

Posaconazole is available in oral and IV formulations. The oral form has 2 different preparations: the oral solution, which requires administration with food (high-fat meals) for better absorption, and the delayed-release tablets, which are less affected by the presence of food. The oral solution has a saturable absorption for which multiple dosing is required. This is avoided with the use of delayed-release tablets. Since 2014, an IV formulation is also available and preferred for those with abnormal gastrointestinal absorption. It is important to take into consideration that the IV form uses a cyclodextrine vehicle for solubility, which can accumulate and cause renal dysfunction.[26] Monitoring of renal function is indicated with the IV formulation. Dose adjustment is not necessary for patients on hemodialysis.[27]

Therapeutic drug monitoring is recommended due to potential suboptimal absorption, particularly in patients with mucositis and graft-versus-host disease of the gut. Highly variable concentrations of posaconazole have been shown to affect the efficacy and response rates for invasive fungal infections. Because the concentration of posaconazole tends to increase steadily during the first week and then remain stable, it is recommended to obtain trough levels between days 4 and 7 of therapy, and at interval periods thereafter. The recommended trough concentrations for prophylaxis is 0.7 μg/mL or more, and for treatment it is 1.0 μg/mL or more.[28]

Although posaconazole has similar activity to voriconazole against Aspergillus spp and Candida spp, clinical data are still limited and, therefore, posaconazole does not have a primary recommendation for the treatment of any of these fungal infections, with the exception of oropharyngeal candidiasis (including human immunodeficiency virus patients).[19] The FDA-approved indications for posaconazole are, therefore, prophylaxis of invasive aspergillosis and disseminated candidiasis in the severely immunocompromised host.[13,29,30] Additionally, posaconazole has proved to be effective as step-down or salvage therapy for mucormycosis,[31] salvage therapy in invasive aspergillosis in those patients refractory or intolerant to voriconazole, and step-down therapy for intravascular Candida infections susceptible to posaconazole but resistant to fluconazole.[13,19] Other potential uses are Scedosporium and Fusarium infections.[32]

Drug-drug interactions need to be considered with posaconazole because it inhibits CYP3A4 activity, requiring dosage adjustment of drugs metabolized via this pathway (rifabutin, phenytoin, efavirenz, cimetidine, and esomeprazole are among the most common). Calcineurin inhibitor toxicity (cyclosporine and tacrolimus) and vincristine toxicity resulting in neurotoxicity and other adverse reactions have been described.[26]

Voriconazole

Voriconazole compared with other triazoles has enhanced activity against *Candida* spp and *Aspergillus*, including *A terreus*, and is also effective against *Cryptococcus* spp, *Fusarium* spp, and endemic fungi. However, voriconazole has very little activity against *Zygomycetes* (see **Table 1**).

Like most of the triazoles, voriconazole is metabolized in the liver by the CYP450, particularly by the subenzymes 2C19, 2C9, and 3A4. Genetic polymorphisms in 2C19 and 3A4 have been described as affecting the metabolism of voriconazole and, therefore, are responsible for some of the variability observed among individuals. This fact, and that adults treated with voriconazole demonstrate nonlinear metabolism kinetics, may together explain the unpredictable bioavailability of voriconazole. Therapeutic drug level monitoring is, therefore, recommended and trough concentrations should be checked 4 to 7 days after initiation of therapy and at regular intervals thereafter. A target of greater than 1 mg/L is recommended for patients either on prophylaxis or receiving treatment of invasive fungal infections. Because clinical outcome has been shown to correlate with higher concentrations, an increased target (eg, 2 mg/L) may need to be set for those with very severe infection or poor prognosis (eg, CNS infection, multifocal disease). However, to minimize toxicity, the trough should be kept to less than 4 to 6 mg/L.[28]

Voriconazole, like other azoles, contains cyclodextrin and, therefore, the IV formulation should be used with caution in patients with renal impairment (creatinine clearance <50 mL/min) because it can accumulate. Creatinine monitoring is recommended. Removal of the drug during 4-hour hemodialysis does not require redosage.[33]

The main indications for voriconazole are treatment of invasive and CNS aspergillosis, non-neutropenic candidemia, candidiasis of the esophagus, disseminated candidiasis, and serious infections due to *F* spp and *Scedosporium apiospermum*. In patients with neutropenic candidemia, echinocandins are preferred. However, voriconazole can be used if additional mold coverage is desired or as a step-down therapy if there is clearance of blood cultures and susceptible isolates.[13,19,23]

Voriconazole is usually well-tolerated. The most common adverse effects are visual disturbances (eg, altered perception of light, achromatopsia, and photophobia) and hallucinations. These events are usually mild and transitory. Elevation of liver enzymes is also seen. They tend to be dose-dependent and usually transitory, with only a few cases of hepatic failure and death reported. It is, therefore, recommended to monitor liver function test, including bilirubin at baseline and weekly during the first month of therapy, and regularly thereafter if significant changes occur. Visual function needs to be monitored for treatments longer than 28 days.[33] Drug-drug interactions are also frequent with voriconazole and should always been assessed before and during treatment.[33]

Isavuconazole

Isavuconazole is the newer member of the triazole family. It has a broad spectrum of activity with excellent bioavailability and tolerability. Isavuconazole is active against yeast, molds, and dimorphic-fungi (see **Table 1**). It has been FDA approved for the use of invasive aspergillosis and mucormycosis.

Isavuconazole, like other azoles, affects the synthesis of ergosterol by inhibiting the 14α-lanosterol demethylation, favoring the accumulation of toxic methylated precursors, causing fungal cell death. Isavuconazole specifically binds to CYP51 protein, conferring broader antifungal spectrum even to pathogens resistant to other azoles.[34,35] It is metabolized in the liver by the CYP3A4 and CYP3A5 isoenzymes. Therefore, drugs that affect these enzymes can alter isavuconazole levels, including lopinavir or ritonavir (increased isavuconazole levels), rifampin, carbamazepine, long-acting barbiturates, and St John's wort (decreased levels). In addition, isavuconazole can also increase levels of sirolimus, everolimus, cyclosporine, mycophenolate mofetil, and digoxin and decrease levels of bupropion. These are just a few examples and therefore it is important to review drug interactions in detailed when used in clinical practice.

Isavuconazole is otherwise usually well tolerated. The most common side effects are nausea, vomiting, diarrhea, rash, and peripheral edema. Rarely hepatotoxicity can occur and, therefore, liver enzymes should be monitored. No dose adjustments are necessary in mild-to-moderate liver dysfunction. However, it should not be used in patients with severe liver disease. Unlike voriconazole and posaconazole, renal toxicity is not a main issue with isavuconazole because the IV formulation does not contain cyclodextrin, which accumulates in renal failure. QT prolongation is not usually an issue with Isavuconazole. However, QT shortening has been occasionally described and, therefore, its use is contraindicated in those with familiar short QT syndrome. The implication in other clinical scenarios is not clearly known.

Available in oral and IV formulations, isavuconazole is the drug of choice for patients who do not tolerate voriconazole, in invasive aspergillosis, and as an alternative to posaconazole as step-down therapy from lipid AmB in the treatment of mucormycosis. Isavuconazole has also in vitro activity against *Cryptococcus* spp and endemic mycosis and available clinical studies suggest that it may be an alternative treatment.[36] However, there are relatively few studies and limited numbers of subjects, and further studies are needed before its use can be generally recommended.

Echinocandins

The echinocandins are a new class of antifungals that work by disrupting the fungal cell wall because they inhibit the (1,3)-β-D-glucan synthase complex important for β-glucan synthesis. The distribution of β-glucan varies among the different fungi and while in yeast, β-glucan account for 30% to 60% of the cell wall, in filamentous fungi, they are found at the hyphae. This is important because depletion of β-glucan in yeast (eg, *Candida*) causes loss of resistance to osmotic forces, contributing to cells lysis and, therefore, achieves a fungicidal effect. In filamentous fungi (eg, *Aspergillus*) they inhibit the growth of the hyphae, resulting in a fungistatic effect. In contrast, because there are no β-glucans or β-glucan synthases in humans, these agents are less toxic than other antifungals.

There are 3 echinocandins currently available in the United States: caspofungin, micafungin, and anidulafungin. They all have similar spectrums of activity but differ in the metabolic pathways, dosing, drug interactions, and safety profiles.

Echinocandins are fungicidal against *Candida* spp, including the triazole resistants *Candida glabrata* and *Candida krusei*. They have good activity against *Aspergillus* spp and *Cryptococcus* spp with the exception of *Cryptococcus neoformans* and *Cryptococcus gattii*. They exhibit modest activity against dimorphic fungi and non-*Aspergillus* molds, but no activity against *Mucorales*, *Fusarium* spp, and *Scedosporium* spp (see **Table 1**). Regarding *Pneumocystis jirovecii*, clinical data are limited but experimental models suggest that they may be useful for prophylaxis but not for treatment. This is likely because only the cyst, and not the trophic forms, expresses glucan synthase.[37–39]

Among the major advantages of using echinocandins versus other antifungals is their activity against *Candida* spp. They are, therefore, the agents of choice to treat invasive candidiasis (particularly in very ill and neutropenic patients) and have activity against *Candida* biofilms, making them very useful for catheter and prosthetic infections.[19]

Because they have a different mechanism of action, echinocandins seem to have an additive effect when used in combination with other antifungal agents.[40] Furthermore, it is thought that as echinocandins cause injury to the fungi they release β-glucans, which can have some immunomodulatory and inflammatory effect, important to some extent for clearing of the infection.

Echinocandins are poorly absorbed after oral administration and are only available as IV formulation. They bind highly to plasma proteins and, therefore, low concentrations are found in CNS, urine, and eye. With the exception of anidulafungin, these agents are metabolized in the liver. Their renal clearance is minimal and these agents are not dialyzable. Therefore, dose adjustments are not necessary in renal failure or in patients undergoing hemodialysis. Regarding their use during pregnancy and lactation, the FDA considers caspofungin and micafungin as class C and, therefore, not safe during pregnancy.[41] Lactation should also be avoided because infant risk cannot be ruled out. Anidulafungin is, however, a class B agent and, based on the World Health Organization, is compatible with breastfeeding. Monitoring infants for side effects is recommended.[15,39] Although the spectrum of activity is similar among echinocandins, there are some important differences.

Caspofungin
The main FDA-approved indications for caspofungin are the treatment of esophageal candidiasis, candidemia, and disseminated candidiasis. It is also approved for empiric treatment of febrile neutropenia and for salvage therapy for invasive aspergillosis in patients who have failed or are intolerant of other antifungal agents.[19]

A loading dose is required because the drug diffuses into the tissues on initial dose. Metabolized by the liver, it is recommended that the dose be reduced in patients with severe hepatic insufficiency. Echinocandins, unlike other antifungals, are not primarily metabolized by CYP450 and, although the exact mechanism of action is not clearly stablished, data suggest that OATP-1B1, an anion-transporting polypeptide, is needed for the uptake by hepatocytes. Therefore, drugs that interact with OATP-1B1, such as cyclosporine and rifampin, may affect caspofungin levels.[42]

Tacrolimus, dexamethasone, and carbamazepine are among others drugs that interact with caspofungin. Thorough evaluation of drug-drug interactions need to be assessed before and during therapy with caspofungin.

Micafungin

Micafungin is indicated for the treatment of candidemia, esophageal and disseminated candidiasis, and for prophylaxis of disseminated candidiasis in hematopoietic stem cell transplant patients.

Micafungin has linear elimination and does not require a loading dose. It also does not require dose reduction in liver impairment, but it is advised to monitor creatinine and liver enzymes.[43] It has less drug-drug interactions than caspofungin. It does not seem to interact with tacrolimus, cyclosporine, or mycophenolate mofetil; and only mild interactions are described with sirolimus, nifedipine, and Itraconazole.[43]

Most common adverse reactions include diarrhea, nausea, vomiting, pyrexia, thrombocytopenia, and headache. Histamine-mediated symptoms are also described and include rash, pruritus, facial, swelling, and vasodilatation.

Anidulafungin

Anidulafungin is a semisynthetic polypeptide synthesized from the fermentation product of *Aspergillus nidulans*. It has been FDA-approved to treat candidemia and esophageal and disseminated candidiasis. Anidulafungin undergoes slow biochemical degradation and is not metabolized by the liver. Isolated cases of hepatic dysfunction have been reported, although a causal relationship to anidulafungin has not been established. Monitoring of liver enzymes is recommended. Infusion-related adverse events are rare and include rash, urticaria, flushing, pruritus, dyspnea, bronchospasm, and hypotension. No significant drug-drug interactions have been seen in the drugs investigated.

Fluocytosine

Fluocytosine (5FC) is an antimetabolite with antifungal properties. It works by interfering with DNA and protein synthesis. 5FC is transported into the fungi and deaminated to 5-fluorouracil (5-FU) by cytosine deaminase (not present in mammalian cells). Then it gets incorporated into the DNA, where it interferes with DNA synthesis. In addition, 5FC can be converted into 5-fluorouridine triphosphate by 5-fluorouridine monophosphate and 5-fluorouridine diphosphate. Then gets incorporated into fungal RNA, where it disrupts the amino acid pool and prevents protein synthesis. 5FC can be fungicidal or fungistatic depending on the fungi. 5FC has activity against *Candida* spp,

Cryptococcus spp, and *Saccharomyces* spp, although the endemic fungi *Aspergillus* spp and *Zygomycetes* are generally resistant (see **Table 1**).

In the United States, 5FC is available only in oral formulation, but it has excellent bioavailability with good penetration into bone, peritoneal, and synovial fluid. It penetrates well into CSF and is excreted by urine. It is important to monitor drug concentrations, particularly in patients with renal impairment, because high concentrations (>100 mg/mL) have been associated with thrombocytopenia and hepatotoxicity.[44]

Drug levels should be measured between days 3 and 5 of initiation of therapy, usually 2 hours after administration. In cases of renal failure, toxicity or increased concentration levels have been reported. CBC should be monitored for leukopenia and thrombocytopenia.

5FC is mostly used in combination with other therapies because resistance commonly occurs during treatment of initially susceptible strains. In the setting of *Candida* infections, 5FC is used in combination with AmB, particularly in refractory *Candida* infections such as endocarditis, endophthalmitis, and meningitis.[19] It is also recommended for cryptococcosis, especially if there is CNS involvement.[12]

It should be avoided during pregnancy and is considered class C by the FDA. Breast feeding is not recommended while receiving 5-FU.

The most common side effects include rash, diarrhea, and elevation of liver enzymes. Bone marrow suppression is more commonly associated with prolonged therapy (>7 days) and blood levels more than 100 μg/mL.[18]

REFERENCES

1. Limper AH, Offord KP, Smith TF, et al. *Pneumocystis carinii* pneumonia. Differences in lung parasite number and inflammation in patients with and without AIDS. Am Rev Respir Dis 1989;140(5):1204–9.
2. Vassallo R, Standing JE, Limper AH. Isolated *Pneumocystis carinii* cell wall glucan provokes lower respiratory tract inflammatory responses. J Immunol 2000;164(7):3755–63.
3. Lenardon MD, Munro CA, Gow NA. Chitin synthesis and fungal pathogenesis. Curr Opin Microbiol 2010; 13(4):416–23.
4. Drew RH. Pharmacology of amphotericin B. In: Kauffman CA, ed. UpToDate. Waltham (MA): UpToDate. Available at: https://www.uptodate.com/contents/pharmacology-of-amphotericin-b?source=search_result&search=amphotericin%20b&selectedTitle=4~146. Accessed August 18, 2016.
5. Anderson TM, Clay MC, Cioffi AG, et al. Amphotericin forms an extramembranous and fungicidal sterol sponge. Nat Chem Biol 2014;10(5):400–6.

6. Johnson PC, Wheat LJ, Cloud GA, et al. Safety and efficacy of liposomal amphotericin B compared with conventional amphotericin B for induction therapy of histoplasmosis in patients with AIDS. Ann Intern Med 2002;137(2):105–9.

7. Borro JM, Sole A, de la Torre M, et al. Efficiency and safety of inhaled amphotericin B lipid complex (Abelcet) in the prophylaxis of invasive fungal infections following lung transplantation. Transplant Proc 2008;40(9):3090–3.

8. Rijnders BJ, Cornelissen JJ, Slobbe L, et al. Aerosolized liposomal amphotericin B for the prevention of invasive pulmonary aspergillosis during prolonged neutropenia: a randomized, placebo-controlled trial. Clin Infect Dis 2008; 46(9):1401–8.

9. AmBisome (amphotericin B) liposome for injection [package insert]. Gilead Sciences, Inc; 2012. Available at: https://www.astellas.us/docs/ambisome.pdf. Accessed September 27, 2016.

10. Barcia JP. Hyperkalemia associated with rapid infusion of conventional and lipid complex formulations of amphotericin B. Pharmacotherapy 1998;18(4): 874–6.

11. Wright DG, Robichaud KJ, Pizzo PA, et al. Lethal pulmonary reactions associated with the combined use of amphotericin B and leukocyte transfusions. N Engl J Med 1981;304(20):1185–9.

12. Perfect JR, Dismukes WE, Dromer F, et al. Clinical practice guidelines for the management of cryptococcal disease: 2010 update by the infectious diseases society of America. Clin Infect Dis 2010; 50(3):291–322.

13. Patterson TF, Thompson GR 3rd, Denning DW, et al. Practice guidelines for the diagnosis and management of aspergillosis: 2016 update by the infectious diseases society of America. Clin Infect Dis 2016; 63(4):e1–60.

14. Amphotericin B. 2016. Available at: http://www. micromedexsolutions.com/micromedex2/librarian/PF DefaultActionId/evidencexpert.DoIntegratedSearch# close. Accessed September 27, 2016.

15. UNICEF WHO. Anon: breastfeeding and maternal medication. Geneva (Switzerland): World Heath Organization; 2002.

16. J.R. AEDaP. Pharmacology of azoles. In: Kauffman CA, ed. UpToDate. Walthman (MA): UpToDate. Available at: https://www.uptodate.com/contents/pharmacology-of-azoles?topicKey=ID%2F495&elapse. Accessed August 18, 2016.

17. Toon S, Ross CE, Gokal R, et al. An assessment of the effects of impaired renal function and haemodialysis on the pharmacokinetics of fluconazole. Br J Clin Pharmacol 1990;29(2):221–6.

18. Thompson GR 3rd, Cadena J, Patterson TF. Overview of antifungal agents. Clin Chest Med 2009; 30(2):203–15, v.

19. Pappas PG, Kauffman CA, Andes DR, et al. Clinical practice guideline for the management of candidiasis: 2016 update by the Infectious Diseases Society of America. Clin Infect Dis 2016;62(4):e1–50.

20. Galgiani JN, Ampel NM, Blair JE, et al. 2016 Infectious Diseases Society of America (IDSA) clinical practice guideline for the treatment of coccidioidomycosis. Clin Infect Dis 2016;63(6):e112–46.

21. Grant SM, Clissold SP. Itraconazole. A review of its pharmacodynamic and pharmacokinetic properties, and therapeutic use in superficial and systemic mycoses. Drugs 1989;37(3):310–44.

22. Boelaert J, Schurgers M, Matthys E, et al. Itraconazole pharmacokinetics in patients with renal dysfunction. Antimicrob Agents Chemother 1988; 32(10):1595–7.

23. Limper AH, Knox KS, Sarosi GA, et al. An official American Thoracic Society statement: treatment of fungal infections in adult pulmonary and critical care patients. Am J Respir Crit Care Med 2011; 183(1):96–128.

24. Wheat LJ, Freifeld AG, Kleiman MB, et al. Clinical practice guidelines for the management of patients with histoplasmosis: 2007 update by the Infectious Diseases Society of America. Clin Infect Dis 2007; 45(7):807–25.

25. Chapman SW, Dismukes WE, Proia LA, et al. Clinical practice guidelines for the management of blastomycosis: 2008 update by the Infectious Diseases Society of America. Clin Infect Dis 2008;46(12): 1801–12.

26. NOXAFIL® (posaconazole) injection, for intravenous use. NOXAFIL ® (posaconazole) delayed-release tablets, for oral use. NOXAFIL ® (posaconazole) oral suspension [package insert]. Merck Sharp & Dohme Corp; 2016. Available at: https://www.merck. com/product/usa/pi_circulars/n/noxafil/noxafil_pi.pdf. Accessed September 27, 2016.

27. Courtney R, Sansone A, Smith W, et al. Posaconazole pharmacokinetics, safety, and tolerability in subjects with varying degrees of chronic renal disease. J Clin Pharmacol 2005;45(2):185–92.

28. Ashbee HR, Barnes RA, Johnson EM, et al. Therapeutic drug monitoring (TDM) of antifungal agents: guidelines from the British Society for medical mycology. J Antimicrob Chemother 2014;69(5): 1162–76.

29. Ullmann AJ, Lipton JH, Vesole DH, et al. Posaconazole or fluconazole for prophylaxis in severe graft-versus-host disease. N Engl J Med 2007;356(4): 335–47.

30. Cornely OA, Maertens J, Winston DJ, et al. Posaconazole vs. fluconazole or itraconazole prophylaxis in patients with neutropenia. N Engl J Med 2007; 356(4):348–59.

31. Vehreschild JJ, Birtel A, Vehreschild MJ, et al. Mucormycosis treated with posaconazole: review of

96 case reports. Crit Rev Microbiol 2013;39(3): 310–24.

32. Dekkers BG, Bakker M, van der Elst KC, et al. Therapeutic drug monitoring of posaconazole: an update. Curr Fungal Infect Rep 2016;10:51–61.

33. VFEND- voriconazole tablet, film coated. VFEND-voriconazole injection, powder, lyophilized, for solution. VFEND- voriconazole powder, for suspension [package insert]. New York: Roerig, division of Pfizer, Inc; 2015. Available at: http://labeling.pfizer.com/ShowLabeling.aspx?id=618. Accessed September 27, 2016.

34. Livermore J, Hope W. Evaluation of the pharmacokinetics and clinical utility of isavuconazole for treatment of invasive fungal infections. Expert Opin Drug Metab Toxicol 2012;8(6):759–65.

35. Miceli MH, Kauffman CA. Isavuconazole: a new broad-spectrum triazole antifungal agent. Clin Infect Dis 2015;61(10):1558–65.

36. Thompson GR 3rd, Rendon A, Ribeiro Dos Santos R, et al. Isavuconazole treatment of cryptococcosis and dimorphic mycoses. Clin Infect Dis 2016; 63(3):356–62.

37. Kottom TJ, Limper AH. Cell wall assembly by *Pneumocystis carinii*. Evidence for a unique gsc-1 subunit mediating beta -1,3-glucan deposition. J Biol Chem 2000;275(51):40628–34.

38. Schmatz DM, Powles M, McFadden DC, et al. Treatment and prevention of pneumocystis carinii pneumonia and further elucidation of the *P. carinii* life cycle with 1,3-beta-glucan synthesis inhibitor L-671,329. J Protozool 1991;38(6):151S–3S.

39. Lewis ER. Pharmacology of echinocandins. In: Kauffman CA, editor. Walthman (MA): UpToDate. Available at: https://www.uptodate.com/contents/pharmacology-of-echinocandins?topicKey=ID%2F 139. Accessed August 18, 2016.

40. Aguilar-Zapata D, Petraitiene R, Petraitis V. Echinocandins: the expanding antifungal armamentarium. Clin Infect Dis 2015;61(Suppl 6):S604–11.

41. FDA) Rp. Product information: ERAXIS(TM) intravenous injection, anidulafungin intravenous injection. New York, 2012. Available at: https://www.accessdata.fda.gov/drugsatfda_docs/label/2006/021632s002lbl.pdf. Accessed May 13, 2017.

42. Sandhu P, Lee W, Xu X, et al. Hepatic uptake of the novel antifungal agent caspofungin. Drug Metab Dispos 2005;33(5):676–82.

43. Mycamine (micafungin sodium) [package insert]. Astellas Pharma Tech Co., Ltd; 2016. Available at: https://www.us.astellas.com/docs/mycamine.pdf. Accessed September 18, 2016.

44. Vermes A, van Der Sijs H, Guchelaar HJ. Flucytosine: correlation between toxicity and pharmacokinetic parameters. Chemotherapy 2000;46(2):86–94.

Clinical Perspectives in the Diagnosis and Management of Histoplasmosis

Marwan M. Azar, MD[a], Chadi A. Hage, MD[b],*

KEYWORDS

- Histoplasmosis • Endemic • Diagnosis • Treatment

KEY POINTS

- Histoplasmosis, caused by the dimorphic fungus *Histoplasma capsulatum*, is endemic to certain regions within the United States, as well as other parts of the world.
- Pneumonia is the most common disease presentation but extrapulmonary dissemination can occur, especially in immunocompromised patients.
- A multipronged approach is recommended for diagnosis, including laboratory, radiographic, histopathologic, microbiologic, and serologic evaluation.
- Manifestations that are always treated include moderate-to-severe acute pulmonary histoplasmosis, disseminated disease, and histoplasmosis in immunocompromised individuals.
- Amphotericin B is the drug of choice for moderate-to-severe and disseminated presentations, whereas itraconazole is appropriate for mild disease and as step-down therapy.

INTRODUCTION

Histoplasma capsulatum, the etiologic agent of histoplasmosis, is a dimorphic fungus highly endemic to the Mississippi and Ohio River valleys of North America. In an increasingly interconnected continent, in which millions of travelers migrate through high-prevalence areas, the Ohio River Valley fever has become a disease of international extent, much farther-reaching than the simple geographic confines of its endemicity. Moreover, with increasing numbers of patients receiving immunosuppressive therapies, including solid-organ and bone marrow transplantation and tumor-necrosis-factor inhibitors, the population at risk for histoplasmosis, including severe

disseminated forms, will continue to grow. In terms of disease cadence (acute, subacute, and chronic), onset (primary or reactivation disease), distribution (pulmonary, mediastinal, disseminated, and isolated extrapulmonary) and severity (asymptomatic, mild, and moderate-severe), the clinical spectrum of histoplasmosis is very wide, often contributing to delays in diagnosis. The advent of *Histoplasma* antigen testing has revolutionized the diagnosis of histoplasmosis by providing a convenient and highly sensitive test; however, a multipronged approach is recommended for the diagnosis of histoplasmosis, including laboratory, radiographic, histopathologic, microbiologic, and serologic evaluation. Treatment of

Disclosure Statement: The authors have nothing to disclose.
[a] Pathology Department, Massachusetts General Hospital, Harvard School of Medicine, 55 Fruit Street, GRB 526, Boston, MA 02114, USA; [b] Thoracic Transplantation Program, Department of Medicine, Methodist Professional Center-2, Indiana University Health Methodist Hospital, Indiana University, Suite 2000, 1801 North Senate Boulevard, Indianapolis, IN 46202, USA
* Corresponding author.
E-mail address: chage@iu.edu

Clin Chest Med 38 (2017) 403–415
http://dx.doi.org/10.1016/j.ccm.2017.04.004
0272-5231/17/© 2017 Elsevier Inc. All rights reserved.

histoplasmosis is contingent on the severity and specific manifestation of the disease, but immunocompromised patients and disseminated disease should always be treated. This article details the current concepts in the diagnosis and management of this protean disease.

RISK FACTORS FOR HISTOPLASMOSIS

The primary risk factor for the acquisition of histoplasmosis is living in or traveling to an area endemic for the fungus. The most highly endemic regions of North America have long been known to be the Ohio River and Mississippi River basins.[1] However, based on data from animal infections,[2–4] skin testing for histoplasmin sensitivity,[5] and case reports,[6] areas of previously unrecognized endemicity continue to be elucidated. Since 1938, outbreaks of histoplasmosis have been reported in more than 26 states,[7] widening the presumed geographic distribution of the fungus. Outside of mainland United States, the island of Puerto Rico has been associated with multiple cases of histoplasmosis.[8] H capsulatum var capsulatum is now understood to be endemic to parts of Central and South America, Southern Europe, Southeast Asia, and Oceania,[9] whereas African histoplasmosis caused by H capsulatum var duboisii is prevalent in central and western regions of the continent.[10]

Bird and bat guano are strongly associated with the presence of H capsulatum and their presence is commonly implicated in outbreaks of infection among humans. Disruption of nests and roosting sites, spelunking, and other activities that afford exposure to these animals or their dwellings increase the risk of inhaling fungal spores.[11] In an epidemiologic survey of 105 outbreaks recorded from 1983 to 2013, exposure to birds, bats, or their droppings was reported in 77% of cases.[7] Construction, landscaping, excavation, strong winds, and other natural or anthropogenic phenomena that result in soil aerosolization are other risk factors for acquiring histoplasmosis. Persons involved in work-related or recreational activities that involve the outdoors are, in turn, more likely to be infected.

In addition to epidemiology, host factors play an important role in the susceptibility to histoplasmosis. Immunocompromised patients, particularly those with deficiencies of the cellular immune system, have decreased capacity to contain a burgeoning infection. Such patients are at greater likelihood of developing progressive disseminated disease, even when exposed to smaller fungal inocula.[12] Patients at extremes of age; those infected with human immunodeficiency virus, acquired immune deficiency syndrome (HIV/AIDS); solid-organ transplant recipients[13]; and patients receiving tumor necrosis factor (TNF) inhibitors[14] are populations identified to be at increased risk.[15] However, histoplasmosis may be heterogeneous in different populations of immunosuppressed individuals. After solid-organ transplantation, donor-related infection and reactivation of asymptomatic latent histoplasmosis are the most common mechanisms of infection and occur in a bimodal fashion: within 6 months and after 2 years of transplantation,[16] respectively. On the other hand, almost all patients with HIV/AIDS develop progressive disseminated histoplasmosis secondary to de novo infection.[17] A summary of risk factors for histoplasmosis is found in **Table 1**.

Over the last decade, new at-risk populations have emerged. In a 2001 to 2012 survey of hospitalizations due to histoplasmosis, significant increases in hospital admissions over time were seen with the use of biologic agents, a history of

Table 1
Risk factors for histoplasmosis

Epidemiologic Factor	Host Factors	Pathogen Factors
Endemic area • Ohio and Mississippi River basins (US) • Puerto Rico & Caribbean • Central and South America • Southeast Asia • Oceania • Africa (H var duboisii) Bird and Bat guano exposure • Spelunking Aerosolized soil exposure • Construction • Landscaping • Strong winds	HIV/AIDS (especially CD4 count <150 cells/mm³) TNF-alpha inhibitors Solid organ transplantation Bone marrow transplantation Extremes of age (<2 or>50 y) Other causes of cellular immune suppression or dysfunction	Size of inoculum Inherent virulence

transplantation, and comorbid diabetes, although not with HIV/AIDS,[18] suggesting that antiretroviral therapy may have mitigated the risk of histoplasmosis in this group. Though infections in individuals on TNF-inhibitors are increasingly common, outcomes seem to be favorable.[15] Due to age-associated alterations in cellular immunity, elderly patients may be at higher risk for histoplasmosis. In the aforementioned series, persons older than the age of 65 years were more likely to be hospitalized for their disease than younger persons.[18]

APPROACH TO DIAGNOSIS OF HISTOPLASMOSIS

Histoplasmosis can present in distinct clinical syndromes that vary by clinical course, severity, disease extent, and radiographic findings. Defining the clinical syndrome at hand is key because available diagnostics are not equally sensitive and specific for all manifestations of the disease,[19,20] and because certain tests may be preferred in certain clinical scenarios. For example, although antigen detection in serum and urine is a very useful test in patients with severe acute or disseminated histoplasmosis, it is less sensitive than serology for the diagnosis of subacute and chronic pulmonary histoplasmosis.[20,21] Conversely, serology is unreliable in patients with a reduced ability to produce antibodies. In addition, both the need and selection of antifungals are contingent on the clinical syndrome. Indeed, inflammatory manifestations, such as pericarditis and arthritis, or asymptomatic pulmonary nodules most often do not require treatment, whereas severe or disseminated disease always does. Understanding the underlying host factors that predispose the patient to infection is critical in formulating an effective treatment strategy.[12] Immunocompromised individuals are at increased risk for both severe and disseminated forms of the disease.[21] In addition to appropriate antifungals, reconstituting the cellular immune system by reducing or withdrawing immunosuppressive medications, or by instituting antiretroviral therapy in patients with HIV/AIDS, is usually required to achieve a successful outcome. Knowledge of the pathogen itself, including its ability to reactivate from latent granulomas decades after initial infection, will inform the clinician about the patient's underlying disease pathogenesis, particularly in cases in which no recent exposure can be identified.

CLINICAL SYNDROMES
Acute Pulmonary Histoplasmosis

Symptomatic acute pulmonary histoplasmosis occurs in approximately 10% of persons after inhalation of fungal spores. Almost all patients develop an asymptomatic or self-limited infection that is often undetected. Factors that increase the likelihood for symptomatic disease include being at the extremes of age, having an immunocompromising condition (particularly those affecting the cellular immune system), and exposure to a large inoculum.[22] The most common symptoms reported include cough, dyspnea, malaise, fever, and chills. Less common manifestations include chest pain due to concurrent mediastinal lymph node enlargement and rheumatologic complaints, including arthralgias, arthritis, erythema nodosum, and erythema multiforme.[23,24] Symptoms last less than 2 weeks and are often misdiagnosed as a bacterial pneumonia or viral respiratory illness. Diffuse patchy infiltrates or focal infiltrates are common findings on chest roentgenograms, whereas computed tomography (CT) of the chest often demonstrates enlarged mediastinal and hilar lymph nodes (**Fig. 1**). When present, pancytopenia, and elevated liver function tests should prompt a workup of disseminated infection (**Table 2**).

Subacute Pulmonary Histoplasmosis

Exposure to smaller inocula of *H capsulatum* may lead to the development of a slowly progressive infection over several weeks to months. This subacute form of pulmonary histoplasmosis is characterized by milder but more persistent respiratory and constitutional symptoms. On chest imaging, focal opacities predominate and mediastinal and hilar adenopathy are common findings[25] (see **Table 2**).

Chronic Pulmonary Histoplasmosis

Chronic pulmonary histoplasmosis follows a more protracted course than the subacute form, smoldering over a period of months to years.[26] This

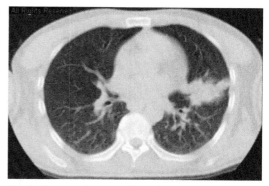

Fig. 1. Acute pulmonary histoplasmosis presenting as a community-acquired pneumonia.

Table 2
Pulmonary and mediastinal histoplasmosis

Entity	Risk Factor	Clinical Time-Course	Chest Imaging	Diagnostic Test	Indication for Treatment	Treatment	Antifungal Duration
Progressive disseminated histoplasmosis	Immuno-suppression	1–2 wk	Diffuse reticulonodular infiltrates	• Histoplasma antigen (urine, serum, CSF) • Culture (blood, bone marrow, CSF) • Bone marrow or adrenal biopsy	Always	Amphotericin B (severe) 1–2 wk followed by itraconazole Itraconazole (mild and as step-down)	12 mo followed by maintenance antifungal suppression until immune recovery
Acute Pulmonary Histoplasmosis	High inoculum exposure	1–2 wk	Diffuse infiltrates	• Histoplasma antigen (serum, urine, BAL) • BAL cytopathology and culture	Moderate or severe disease Immunosuppressed patient	Amphotericin B (severe)1–2 wk followed by itraconazole Itraconazole (mild and as step-down)	12 wk
Subacute Pulmonary Histoplasmosis	Low inoculum exposure	Weeks to months	Focal infiltrates	• Histoplasma serology • Histoplasma antigen (BAL) • BAL cytopathology and culture	If symptoms last>1 mo Immunosuppressed patient	Itraconazole	6–12 wk
Chronic Pulmonary Histoplasmosis	Chronic obstructive pulmonary disease and other lung diseases Smoking	Months to years	Cavities Fibrosis Pleural Thickening Calcifications	• Histoplasma serology • Sputum cytopathology and culture • Histoplasma antigen (BAL) • BAL cytopathology and culture	Always	Itraconazole	1–2 y and until radiologic resolution or stabilization

Diagnosis and Management of Histoplasmosis 407

Mediastinal Adenitis	Reactive and enlarged mediastinal lymph nodes	Early complication	Homogenous enhancement of mediastinal lymph nodes on computed tomography (CT)	• Histoplasma serology	If compressive symptoms present or adenitis last>1 mo	Itraconazole and steroids	6–12 wk
Mediastinal Granuloma	Coalesced necrotic mediastinal lymph nodes	Early or late complication	Heterogeneous enhancement of confluent mediastinal lymph nodes on CT. Calcifications if late	• Histoplasma serology	If compressive symptoms present	Surgery and itraconazole	6–12 wk
Mediastinal Fibrosis	Fibrosis of mediastinal structures	Late complication	Homogenous enhancement of mediastinal mass, with constriction points on CT. Calcifications	• Histoplasma serology	If compressive symptoms present	Stenting Arterial embolization Surgery	Not applicable

entity occurs in patients with abnormal lung architecture, often from years of tobacco abuse, or in patients with emphysema or pneumoconioses, and is thought to be the result of immune dysregulation in the face of fungal antigens.[27] The natural course is one of repeated exacerbations but with an overall arc of slow respiratory decline. Shortness of breath and productive cough are accompanied by fever, weight loss, and night sweats. Chest radiographs show calcified mediastinal and hilar lymph nodes of normal size. Infiltrates seen on chest imaging evolve over time, first from focal or diffuse infiltrates to consolidations, cavitation, interstitial fibrosis, and pleural thickening, mimicking pulmonary tuberculosis[28] (see **Fig. 2** and **Table 2**).

Pulmonary Nodules

Pulmonary nodules are a common incidental finding on chest imaging of patients who reside or have previously lived in endemic regions. In asymptomatic patients, pulmonary nodules most commonly represent old disease that has been effectively controlled. Differentiating these nodules from malignancy is difficult, often requiring pathologic examination obtained through biopsies or excisional procedures. Cultures and stains are often negative but finding granulomas on histopathology is suggestive. There is some evidence that histoplasmosis-associated nodules have decreased radionuclide uptake on PET scanning compared with malignancy.[29]

Mediastinal Histoplasmosis

There are 3 mediastinal manifestations of histoplasmosis: (1) mediastinal adenitis, (2) mediastinal granuloma, and (3) mediastinal fibrosis. Mediastinal adenitis consists of enlarged mediastinal lymph nodes that develop in response to acute pulmonary infection.[27] Mediastinal granuloma is characterized by enlarged mediastinal lymph nodes that become slowly necrotic and coalesce into a semisolid mediastinal mass.[19] Although mediastinal adenitis is usually an early complication after pulmonary infection, mediastinal granuloma may also occur decades later (**Fig. 3**). Both syndromes are most commonly subclinical but occasionally the nodes may become large enough to compress nearby structures, leading to chest pain. Excessive compression can lead to impingement of the esophagus, airways, and superior vena cava (SVC), leading to chronic dysphagia, chronic cough and lung collapse, and SVC syndrome, respectively.[30,31] In mediastinal granuloma, fistula to adjacent anatomic structures may rarely develop, expelling necrotic contents into bronchi or into the esophagus. Recurrent coughing fits

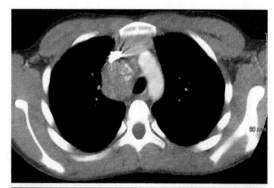

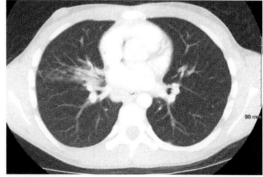

Fig. 3. A 16-year-old boy with a history of acute histoplasmosis 4 years prior, presents with recurrent right middle lobe following obstructive pneumonia (*bottom*) with bronchoscopy showing airway impingement. Chest CT shows a large mediastinal granuloma with calcifications (*top*).

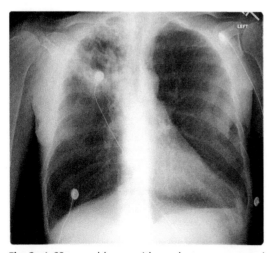

Fig. 2. A 68-year-old man with emphysema presented with persistent productive cough, low-grade fever, and weight loss, diagnosed with chronic pulmonary histoplasmosis. Sputum culture grew *Histoplasma capsulatum*, serology was positive for CF, 1:128 and 1:64 for mycelia, and M band was positive on ID.

accompanied by fevers, chills, diaphoresis, and other constitutional symptoms may occur as a result of bronchial obstruction. However, when contents are deposited into the mediastinal esophagus, debris is uneventfully swallowed and patients usually remain asymptomatic. Bacterial superinfection of necrotic lymph nodes is a potentially devastating complication of mediastinal granuloma and manifests with a sepsis syndrome.[32]

Mediastinal fibrosis is a late complication of histoplasmosis in which mediastinal tissues become increasingly fibrotic over time, leading to progressive encasement of enclosed anatomic structures. This syndrome may be initially asymptomatic but usually progresses until impingement of vital structures leads to obstructive symptomatology, the most dreaded of which are obstruction of the pulmonary artery or SVC.[33] The underlying pathophysiology is thought to be secondary to immune over-reaction to fungal antigens found in mediastinal tissues and, as a result, it occurs more frequently in younger individuals with a more robust cellular immunity.

On CT scanning, mediastinal adenitis manifests as enlarged lymph nodes that are solid in appearance and with homogenous enhancement (**Fig. 4**), whereas in mediastinal granuloma, lymph nodes are heterogeneous and may include septations.[34] Mediastinal fibrosis is characterized by a fibrotic, calcified mediastinum with evidence of compression points on nearby airways or vessels.[35] Mediastinal granuloma may be confused with malignancy because it appears as a heterogeneous mediastinal mass on imaging. Obtaining mediastinal tissue is often needed to identify the underlying cause (infectious vs malignant vs connective tissue disorder). Tissue examination

usually reveals evidence of necrosis and granulomatous inflammation. Cultures are usually negative but dead organisms may sometimes be noted on stains. In contrast, a tissue diagnosis is not indicated in mediastinal fibrosis because fibrotic tissue will yield fibrotic tissue that cannot effectively differentiate between various potential causes. In addition, the fibrotic mediastinum becomes hardened and is highly susceptible to injury during diagnostic procedures. Antigen testing is poorly sensitive for the diagnosis of mediastinal histoplasmosis, especially mediastinal fibrosis, because the burden of fungal infection is low.[36] However, serology is a useful indicator of past infection and is an important part of solving this diagnostic puzzle (see **Table 2**).

Pericarditis

Acute pericarditis follows acute pulmonary histoplasmosis in few cases (5%) and is thought to be secondary to pericardial irritation from nearby mediastinal node inflammation. As such, it is considered to be an inflammatory-immune process rather than a consequence of fungal invasion into the pericardium. The syndrome occurs 2 to 6 weeks after pulmonary infection and is characterized by chest pain, typical electrocardiogram change, and sometimes a pericardial rub.[37,38]

Progressive Disseminated Histoplasmosis

Progressive disseminated histoplasmosis develops when inhaled yeast successfully break through the immune system's defenses and disseminate hematogenously to various parts of the body. Patients with compromised cellular immune systems (see previous discussion of risk factors) and patients younger than 1 year or older than 50 years are at significantly increased risk for disseminated histoplasmosis.[21] This syndrome can be primary progressive, following an acute pulmonary infection or developing many years after a previously arrested infection (latent disease), once a patient has become newly immunocompromised. Acute progressive disseminated histoplasmosis occurs in the most highly immunocompromised patients (including infants) and is typified by a sudden onset and a systemic inflammatory response syndrome leading to rapid clinical deterioration.[39] In the subacute form, patients experience persistent symptoms, including fever, weight loss, night sweats, cough, and shortness of breath.

The reticuloendothelial system (liver, spleen, bone marrow, and lymph nodes), the gastrointestinal tract (especially the oral mucosa), the central nervous system (CNS; may produce focal lesion or

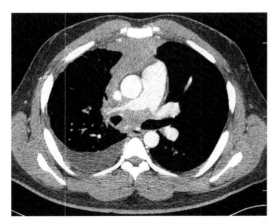

Fig. 4. Fibrosing mediastinitis with narrowing on pulmonary arteries causing right heart failure and persistent hypoxia in a middle-aged man from Indiana.

diffuse meningitis), and the adrenal glands (may lead to adrenal insufficiency) are the most common sites of dissemination.[40–43] In contrast to other endemic fungal infections, the skin is an uncommon extrapulmonary site of infection in histoplasmosis, except in patients with advanced HIV/AIDS.[44]

Diagnosis

The diagnosis of endemic fungal infections has been standardized by the European Organization for Research and Treatment of Cancer Invasive Fungal Infections Cooperative Group and the National Institute of Allergy and Infectious Diseases Mycoses Study Group.[45] Though these definitions were initially generated for research purposes, they can be of use in clinical settings, particularly with atypical presentations. A proven endemic mycosis is contingent on a compatible clinical scenario and a positive culture or histopathology. If culture or pathologic examination is not available or negative, yet the host is immunocompromised, the clinical picture is suggestive and a mycologic laboratory test is present (eg, *Histoplasma* antigen positivity), the diagnosis is considered probable.

Histopathology and Culture

Demonstrating organisms on pathologic examination and/or culture is the gold standard for the diagnosis of histoplasmosis. On histopathology, the presence of caseating or noncaseating granulomas is typical but performing special stains, including Gomori methenamine silver, Giemsa, or periodic acid–Schiff stains, is usually necessary to identify yeast. *H capsulatum* var capsulatum yeast are between 2 to 4 μm in diameter, ovoid shaped, predominantly intracellular (within macrophages and giant cells), and characteristically divide by narrow-based budding. Cytopathologic examination of specimens obtained via fine-needle aspiration or bronchoalveolar lavage (BAL) can also demonstrate yeast cells but is less sensitive than whole tissue pathologic examination.[46] The presence of yeast forms is not pathognomonic of active disease because they may be recovered from healed granulomas or calcified lymph nodes. In these cases, the clinical picture and underlying host factors are key in distinguishing latent from active disease.

H capsulatum requires 4 to 6 weeks to become detectable as a mold on fungal cultures. DNA probes may be used to confirm the presence of *H capsulatum* because diagnosis based on morphology alone may be challenging. Organisms can be recovered from sputum, BAL, blood, bone marrow, and biopsied tissues submitted for culture. The highest sensitivity for culture is in patients with disseminated and chronic pulmonary histoplasmosis.[20] *H capsulatum* cultures pose a potential threat to laboratory personnel and should be handled in a biosafety level 3 laboratory.

Antigen Testing

Though culture and histopathologic diagnosis remain the gold standards for the diagnosis of histoplasmosis, antigen testing provides a reliable, noninvasive, and highly sensitive means for diagnosis. The currently available enzyme immunoassay (EIA)-based assay provides quantitative results and is highly sensitive and specific. A multicenter evaluation of this assay among 218 subjects with histoplasmosis and 229 controls revealed a sensitivity of 91.8%, 87.5%, and 83% for disseminated histoplasmosis, chronic pulmonary histoplasmosis, and acute pulmonary histoplasmosis, respectively. Sensitivity for subacute histoplasmosis was low (30%).[20] A limitation of antigen testing is the significant cross-reactivity of the assay in the presence of other fungal infections, including blastomycosis, paracoccidioidomycosis, penicilliosis, aspergillosis, and coccidioidomycosis.[20]

Combining urine and serum antigen testing increases the overall sensitivity.[47] *Histoplasma* antigen can also be detected in cerebrospinal fluid (CSF) and BAL fluid.[48,49] This is most helpful in patients with CNS histoplasmosis and those with limited pulmonary disease, such as subacute and chronic histoplasmosis, in which serum and urine antigen might be negative. In addition to facilitating diagnosis, monitoring antigen levels is useful to follow response to therapy because antigen levels, particularly in the serum, have been shown to decline with appropriate treatment.[50] Rising antigen levels can also be used as early predictors for clinical relapse or treatment failure.

Serology

Serology is a marker of recent or past infection and, as such, is most useful in the diagnosis of subacute or chronic disease. Anti-*Histoplasma* antibodies appear 4 to 8 weeks after initial infection and persist for decades. There are 3 available methods for detecting antibodies to *H capsulatum*: immunodiffusion (ID), complement fixation (CF), and EIA. ID detects antibodies that bind to H and M fungal antigens and subsequently precipitate on agar gel, producing bands on diffusion. The H band is found in less than 20% of patients but always indicates active infection, whereas the M band is more common (80%) but less specific for active infection.[36] The CF test generates antibody titers. Acute infection is denoted by either a single titer of 1:32 or a fourfold or greater increase in antibody titers between acute and convalescent sera.[51] The EIA is the most sensitive test but suffers from high false-positives and has not been standardized across laboratories, making interpretation difficult.[52] A major limitation of serologic testing is in immunocompromised patients whose ability to mount a humoral immune response is reduced, such as among recipients of organ transplant who are maintained on cell cycle inhibitors.[20] However, serology can be useful in patients with subacute pulmonary histoplasmosis and other populations in whom the sensitivity of antigen testing is suboptimal.[53] Combining serology with antigen testing has been shown to improve the diagnostic yield for acute pulmonary histoplasmosis.

Molecular Diagnostics

Polymerase chain reaction (PCR) testing for *H capsulatum* has historically suffered from poor sensitivity when directly applied to clinical samples. However, newly developed PCR assays have shown improved performance characteristics and may gain a more important role in the diagnosis of histoplasmosis in the near future.[54] In addition, fluorescence in situ hybridization has been successfully applied to blood culture samples of patients with histoplasmosis.[55] DNA probes can be applied to incubating cultures to confirm the diagnosis of histoplasmosis.

TREATMENT
Acute Pulmonary Histoplasmosis

Treatment of acute pulmonary histoplasmosis is indicated when (1) the symptoms are moderate or severe, (2) there is bilateral pulmonary involvement on chest imaging, or (3) the patient is immunocompromised. Itraconazole for 12 weeks is recommended for moderate disease, whereas amphotericin B is indicated for severe manifestations. The liposomal form is preferable due to decreased renal toxicity and evidence of superior efficacy.[56] Step-down therapy to itraconazole can be performed after clinical improvement. In the setting of acute respiratory distress syndrome (ARDS) (**Fig. 5**), adjunctive steroids may be beneficial.[57]

Subacute Pulmonary Histoplasmosis

Subacute pulmonary histoplasmosis is most often self-limited and rarely requires treatment. Therapy with itraconazole for 6 to 12 weeks is indicated if symptoms persist for longer than 1 month.[58]

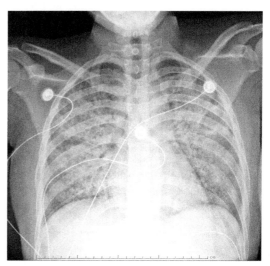

Fig. 5. A 23-year-old man treated with high-dose corticosteroid and intravenous immunoglobulin for refractory immune thrombocytopenia presented with 2 weeks of worsening dyspnea and fevers, leading to respiratory failure and acute respiratory distress syndrome (ARDS) requiring mechanical ventilation. BAL showed *Histoplasma* yeast on Giemsa stain. Urine *Histoplasma* antigen was highly positive. Patient made a complete recovery after timely initiation on liposomal amphotericin B followed by oral itraconazole.

Chronic Pulmonary Histoplasmosis

Treatment of chronic pulmonary histoplasmosis, a slowly destructive pulmonary process, is always warranted. Antifungals have been demonstrated to abrogate progression of the disease radiographically, to enhance microbiologic clearance of respiratory samples, and to improve overall survival. A minimum of 12 to 24 months of itraconazole is recommended; however, treatment should continue until there is no further improvement on serial chest imaging (repeated at 6 month intervals). Cessation of tobacco use is important to maximize recovery of lung function and optimize treatment response.[59] There is up to a 20% rate of relapse after treatment completion, so patients must be followed up for 1 to 2 years posttreatment.[60,61]

Pulmonary Nodules

Treatment of pulmonary nodules is almost never indicated because they represent old, inactive disease.

Mediastinal Histoplasmosis

Mediastinal histoplasmosis is most often asymptomatic, but treatment is indicated when compressive symptoms are present. When mediastinal adenitis presents with chest pain, nonsteroidal anti-inflammatory drugs (NSAIDs) can be pre-scribed to lessen the inflammation. Symptoms that persist for longer than a month can be treated with a tapered course of steroids (over 1–2 weeks) in addition to itraconazole for 6 to 12 weeks due to iatrogenic immunosuppression.[58] Compressive symptoms from mediastinal granuloma should be managed surgically, with partial resection of the offending free wall in the setting of compression, and repair of fistulae when present.[62] Adjunctive itraconazole may be administered, but the benefit of such an intervention is unproven. Bacterial su-perinfection of necrotic lymph nodes requires debridement and antibacterial therapy. For medi-astinal fibrosis, antifungals have not been shown to improve outcomes.[63,64] Additionally, surgery is high-risk due to heavily vascularized and scarred mediastinal tissues that are particularly prone to injury. Treatment should be directed at specific complications of the disease including (1) bron-chial artery embolization for massive or recurrent hemoptysis, (2) placement of pulmonary artery or SVC intravascular stents for vascular obstruction, and (3) placement of bronchial stents for airway obstruction. Unfortunately, the prognosis of medi-astinal fibrosis is poor because progressive dis-ease leads to stent obstruction from tissue overgrowth and new areas of compression. Tar-geting B-lymphocytes with rituximab (anti-CD20 monoclonal antibody) produced favorable thera-peutic results in a small series but larger and controlled studies are necessary to confirm this finding.[65]

Pericarditis

Because pericarditis associated with histoplasmo-sis is an immune manifestation rather than a result of direct fungal invasion, antifungal therapy is usu-ally not indicated. The inflammation can be managed with NSAIDs as with other causes of pericarditis. If symptoms persist for longer than 1 month, a short course of tapered steroids may accelerate resolution. If steroids are prescribed, itraconazole should be administered for 6 to 12 weeks while the patient is iatrogenically immunosuppressed.

Progressive Disseminated Histoplasmosis

Antifungal therapy is always indicated for dissem-inated histoplasmosis because untreated dissem-inated disease is usually fatal. In mild cases, itraconazole can be used, but most cases necessi-tate the use of amphotericin B as initial therapy.[58] As a result of improved deep tissue penetration and better tolerance with less renal toxicity and

infusion-related reactions, the liposomal form is associated with improved outcomes and is recom-mended.[56] Step-down therapy to itraconazole can be performed after 1 to 2 weeks (4–6 weeks for CNS histoplasmosis) if the clinical course is favor-able. Antifungal therapy is recommended for a minimum of 12 months, but the duration is also contingent on clinical, radiographic, and labora-tory improvement. Treatment may be indefinite in the case of immunocompromised patients in whom immunosuppression cannot be reversed. Because of prolonged therapy, therapeutic drug monitoring of itraconazole levels should be done to ensure adequate serum drug concentration. For HIV-positive patients, CD4 count should be greater than 150 cells/μL and HIV viral load less than 50 copies/mL while on a stable antiretro-viral regimen before treatment discontinuation. Urine *Histoplasma* antigen positivity (>2 ng/mL) and evidence of CNS histoplasmosis are indica-tions for continued treatment.[66] Following antigen levels in serum and urine is recommended while on therapy to document clearance and predict relapse and failure.[58]

In immunocompromised patients, clinical deteri-oration can sometimes be secondary to the im-mune reconstitution inflammatory syndrome (IRIS). This syndrome occurs when a reconstituting immune system (as in the setting of newly instituted antiretroviral therapy) mounts a vigorous attack against fungal antigens and is sometimes difficult to distinguish from treatment failure. Repeat anti-gen testing will usually show decreasing levels of antigen despite clinical worsening. Repeat sam-pling of tissues may reveal yeast in tissues but cul-tures are usually negative. A trial of steroids may serve as a diagnostic and therapeutic intervention for IRIS.[32]

SUMMARY

As the number of immunocompromised individ-uals and travelers to and from endemic areas ex-pands, the national and global significance of histoplasmosis will continue to increase. In light of an increasingly interconnected world, physi-cians in both endemic and nonendemic areas should be aware of epidemiologic factors associ-ated with disease acquisition, host factors that in-crease susceptibility to infection, and the varied clinical syndromes with which it can present.

REFERENCES

1. Kwon-Chung KJ, Weeks RJ, Larsh HW. Studies on *Emmonsiella capsulata* (*Histoplasma capsula-tum*). II. Distribution of the two mating types in

1. 13 endemic states of the United States. Am J Epidemiol 1974;99(1):44–9.

2. Burek-Huntington KA, Gill V, Bradway DS. Locally acquired disseminated histoplasmosis in a northern sea otter (*Enhydra lutris kenyoni*) in Alaska, USA. J Wildl Dis 2014;50(2):389–92.

3. Arunmozhi Balajee S, Hurst SF, Chang LS, et al. Multilocus sequence typing of *Histoplasma capsulatum* in formalin-fixed paraffin-embedded tissues from cats living in non-endemic regions reveals a new phylogenetic clade. Med Mycol 2013;51(4):345–51.

4. Johnson LR, Fry MM, Anez KL, et al. Histoplasmosis infection in two cats from California. J Am Anim Hosp Assoc 2004;40(2):165–9.

5. Manos NE, Ferebee SH, Kerschbaum WF. Geographic variation in the prevalence of histoplasmin sensitivity. Dis Chest 1956;29(6):649–68.

6. Pryor HB. Histoplasmosis in California children. J Pediatr 1949;34(1):12–9.

7. Benedict K, Mody RK. Epidemiology of histoplasmosis outbreaks, United States, 1938-2013. Emerg Infect Dis 2016;22(3):370–8.

8. De Jesus LG, Ramos Morales F. Histoplasmosis in Puerto Rico. Three cases with infection from common source. Bol Asoc Med P R 1968;60(10):501–8.

9. Bahr NC, Antinori S, Wheat LJ, et al. Histoplasmosis infections worldwide: thinking outside of the Ohio River valley. Curr Trop Med Rep 2015;2(2):70–80.

10. Gugnani HC, Muotoe-Okafor F. African histoplasmosis: a review. Rev Iberoam Micol 1997;14(4):155–9.

11. Ashford DA, Hajjeh RA, Kelley MF, et al. Outbreak of histoplasmosis among cavers attending the national speleological society annual convention, Texas, 1994. Am J Trop Med Hyg 1999;60(6):899–903.

12. Horwath MC, Fecher RA, Deepe GS Jr. *Histoplasma capsulatum*, lung infection and immunity. Future Microbiol 2015;10(6):967–75.

13. Assi M, Martin S, Wheat LJ, et al. Histoplasmosis after solid organ transplant. Clin Infect Dis 2013;57(11):1542–9.

14. Hage CA, Bowyer S, Tarvin SE, et al. Recognition, diagnosis, and treatment of histoplasmosis complicating tumor necrosis factor blocker therapy. Clin Infect Dis 2010;50(1):85–92.

15. Vergidis P, Avery RK, Wheat LJ, et al. Histoplasmosis complicating tumor necrosis factor-alpha blocker therapy: a retrospective analysis of 98 cases. Clin Infect Dis 2015;61(3):409–17.

16. Kauffman CA, Freifeld AG, Andes DR, et al. Endemic fungal infections in solid organ and hematopoietic cell transplant recipients enrolled in the transplant-associated infection surveillance network (TRANSNET). Transpl Infect Dis 2014; 16(2):213–24.

17. Wheat LJ, Connolly-Stringfield PA, Baker RL, et al. Disseminated histoplasmosis in the acquired immune deficiency syndrome: clinical findings, diagnosis and treatment, and review of the literature. Medicine (Baltimore) 1990;69(6):361–74.

18. Benedict K, Derado G, Mody RK. Histoplasmosis-associated hospitalizations in the United States, 2001-2012. Open Forum Infect Dis 2016;3(1):ofv219.

19. Hage CA, Azar MM, Bahr N, et al. Histoplasmosis: up-to-date evidence-based approach to diagnosis and management. Semin Respir Crit Care Med 2015;36(5):729–45.

20. Hage CA, Ribes JA, Wengenack NL, et al. A multicenter evaluation of tests for diagnosis of histoplasmosis. Clin Infect Dis 2011;53(5):448–54.

21. Wheat LJ, Slama TG, Norton JA, et al. Risk factors for disseminated or fatal histoplasmosis. Analysis of a large urban outbreak. Ann Intern Med 1982; 96(2):159–63.

22. Wheat LJ, Slama TG, Eitzen HE, et al. A large urban outbreak of histoplasmosis: clinical features. Ann Intern Med 1981;94(3):331–7.

23. Rosenthal J, Brandt KD, Wheat LJ, et al. Rheumatologic manifestations of histoplasmosis in the recent Indianapolis epidemic. Arthritis Rheum 1983;26(9): 1065–70.

24. Sizemore TC. Rheumatologic manifestations of histoplasmosis: a review. Rheumatol Int 2013;33(12): 2963–5.

25. Egressy K, Mohammed M, Ferguson JS. The use of endobronchial ultrasound in the diagnosis of subacute pulmonary histoplasmosis. Diagn Ther Endosc 2015;2015:510863.

26. Kennedy CC, Limper AH. Redefining the clinical spectrum of chronic pulmonary histoplasmosis: a retrospective case series of 46 patients. Medicine (Baltimore) 2007;86(4):252–8.

27. Goodwin RA Jr, Owens FT, Snell JD, et al. Chronic pulmonary histoplasmosis. Medicine (Baltimore) 1976;55(6):413–52.

28. Wheat LJ, Wass J, Norton J, et al. Cavitary histoplasmosis occurring during two large urban outbreaks. Analysis of clinical, epidemiologic, roentgenographic, and laboratory features. Medicine (Baltimore) 1984;63(4):201–9.

29. Kadaria D, Archie DS, SultanAli I, et al. Dual time point positron emission tomography/computed tomography scan in evaluation of intrathoracic lesions in an area endemic for histoplasmosis and with high prevalence of sarcoidosis. Am J Med Sci 2013; 346(5):358–62.

30. Micic D, Hogarth DK, Kavitt RT. Mediastinal granuloma: a rare cause of dysphagia. BMJ Case Rep 2016;2016 [pii: bcr2016215536].

31. Chaudhari D, McKinney J, Hubbs D, et al. Mediastinal histoplasmosis presenting as dysphagia: a case report with literature review. Clin J Gastroenterol 2013;6(4):315–8.

32. Wheat LJ, Azar MM, Bahr NC, et al. Histoplasmosis. Infect Dis Clin North Am 2016;30(1):207–27.

33. Parish JM, Rosenow EC 3rd. Mediastinal granuloma and mediastinal fibrosis. Semin Respir Crit Care Med 2002;23(2):135–43.

34. Landay MJ, Rollins NK. Mediastinal histoplasmosis granuloma: evaluation with CT. Radiology 1989; 172(3):657–9.

35. Rossi SE, McAdams HP, Rosado-de-Christenson ML, et al. Fibrosing mediastinitis. Radiographics 2001; 21(3):737–57.

36. Joseph Wheat L. Current diagnosis of histoplasmosis. Trends Microbiol 2003;11(10):488–94.

37. Wheat LJ, Stein L, Corya BC, et al. Pericarditis as a manifestation of histoplasmosis during two large urban outbreaks. Medicine (Baltimore) 1983;62(2): 110–9.

38. Picardi JL, Kauffman CA, Schwarz J, et al. Pericarditis caused by Histoplasma capsulatum. Am J Cardiol 1976;37(1):82–8.

39. Etxeberria-Lekuona D, Hurtado Ilzarbe G, Mendez-Lopez I, et al. Acute progressive disseminated histoplasmosis in a young immunocompetent patient. Rev Clin Esp (Barc) 2013;213(9):e95–6 [in Spanish].

40. Assi MA, Sandid MS, Baddour LM, et al. Systemic histoplasmosis: a 15-year retrospective institutional review of 111 patients. Medicine (Baltimore) 2007; 86(3):162–9.

41. Wheat LJ, Batteiger BE, Sathapatayavongs B. Histoplasma capsulatum infections of the central nervous system. A clinical review. Medicine (Baltimore) 1990; 69(4):244–60.

42. Kumar N, Singh S, Govil S. Adrenal histoplasmosis: clinical presentation and imaging features in nine cases. Abdom Imaging 2003;28(5):703–8.

43. Hariri OR, Minasian T, Quadri SA, et al. Histoplasmosis with deep CNS involvement: case presentation with discussion and literature review. J Neurol Surg Rep 2015;76(1):e167–72.

44. Eidbo J, Sanchez RL, Tschen JA, et al. Cutaneous manifestations of histoplasmosis in the acquired immune deficiency syndrome. Am J Surg Pathol 1993; 17(2):110–6.

45. De Pauw B, Walsh TJ, Donnelly JP, et al. Revised definitions of invasive fungal disease from the European Organization for Research and Treatment of Cancer/Invasive Fungal Infections cooperative group and the National Institute Of Allergy and Infectious Diseases Mycoses Study Group (EORTC/MSG) Consensus Group. Clin Infect Dis 2008; 46(12):1813–21.

46. Gupta N, Arora SK, Rajwanshi A, et al. Histoplasmosis: cytodiagnosis and review of literature with special emphasis on differential diagnosis on cytomorphology. Cytopathology 2010;21(4): 240–4.

47. Swartzentruber S, Rhodes L, Kurkjian K, et al. Diagnosis of acute pulmonary histoplasmosis by antigen detection. Clin Infect Dis 2009;49(12): 1878–82.

48. Hage CA, Davis TE, Fuller D, et al. Diagnosis of histoplasmosis by antigen detection in BAL fluid. Chest 2010;137(3):623–8.

49. Wheat LJ, Musial CE, Jenny-Avital E. Diagnosis and management of central nervous system histoplasmosis. Clin Infect Dis 2005;40(6): 844–52.

50. Hage CA, Kirsch EJ, Stump TE, et al. Histoplasma antigen clearance during treatment of histoplasmosis in patients with AIDS determined by a quantitative antigen enzyme immunoassay. Clin Vaccine Immunol 2011;18(4):661–6.

51. Wheat J, French ML, Kohler RB, et al. The diagnostic laboratory tests for histoplasmosis: analysis of experience in a large urban outbreak. Ann Intern Med 1982;97(5):680–5.

52. Wheat LJ, Kohler RB, French ML, et al. Immunoglobulin M and G histoplasmal antibody response in histoplasmosis. Am Rev Respir Dis 1983;128(1): 65–70.

53. Richer SM, Smedema ML, Durkin MM, et al. Improved diagnosis of acute pulmonary histoplasmosis by combining antigen and antibody detection. Clin Infect Dis 2016;62(7):896–902.

54. Babady NE, Buckwalter SP, Hall L, et al. Detection of Blastomyces dermatitidis and Histoplasma capsulatum from culture isolates and clinical specimens by use of real-time PCR. J Clin Microbiol 2011;49(9): 3204–8.

55. da Silva RM Jr, da Silva Neto JR, Santos CS, et al. Fluorescent in situ hybridization of pre-incubated blood culture material for the rapid diagnosis of histoplasmosis. Med Mycol 2015; 53(2):160–4.

56. Johnson PC, Wheat LJ, Cloud GA, et al. Safety and efficacy of liposomal amphotericin B compared with conventional amphotericin B for induction therapy of histoplasmosis in patients with AIDS. Ann Intern Med 2002;137(2):105–9.

57. Wynne JW, Olsen GN. Acute histoplasmosis presenting as the adult respiratory distress syndrome. Chest 1974;66(2):158–61.

58. Wheat LJ, Freifeld AG, Kleiman MB, et al. Clinical practice guidelines for the management of patients with histoplasmosis: 2007 update by the Infectious Diseases Society of America. Clin Infect Dis 2007; 45(7):807–25.

59. Dismukes WE, Bradsher RW Jr, Cloud GC, et al. Itraconazole therapy for blastomycosis and histoplasmosis. NIAID mycoses study group. Am J Med 1992;93(5):489–97.

60. Sarosi GA, Voth DW, Dahl BA, et al. Disseminated histoplasmosis: results of long-term follow-up. A center for disease control cooperative mycoses study. Ann Intern Med 1971;75(4):511–6.

61. Baum GL, Larkin JC Jr, Sutliff WD. Follow-up of patients with chronic pulmonary histoplasmosis treated with amphotericin B. Chest 1970;58(6): 562–5.

62. Hammoud ZT, Rose AS, Hage CA, et al. Surgical management of pulmonary and mediastinal sequelae of histoplasmosis: a challenging spectrum. Ann Thorac Surg 2009;88(2): 399–403.

63. Goodwin RA, Nickell JA, Des Prez RM. Mediastinal fibrosis complicating healed primary histoplasmosis and tuberculosis. Medicine (Baltimore) 1972;51(3): 227–46.

64. Loyd JE, Tillman BF, Atkinson JB, et al. Mediastinal fibrosis complicating histoplasmosis. Medicine (Baltimore) 1988;67(5):295–310.

65. Westerly BD, Johnson GB, Maldonado F, et al. Targeting B lymphocytes in progressive fibrosing mediastinitis. Am J Respir Crit Care Med 2014;190(9): 1069–71.

66. Myint T, Anderson AM, Sanchez A, et al. Histoplasmosis in patients with human immunodeficiency virus/acquired immunodeficiency syndrome (HIV/ AIDS): multicenter study of outcomes and factors associated with relapse. Medicine (Baltimore) 2014;93(1):11–8.

Diagnosis and Management of Coccidioidomycosis

Luke M. Gabe, MD, Joshua Malo, MD,
Kenneth S. Knox, MD*

KEYWORDS

- Coccidioidomycosis • Fungal infections • Diagnosis • Treatment

KEY POINTS

- Coccidioidomycosis is a primary cause of community-acquired pneumonia in endemic regions.
- The disease burden is rapidly growing within endemic areas secondary to population and environmental changes. Coccidioidomycosis is also seen far outside traditional boundaries in an increasingly mobile society.
- Recent arrival to an endemic area, certain ethnicities, advanced age, pregnancy, and defects in cellular immunity all influence disease severity.
- Coccidioidomycosis is definitively diagnosed when *Coccidioides* is demonstrated on pathology or in culture but is most commonly diagnosed via serology. The use of serology requires an understanding of the testing involved, and results must be interpreted in the context of time and capacity to develop a host immune response.
- Azoles, especially fluconazole, are the mainstay of therapy. The need to treat mild pulmonary disease is controversial but treatment is obligatory in severe or prolonged disease, dissemination, or severe immunosuppression. Treatment duration is months to a year and may be lifelong, depending on the clinical scenario.

INTRODUCTION

Coccidioides spp are a leading cause of community-acquired pneumonia in endemic regions. Although formerly well confined to these endemic areas, broad social and environmental changes have extended the reach of *Coccidioides* beyond traditional geographic boundaries and should be of interest to clinicians worldwide. Its manifestations are protean and many methods of diagnostic testing are available, each with limitations. Treatment, likewise, is commonly tailored to the patient, taking into account the severity and chronicity of the disease as well as the immune status and perceived vulnerability of the host.

HISTORY, ECOLOGY, AND EPIDEMIOLOGY

Coccidioidomycosis was first described in 1892 when an Argentinian medical student discovered spherical organisms resembling the protozoan Coccidia[1,2] in the biopsy specimens of a patient with progressive skin lesions. Similar lesions and biopsy findings were observed from a patient in the San Joaquin Valley of California several years later, and the organism was named *Coccidioides* (resembling Coccidia) *immitis* (not mild). As with *Histoplasma*[3] and *Blastomyces*,[4] *Coccidioides* was initially miscategorized as a protozoan,[1] a mistake perpetuated by its dimorphic nature (**Fig. 1**). Its true identity as a dimorphic fungus

Disclosure Statements: The authors have nothing to disclose.
Division of Pulmonary, Allergy, Critical Care and Sleep Medicine, University of Arizona College of Medicine – Tucson, 1501 North Campbell Avenue, Tucson, AZ 85724, USA
* Corresponding author.
E-mail address: kknox@deptofmed.arizona.edu

Clin Chest Med 38 (2017) 417–433
http://dx.doi.org/10.1016/j.ccm.2017.04.005

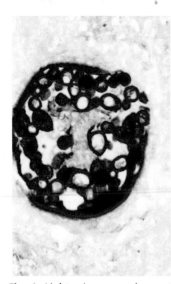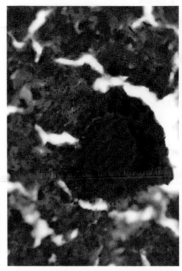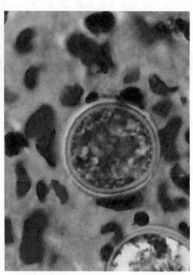

Fig. 1. Light microscopy demonstrating *Coccidioides* in spherular phase, characterized by a circular capsule-bound structure containing numerous small circular endospores. Microscopy findings are demonstrated using Grocott methenamine silver (*left*, original magnification × 400), Papanicolaou (*middle*, original magnification × 100), and hematoxylin-eosin stains (*right*, original magnification × 100).

was later recognized when mycelia were demonstrated to cause disease when injected into animals.[1,5] Subsequent case reports in patients and laboratory workers noted dissemination during the course of infection and emphasized the lungs as the portal of entry with development of lobar pneumonia, pleuritic chest pain, and often erythema nodosum.[1,6] This syndrome, now known in California as San Joaquin fever or valley fever, led to the identification of *Coccidioides* as the cause. A second species, *C posadasii*, was eventually identified.[7] *C immitis* mostly inhabits the San Joaquin Valley of California whereas *C posadasii* inhabits all other endemic regions. Overlap of these endemic regions is now known to exist and the clinical manifestations are indistinguishable between species.

Coccidioides spp are endemic to arid regions of the American Southwest, Northern Mexico, and several desert regions of Central and South America (**Fig. 2**). The organism tends to grow in sandy soil 10 cm to 30 cm below the surface,[8,9] where in wet conditions it grows as a mold with septate hyphae. In dry conditions, the hyphae desiccate to form small arthroconidia, or spores, 3 μm to 5 μm in diameter, later to be dispersed by aerosolization when the soil is disturbed by weather or commercialization. Spores are then inhaled, the route via which virtually all human disease occurs, although direct inoculation through broken skin is occasionally reported.[10] Once deposited in the periphery of the lungs the organism progresses to form much larger spherules, 20 μm to 100 μm in diameter, which eventually contain hundreds of 2 μm to 4 μm endospores; the spherule ruptures and releases these endospores, each of which is capable of creating a new spherule.

Rising Incidence in Endemic Areas

Arizona and California are the 2 states where the burden of coccidioidomycosis permits an estimation of incidence. Data for other areas are largely limited to coccidioidin skin testing surveys: positive skin reactivity in Mexican endemic regions ranges from 10% of the population (Baja California) to 93% (Coahuila).[10–12] Based on skin testing, 3% of endemic inhabitants seem to be newly infected each year.[13,14] Reports increasingly occur after dust storms,[15] military exercises,[16] earthquakes and landslides,[17] and outdoor recreation and during the dry season.[18,19] Consequently, up to 30% of cases of community-acquired pneumonia in Arizona may be due to coccidioidomycosis.[20]

Within Arizona and California, available data suggest a dramatic increase in disease burden. Although recent changes in laboratory-based case reporting in Arizona may partially be responsible for the increased incidence, from 2001 to 2010, the incidence of coccidioidal infection in Arizona increased from 12 cases to 58.2 cases per 100,000.[21,22] *Coccidioides*-specific diagnostic testing is only performed in a minority of patients presenting for care with compatible symptoms, suggesting that even these data are underestimates of true incidence.[23]

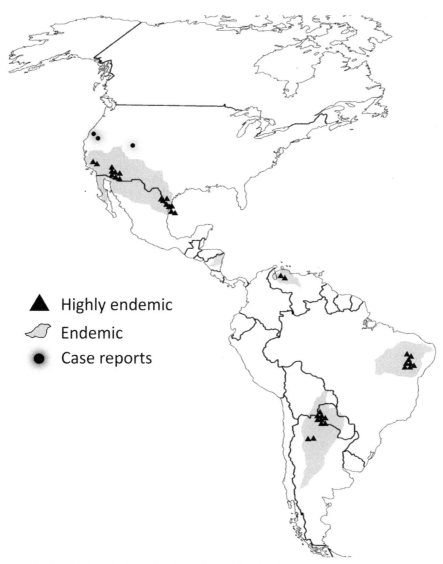

Fig. 2. Geographic distribution of the endemic region of *Coccidioides*. Case report markers denote areas with outbreaks and evidence of the organism in the local environment, and may represent new or previously undiscovered endemic zones.

Nonendemic Areas

The increasingly mobile, globalized population as well as the discovery of *Coccidioides* outside traditional boundaries has made coccidioidomycosis an increasingly relevant disease on national and global scales.[24–27] An estimated 10% of United States coccidioidomycosis cases occur outside of California and Arizona. Outbreaks in distant locations are reported in groups that have traveled to endemic regions, even briefly,[28,29] as has reactivation in immunosuppressed patients months to years after travel to an endemic region.[9,30] Dry arthroconidia have been shown viable for at least 6 months and fomite transmission via

dust on objects from the endemic region can occur.[31,32]

In 2001, an outbreak at an archaeological dig site at Dinosaur National Monument in northern Utah extended the reach of the known endemic territory in that state by approximately 200 miles.[33] In 2010 to 2011, 3 acute cases of coccidioidomycosis were diagnosed in southern Washington state[34] in patients without any recent travel history to a recognized endemic region (see **Fig. 2**). Finally, a healthy teenager in China with no history of travel or discernable fomite exposure was diagnosed with acute coccidioidomycosis[26]; the only possible exposure gleaned from investigators was that he had previously choked on seawater, in which *Coccidioides* is known to be able to survive.[35,36]

Susceptible Populations

The risk of acquiring symptomatic coccidioidomycosis seems to decline by 5% per year,[37] suggesting that this may be due to acquired subclinical disease with subsequent immune protection. As observed since the 1930s, recurrent disease through subsequent environmental exposure, as opposed to reactivation, remains a rare event.

Men have a higher incidence of coccidioidomycosis than women, historically attributed to outdoor occupational and recreational activities. Men may also be at increased risk of dissemination and severe disease, however, due to differences in comorbidities and sex hormones.[22,37–39] Pregnancy confers special risk, both to infection and dissemination. The risk is augmented when infection is acquired in the later stages of pregnancy and may be due to changes in sex hormones and decreases in cell-mediated immunity.[39–41]

Although the role of ethnicity is controversial in conferring risk for acquiring coccidioidomycosis, it is implicated in the risk of progression to severe or disseminated disease. Those of African or Filipino descent disproportionately develop disseminated disease with greater frequency than whites.[42] Blood groups A and B and various class II HLA alleles, which are more common in those of African and Filipino descent, are associated with severe and disseminated disease.[42,43]

Immunosuppression has become an increasingly important feature in the aging, comorbid population of the Southwest. Diabetics seem at increased risk of severe pulmonary disease; those with especially poor glycemic control are at increased risk of dissemination.[43,44] Patients with inflammatory arthropathies have an elevated risk that is mediated by both immunosuppressive medications (in particular biologics) and the underlying disease.[45–47] Patients with hematologic malignancies are observed to have a striking risk of dissemination (20%) once infected, with associated high mortality (50%).[48]

Coccidioidomycosis has long been recognized as an opportunistic infection in HIV patients. As seen in other opportunistic diseases in HIV, CD4 counts seem the most important predictor of disease acquisition as well as dissemination. Studies from an Arizona HIV clinic in 1988[49] and then from 2003 to 2008[50] demonstrated a marked decline in annual incidence of active coccidioidomycosis from 7.3% to 0.9%, in step with the advent and improvement of combination antiretroviral therapy.

Coccidioidomycosis is the most common endemic mycosis to cause disease in North American solid organ transplant recipients.[51] Among transplant patients in endemic areas, a known history of coccidioidomycosis, positive serology at transplantation, and use of antirejection therapy are risk factors for post-transplant coccidioidomycosis.[52–56] Coccidioidomycosis rates in transplant patients in the 1970s to 1980s reached approximately 9% in some populations, with 75% dissemination and 63% mortality.[57] These numbers have declined with time due to antifungal prophylaxis in selected high-risk patients. Donor-derived coccidioidomycosis also remains a significant concern for the transplant community. Because post-transplant coccidioidomycosis is frequently assumed to represent reactivation of latent disease in the recipient, this phenomenon is likely under-recognized within endemic areas. Reports of donor-derived infection are, therefore, limited to recipients with no previous exposure to endemic areas and frequently describe disseminated disease.[58–64]

CLINICAL PRESENTATION

Once inhaled, the arthroconidia of *Coccidioides* are highly virulent with as low as 1 spore able to cause disease in animal experiments. The organism is so highly infectious when aerosolized that it is listed as a potential bioterror agent and represents a serious threat to laboratory personnel who are not properly trained to take the necessary precautions.[2] Nevertheless, the majority experiences a self-limited or even asymptomatic infection with subsequent resolution and long-lived immunity; 60% of patients with positive skin tests in epidemiologic surveys have no recollection of their symptoms.[65] After exposure, incubation time prior to symptoms is 7 days to 28 days. Among those with symptomatic disease, 90% experience a self-limited respiratory illness, with only 1% to 10% progressing to severe or disseminated disease.[42]

Patients with primary pulmonary coccidioidomycosis commonly develop a flulike syndrome with cough and fever in 75%, often with pleurisy. Individuals may develop a skin reaction after several weeks, most commonly erythema nodosum or erythema multiforme. These skin reactions are immunologic phenomena and not a manifestation of disseminated disease; their presence is associated with a lower likelihood of disease progression.[10] Although its individual components of fever, arthralgia, and erythema nodosum are common, the classically described triad of desert rheumatism manifests in only a minority of *Coccidioides* infections. Overall, fatigue, presence of skin findings, arthralgias, and a subacute time course each favor coccidioidomycosis rather than bacterial pneumonia. Symptoms, such as rash and arthralgia, may be misleading and trigger administration of corticosteroids. Although not recommended, short courses early in the disease process fortunately do not seem to elevate risk of progression.[66]

Pulmonary Manifestations and Chest Imaging

Coccidioidomycosis most commonly manifests as a lobar or segmental pneumonia (**Figs. 3** and **4**), although a multifocal pneumonia is also possible. Chest imaging may also demonstrate hilar lymphadenopathy and a tree-in-bud pattern.[67] As the infection progresses to resolution, the most common pulmonary sequelae are a residual pulmonary nodule (coccidioidoma) or a small cavity. As with other endemic mycoses, nodules from old *Coccidioides* infections are common incidental findings on chest imaging and represent a substantial health care burden when, depending on their appearance and patient risk factors, they require differentiation from malignancy via serial imaging or invasive procedures.[68] Because of this, it is recommended to follow coccidioidal pneumonia radiographically to resolution to document nodules and prevent downstream work-up. In contrast to histoplasmosis, *Coccidioides* nodules usually do not calcify.

Cavities are thought to form either by liquefaction of a nodule with drainage into the bronchial tree or by ballooning surrounding the original infectious site.[2] They usually demonstrate a thin-walled or grapeskin appearance, a marker that helps distinguish them from other processes (**Fig. 5**). Occasionally, pneumothorax may be the initial presentation of a coccidioidal infection. Cavities may erode or rupture to cause a bronchopleural fistula. Cavities may also progress to a chronic fibrocavitary pneumonia,[67] which is more common in diabetics and is manifested clinically as chronic constitutional and respiratory symptoms, including weight loss, fevers, night sweats, chronic cough, and sputum production.[65] Cavities may be complicated by a mycetoma, usually aspergillus; rarely, a *Coccidioides* cavity hosts a *Coccidioides* fungal ball.[69,70]

Pleural effusion is estimated to complicate 5% to 15% of primary pulmonary coccidioidomycosis. Effusions are of variable size, and size does not correlate with dissemination risk. Fluid analysis usually demonstrates an increased presence of lymphocytes and eosinophils. Effusions may be either transudative or exudative with variable chemistries; 22% meet criteria for complicated parapneumonic effusion or empyema and drainage may be indicated.[2,71] However, in contrast to parapneumonic bacterial effusions, even large *Coccidioides* effusions are likely to resolve spontaneously. Pleural fluid serology performed well in discriminating coccidioidal effusions in 1 series.[72] Microbiologic isolation of *Coccidioides* spp from the pleural space is rare.[71,72] In cases requiring surgical intervention or biopsy of the pleural space, pathology demonstrates granulomatous infiltration.[73]

Airway coccidioidomycosis is an unusual presentation that is also considered severe; it can present in both immunocompetent and immunocompromised patients and can result in airway obstruction. It is more commonly due to direct endobronchial infection than to erosion from a structure external to the airway, such as a lymph node.[74]

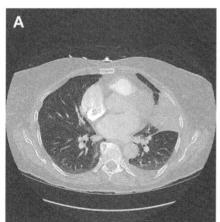
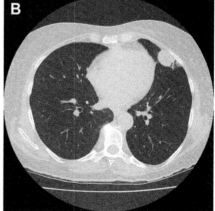

Fig. 3. (*A*) Chest CT demonstrating acute coccidioidal lobar pneumonia and associated small pleural effusion. (*B*) Follow-up imaging 2 months later demonstrates resolution of much of the airspace opacity with residual disease coalescing into a nodule and resolution of the effusion.

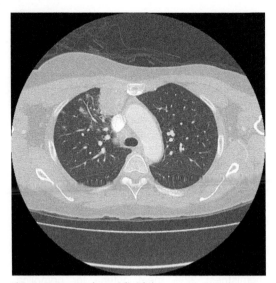

Fig. 4. Segmental coccidioidal pneumonia presenting as a masslike consolidation with several associated nodular opacities.

Acute respiratory failure is rare and usually seen in patients with significant immunosuppression or massive organism exposure. The disease rarely can progress to acute respiratory distress syndrome (ARDS), in which mortality approaches 100%. Acute eosinophilic pneumonia may also contribute to respiratory failure.[75]

A significant proportion of those infected, as high as 84%, report fatigue severe enough to interfere with activities of daily living for a mean 96 days after illness onset. The economic impact is remarkable—82% in a single coccidioidomycosis cohort missed a median 10 working days.[76] Fatigue may take months to resolve.[76,77]

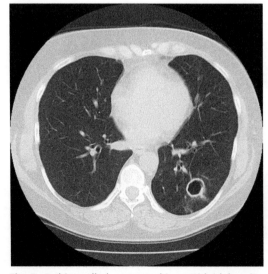

Fig. 5. A thin-walled, or grapeskin coccidoidal cavity.

Disseminated Disease

Overall, dissemination occurs in 1% of immunocompetent patients. The skin, central nervous system (CNS), musculoskeletal system, and lymph nodes are most common; however, involvement of any tissue or organ is possible with occurrences documented within serosal spaces (eg, pericardium and peritoneum) as well as the genitourinary tract and retropharyngeal space.[78,79] Vigilance for exploring new symptoms in patients with known coccidioidomycosis is required. Occasionally, the manifestations of disseminated disease represent the initial presenting complaint.

Skin involvement by dissemination most commonly manifests as nodules. Papules, gummas, acneiform pustular lesions, verrucous plaques, and abscesses with fistulae have also been described.[10] These usually involve the face, neck, scalp, and chest wall. In addition to organisms, pathology typically demonstrates necrotizing granulomas. Given the impact of disseminated disease on prognosis and management, it is important to distinguish these manifestations from the immune-mediated skin findings of an acute pulmonary infection, which are much more common.[80]

Musculoskeletal dissemination is usually in the form of monoarticular or vertebral joint infections. Skeletal involvement is most frequently osteomyelitis of axial structures and vertebral bodies. Appendicular bone involvement is less common but when present usually involves the lower extremities, especially the knees. Tenosynovitis is rare but reported, with frequent relapse when medical therapy is discontinued.[81]

CNS involvement is a highly morbid complication of disseminated disease. It usually develops within months of the initial infection but can occur years later; its development does not seem affected by medical therapy during the primary acute infection.[65,82] Rapid onset is possible but a chronic course with insidious onset is more typical; 30% to 50% of patients develop obstructive hydrocephalus requiring urgent neurosurgical intervention. Up to 50% of patients develop a vasculitis with cerebral infarction.[82,83] Complaints of chronic persistent headaches, nausea, vomiting, or vision changes in patients with a known coccidioidal infection should prompt consideration of brain imaging and lumbar puncture. Spinal fluid analysis usually demonstrates a lymphocytic predominance, sometimes with eosinophils, and a low glucose. Organism isolation is rare and spinal fluid serologic testing is useful. Consultation with coccidioidomycosis experts is prudent in these difficult cases.

As with other endemic fungi, isolation of *Cocci-dioides* from the blood is rare but portends a poor prognosis. In the largest available case series, drawn primarily from untreated HIV patients with low CD4 counts, 22 of 33 patients with fungemia died,[84] with a mean survival of less than 2 weeks from presentation. Miliary coccidioidomycosis seems indistinguishable from miliary tuberculosis on chest imaging and may represent underlying fungemia with hematogenous spread (**Fig. 6**).

LABORATORY TESTING

Demonstration of spherules on pathology or isolation of *Coccidioides* in culture is the gold standard for diagnosis of coccidioidomycosis but is infrequent compared with the large number of actual cases that present for care. Serology is the most commonly used method of diagnosis.[85] Eosinophilia from blood and affected body fluids is suggestive of the diagnosis. Galactomannan antigen testing is also available and is useful in select patients.

Serology

Serologic testing is the most widely used method in practice to diagnose coccidioidomycosis, but the nuances of the many available tests are daunting. These nuances, perhaps along with the knowledge that most coccidioidomycosis cases are self-limited, may be why many patients presenting with community-acquired pneumonia in endemic areas do not routinely undergo *Coccidioides*-specific testing.[23] The presence and profile of *Coccidioides*-specific antibodies depend on both the

ability of the host to mount a serologic response and the time since initial infectious exposure (**Fig. 7**). Antibody production lags behind illness onset by several weeks, with serologic response potentially weaker and more delayed in immunocompromised patients.[86] For this reason, serial testing is frequently required to avoid false-negative results. In contrast to other infections, antibody concentrations usually decrease over time to undetectable levels on resolution of the existing infection; positive antibody assays, therefore, represent recent infection, chronic disease activity, or reactivation.[87] The characteristics of serologic tests for *Coccidioides* also depend on the characteristics of the population and the reason for their performance,[88] demonstrating better diagnostic yield when drawn to investigate acute illness compared with case-finding or screening approaches.

Enzyme immunoassay (EIA) (Premier, Meridian Bioscience, Cincinnati, Ohio; and OMEGA, IMMY, Norman, Oklahoma) is a qualitative test for *Coccidioides*-specific IgM or IgG and is readily available outside of reference laboratories. Testing for both IgM and IgG is suggested to maximize sensitivity,[89] and both are run as a panel. Controversy exists in the literature regarding false-positive rates with an isolated EIA IgM. One study found that 82% of isolated positive EIA IgM tests were falsely positive.[90] In contrast, a study by Blair and Currier[91] concluded that false-positive EIA IgM tests were uncommon and should prompt evaluation. These disparate findings may be due to methodological differences and unaccounted bias. A positive EIA IgG, whether in isolation or together with a positive EIA IgM, should be sent to a reference laboratory for confirmation and

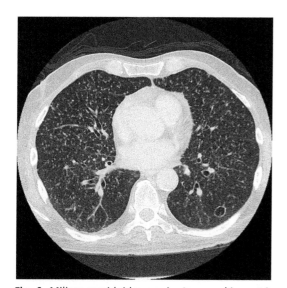

Fig. 6. Miliary coccidoidomycosis. A grapeskin cyst is also demonstrated in the left lower lobe.

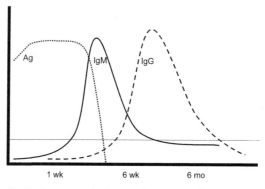

Fig. 7. Conceptual schema of presence of coccidioidal antigen (Ag) and anticoccidioidal antibodies in the serum as a function of time. Exact details of each curve vary according to the individual host immune response. In contrast to other infections, anticoccidioidal IgG becomes undetectable by laboratory assay over time.

quantification. This is usually done by immunodif-fusion-complement fixation (discussed later). A negative EIA panel does not require confirmation by other testing modalities, but serial testing may be required because testing may have occurred prior to seroconversion or in a functionally immu-nosuppressed patient. Additionally, early initiation of fluconazole treatment may lessen the IgG response.[92] EIA panels, in comparison to immuno-diffusion methods, offer the advantage of rapid turnaround and higher sensitivity, although they are less specific.

IDTP (immunodiffusion-tube precipitin) and IDCF (immunodiffusion-complement fixation) may be performed either as initial tests in reference labora-tories, or IDCF may be performed to confirm a pos-itive EIA IgG test. If EIA or IDCF is positive, the traditional CF test is often performed as a reflex test to provide quantitative information in the form of a titer. High titers (>1:16) are suggestive of dissemination. In 1 cohort, however, 24% of pa-tients with disseminated disease had initial titers less than or equal to 1:16, and 12% of patients had higher titers but no evidence of dissemina-tion.[93] CF titers are commonly followed over time in patients with severe or disseminated disease to assess for response to therapy. Serology requires positive testing in the context of a compatible clin-ical presentation (**Fig. 8**) to secure a diagnosis.[85]

Eosinophilia

Eosinophilia is noted on white blood cell differen-tial of peripheral blood in 25% to 30% of cases.[94] The lack of peripheral eosinophilia in bacterial community-acquired pneumonia makes this feature, when present, helpful in distinguishing community-acquired pneumonia as coccidioidal rather than bacterial. The presence of eosinophilia in bronchoalveolar lavage (BAL) of coccidioido-mycosis patients has been recognized for de-cades,[74,95] although its exact predictive value is unknown. The similarity of this feature of coccidioi-dal pneumonia with eosinophilic pneumonia poses a potential for diagnostic error, especially outside of the endemic regions.[96,97]

Pathology and Microbiology

Histopathologic assessment of biopsies or cyto-logic examination of body fluids, such as BAL

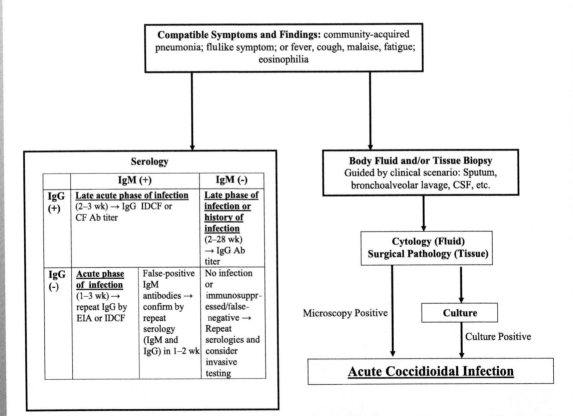

Fig. 8. Simplified diagnostic algorithm for investigation of potential acute coccidioidomycosis. Ab, antibody. (*Adapted from* Malo J, Luraschi-Monjagatta C, Wolk DM, et al. Update on the diagnosis of pulmonary coccidioi-domycosis. Ann Am Thorac Soc 2014;11(2):249; with permission.)

and sputum, almost exclusively yields spherules, although mycelia have been reported, especially in patients with chronic disease and diabetics,[98–100] and can be misdiagnosed. Papanicolaou and calcofluor white stains are the most sensitive to detect the often elusive spherules,[101,102] although they may also be seen with potassium hydroxide, periodic acid–Schiff, Grocott methenamine silver, and hematoxylin-eosin stains. In the event of negative cytology or histopathology, culture of the specimen may yield a diagnosis. *Coccidioides* grows better in culture than other endemic fungi and may grow to an identifiable state in less than 1 week.[65] Confirmation of culture results is often performed via a chemiluminescent DNA probe (Accuprobe, Gen-Probe Inc, San Diego, California)[103,104] or DNA sequencing[105,106] in a reference laboratory.

In disseminated disease, fluid and tissue samples by lumbar puncture, needle biopsy, or surgical excision may be required depending on the presentation. In pulmonary coccidioidomycosis, bronchoscopy can be particularly helpful in the presence of parenchymal infiltrates, cavitary disease, or bronchopleural fistula, although not in solitary pulmonary nodules. Bronchoscopy yielded a rapid diagnosis on BAL in 30% to 64% of cases[107,108] and in 1 study was the first procedure to produce a diagnostic specimen in 33%.[107] The use of all available diagnostic procedures, including brushings and transbronchial biopsy, may increase diagnostic yield.

Antigen Testing

Protein antigen testing for *Coccidioides* is not available. Polysaccharide-based antigen testing has been explored, with a *Coccidiodes*-specific galactomannan test now commercially available (MVista, MiraVista Diagnostics, Indianapolis, Indiana). This assay detected antigenemia in up to 73% of immunosuppressed subjects with moderate to severe or disseminated disease,[109,110] a population in whom serologic testing is less reliable. The *Coccidioides*-specific galactomannan test exhibits cross-reactivity with sera from patients with histoplasmosis and blastomycosis and its utility in immunocompetent patients with mild disease is not well defined.

The use of the $(1\rightarrow3)$-β-D glucan assay in coccidioidomycosis has not been well defined. In 1 study it seemed to perform with similar test characteristics (sensitivity 44% in hospitalized subjects and specificity 91%) as in other fungal infections.[111] Although potentially useful, the test is nonspecific due to positive results with other fungi, especially *Aspergillus* and *Pneumocystis*.[112]

Skin Testing

Skin reaction tests to coccidiodin or spherulin historically played a vital role in epidemiologic research on coccidioidomycosis. A newly approved agent is now commercially available (Spherusol, Nielsen Biosciences, San Diego, California)[113] solely for detection of delayed-type hypersensitivity in patients with a known history of pulmonary coccidioidomycosis. Other clinical applications may prove useful but are currently theoretic.[114]

Immunodiagnosis

Cellular immunity to *Coccidioides* may be assessed by a test akin to the interferon-γ release assay used in latent tuberculosis, with a robust correlation between skin test induration and cytokine release from stimulated leukocytes.[115] Measurement of interleukin 17 may also prove useful in blood and BAL.[115,116] The use of immunodiagnosis remains an area of research interest with no commercially available assays.

Molecular Testing

Clinically, polymerase chain reaction (PCR)-based testing is largely used for speciation after culture growth. Promising results have been demonstrated when applying the technology to respiratory samples,[117,118] although PCR was less sensitive when applied to cerebrospinal fluid (CSF) and pleural fluid.[72,118] PCR seems to have a similar performance to fungal culture.[118] The optimal nucleotide sequence targets are still under investigation.

MANAGEMENT

It has been known since the 1930s that most cases of coccidioidomycosis are self-limited and resolve without antifungal therapy. Although it is agreed that severe and disseminated disease merits treatment, it is less clear which patients with mild pulmonary coccidioidomycosis benefit (**Box 1**). The risk/benefit ratio of oral azole treatment has shifted most clinicians in favor of therapy, with a goal of hastening recovery and preventing progression to severe or disseminated disease. This approach is not well supported, however, by the available evidence. Guidelines regarding treatment rely largely on expert opinion and updated guidelines were recently published.[119]

The Immunocompetent Patient: Primary Pulmonary Disease and Its Sequelae

The decision to treat primary pulmonary disease is informed by only few data from small studies, which do not demonstrate a clear benefit to treatment. In a small prospective 2009 study, outpatients were randomly assigned to receive treatment or no treatment. Of 36 untreated patients, no adverse effects were observed; furthermore, no difference in rate of improvement was observed between treated and untreated groups.[120] In a small 2012 outpatient observational study in which the decision to treat was determined by individual clinicians, treated and untreated groups did not differ significantly in time to symptom resolution.[13] It is generally agreed that patients with elements suggestive of more severe disease, progressive symptoms for weeks or those with a high-risk phenotype should be treated. There is no literature comparing antifungal agents or duration of therapy; fluconazole (usually 400 mg/d) is typically preferred compared with other azoles due to good absorption and few side effects. Therapy should be continued for a duration of 3 months to 6 months. Regardless of the decision to treat, patients should be followed clinically with titers and chest imaging to resolution. Guidelines also recommend that all patients receive education regarding their expected clinical course as well as guided physical reconditioning.[119]

Pulmonary nodules known to be sequelae of coccidioidomycosis do not require treatment. Pulmonary cavities are usually asymptomatic; they occasionally are implicated in cough or hemoptysis, which may be managed with observation, several months of fluconazole, or surgical therapy depending on the severity. Expert opinion suggests that cavities greater than 3 cm may benefit from surgical excision.[121] The rare development of a bronchopleural fistula and pyopneumothorax due to a cavity rupture generally requires surgical and medical management.[122,123]

Chronic coccidioidal pneumonia is treated with azole therapy for at least a year,[121] and some patients may require lifelong treatment.[65] Overwhelming pulmonary disease, such as that with diffuse infiltrates or severe hypoxia, is usually treated with amphotericin B induction, possibly concomitantly with an azole, and with eventual discontinuation of the amphotericin after clinical improvement. In patients with diffuse infiltrates and who are acutely ill, concomitant administration of corticosteroids, as may be considered in *Pneumocystis* pneumonia or ARDS, has been reported[75] but is controversial and unproved in coccidioidal disease. Severe, refractory coccidioidal ARDS has been successfully managed with extracorporeal membrane oxygenation.[124]

Disseminated Disease

All cases of dissemination require therapy. As in very severe pulmonary disease, severely ill patients are treated with amphotericin; those who are less ill, including outpatients, may be treated with azole therapy.[119] Duration of therapy is at least 1 year and could be lifelong; if there is no CNS involvement, clinical assessment and a declining CF titer (eg, to <1:4) suggest infection control and may be useful to guide therapy duration. Up to 30% of patients relapse after treatment discontinuation, emphasizing the need for vigilant continued follow-up.

Itraconazole is preferred for bone and joint involvement, although its use is sometimes limited by medication interactions and decreased absorption in the setting of gastric acid suppression.[65,119,125] Vertebral involvement frequently requires surgical stabilization and surgical consultation is suggested in all cases. Amphotericin is preferentially recommended by some experts in severe, function-threatening skeletal disease until control of the infection.[119]

CNS involvement by Coccidioides most commonly manifests as meningitis, is fraught with potential complications, and is uniformly fatal if untreated. Amphotericin B is ineffective intravenously and requires intrathecal administration. The introduction of azoles revolutionized treatment of CNS disease.[126] Therapy is initiated at a daily dose of 400 mg to 800 mg of fluconazole. In 1 series, 14 of 18 patients presumed cured of CNS disease went on to relapse after being taken off azole therapy, suggesting that CNS disease is only suppressed and never cured and that lifelong therapy is warranted.[127] Beyond antifungal therapy, close attention is warranted for the development of obstructive hydrocephalus, which requires urgent neurosurgical evaluation for placement of a CSF shunt. Vasculitis, infarction, and abscess are also potential complications and are managed on a case-by-case basis. Posaconazole and voriconazole have been used with some success as salvage therapy.[128] The new antifungal agent isavuconazole has a similar minimum inhibitory concentration against C posadasii as other azoles and good CNS penetration,[129] but as yet there are no clinical data to support its use. Echinocandins are not recommended. Consultation with an expert in coccidioidomycosis is recommended and resources are available online (Table 1).[130]

The Immunodeficient Patient

Neither amphotericin B nor the azoles are fungicidal against Coccidioides,[131] underscoring the necessity of an intact cellular immune response in controlling and clearing the infection. Modulating the degree of immunosuppression may be possible as an adjunct to antifungal therapy in some cases. Because serology may be negative in the immunosuppressed patient, an aggressive diagnostic approach, including repeated serology and often bronchoscopy or biopsy, is commonly required in this population.[132]

In HIV patients, treatment with antifungals should not overshadow the importance of antiretroviral therapy. Skin testing and in vitro data suggest that patients with a peripheral CD4 count greater than 250/μL maintain a cellular immune response to Coccidioides antigens[133] and may be treated under the same paradigm as an immunocompetent patient.[121] In those with lower counts, azole monotherapy versus combination amphotericin B and azole is used, depending on the severity of the presentation.

Coccidioidomycosis patients taking immunosuppressives, including corticosteroids, disease-modifying medications, or biologics for autoimmune disease, are treated in all circumstances. Depending on individual circumstance, immunosuppressive therapy may be discontinued or lessened during active infection. Reintroduction of immunosuppressive therapy is possible after control of the infection and cessation of antifungal therapy is sometimes possible.[134]

All forms of active coccidioidomycosis are treated in solid organ transplant patients. Given the necessity of continued immunosuppression, treatment is commonly lifelong; maintenance therapy may sometimes be at a reduced fluconazole dose of 200 mg daily at the discretion of the clinician. Because of the previously discussed risk of reactivation of dormant disease post-transplant, it is recommended that all transplant candidates in endemic regions be screened prior to transplant. Given available case reports,[135–138] this also seems prudent for patients with a history of residence in an endemic area. In the approach of 1 institution,[139] those with a previous history of active coccidioidomycosis are treated with 200 mg daily fluconazole for at least 6 months, those with positive serology are treated with 400 mg daily for 1 year followed by lifelong suppression, and transplant is delayed until adequate control of any active infection is demonstrated. Beyond noting that azoles increase tacrolimus levels via inhibition of cytochrome P450 3A4, adverse events are expected to be low. The high incidence of coccidioidomycosis in endemic transplant recipients, especially after the first year, has raised the question of universal prophylaxis.[140]

Approximately 2.6% of endemic hematopoietic stem cell transplant patients are diagnosed with coccidioidomycosis[132]; the similarity of this incidence to the endemic population at large may be due to universal prophylaxis protocols in the first 100 days post-transplant. When diagnosed, however, the disease tends to be abrupt, rapidly progressive, and with high morbidity and mortality. Care centers on aggressive diagnostic strategies and prompt initiation of an azole, or amphotericin

Table 1
Commonly encountered clinical scenarios and suggested management strategies

Clinical Scenario	Radiographic Findings	Laboratory Findings	Interpretation
Asymptomatic endemic resident	Pulmonary nodule on pre-employ chest radiograph	(−) Serology	Possible coccidioidoma vs malignancy. No antifungal therapy. Imaging follow-up according to individual malignancy risk (patient history, nodule appearance).
Asymptomatic endemic resident	Pulmonary nodule found on screening CT	(+) Serology	Likely coccidioidoma vs malignancy. No antifungal therapy. Imaging follow-up according to individual malignancy risk.
Asymptomatic endemic resident anticipating initiation of biologic therapy or organ transplantation	No findings	(+) Serology	Past, likely recent, coccidioidal infection at risk for reactivation on immunosuppression. Treatment course recommended prior to immunosuppression.
Endemic resident with cough, pleurisy, fatigue ± skin findings	Lobar infiltrate	(+) Serology	Probable coccidioidal pneumonia. Consider treatment depending on severity of illness and risk of complications. Follow radiographically to resolution.
Endemic resident with cough, pleurisy, fatigue ± skin findings	CT scan with small infiltrate and satellite small nodules	(−) Serology	Possible to probable acute coccidioidal pneumonia. Consider empiric treatment based on severity of illness and risk of dissemination. Repeat serologies in follow-up. Follow radiographically to resolution.
Endemic resident with severe community-acquired pneumonia (significant hypoxia and/or critical illness)	Lobar infiltrate and areas of diffuse airspace disease	Serology pending but with peripheral eosinophilia	Severe community-acquired pneumonia with probable risk of coccidioidal infection. Include azole antifungal in empiric antimicrobial regimen pending clinical evolution.

in severe disease, with indefinite maintenance therapy thereafter.

Pregnancy

An infected pregnant patient represents a treatment dilemma. Although azoles were classically thought highly teratogenic at any point in pregnancy, this view has been refined over time such that their risk seems confined to the first trimester. Because of this new view, a management strategy centered on surveillance versus amphotericin B in the first trimester depending on disease severity, and azole-based therapy in the second and third trimesters, has been suggested.[41,119] Increased risk of dissemination extends into the postpartum period and may be greatest at that time.

SUMMARY

Coccidioidomycosis is one of the primary causes of community-acquired pneumonia in endemic regions with myriad pulmonary and extrapulmonary manifestations. Infections are increasingly recognized outside endemic areas given the mobile society. Diagnostic testing is varied and each modality has limitations, with serology the most commonly used diagnostic test in everyday practice. Azoles are the mainstay of therapy in most cases. Primary pulmonary coccidioidomycosis, although the most common manifestation of disease, bears the most uncertainty regarding the decision to treat. Invasive procedures or surgical biopsy is indicated when diagnosis is not secured, particularly in patients with severe or progressive disease. As always, expert consultation is prudent when diagnosed outside the endemic area or when confronted with a treatment dilemma.

REFERENCES

1. Hirschmann JV. The early history of coccidioidomycosis: 1892-1945. Clin Infect Dis 2007;44(9): 1202–7.
2. Thompson GR 3rd. Pulmonary coccidioidomycosis. Semin Respir Crit Care Med 2011;32(6): 754–63.
3. Darling S. A protozoan general infection producing pseudo tubercles in the lungs and focal necrosis in teh liver, spleen, and lymph nodes. JAMA 1906;46: 283–5.
4. Gilchrist TC. A case of blastomycetic dermatitis in man. Johns Hopkins Hosp Rep 1896;1:269–83.
5. Ophuls W. Further observations on a pathogenic mould formerly described as a protozoon(Coccidioides immitis, Coccidiodes pyogenes). J Exp Med 1905;6(4–6):443–85.
6. Smith C. Reminiscences of the flying chlamydospore and its allies. In: Ajello L, editor. Symposium on coccidioidomycosis. Tucson (AZ): University of Arizona Press; 1967. p. xiii–xxii.
7. Fisher MC, Koenig GL, White TJ, et al. Molecular and phenotypic description of Coccidioides posadasii sp. nov., previously recognized as the non-California population of Coccidioides immitis. Mycologia 2002;94(1):73–84.
8. Fisher FS, Bultman MW, Johnson SM, et al. Coccidioides niches and habitat parameters in the southwestern United States: a matter of scale. Ann N Y Acad Sci 2007;1111:47–72.
9. Brown J, Benedict K, Park BJ, et al. Coccidioidomycosis: epidemiology. Clin Epidemiol 2013;5: 185–97.
10. Garcia Garcia SC, Salas Alanis JC, Flores MG, et al. Coccidioidomycosis and the skin: a comprehensive review. An Bras Dermatol 2015;90(5):610–9.
11. Mondragón-González R, Méndez-Tovar LJ, Bernal-Vázquez E, et al. Detección de infección por Coccidioides immitis en zonas del estado de Coahuila, México. Rev Argent Microbiol 2005;37(3):135–8.
12. Laniado Laborin R, Cardenas Moreno RP, Alvarez Cerro M. Tijuana: endemic zone of Coccidioides immitis infection. Salud Publica Mex 1991;33(3): 235–9 [in Spanish].
13. Blair JE, Chang YH, Cheng MR, et al. Characteristics of patients with mild to moderate primary pulmonary coccidioidomycosis. Emerg Infect Dis 2014;20(6):983–90.
14. Tsang CA, Anderson SM, Imholte SB, et al. Enhanced surveillance of coccidioidomycosis, Arizona, USA, 2007-2008. Emerg Infect Dis 2010; 16(11):1738–44.
15. Flynn NM, Hoeprich PD, Kawachi MM, et al. An unusual outbreak of windborne coccidioidomycosis. N Engl J Med 1979;301(7):358–61.
16. Crum N, Lamb C, Utz G, et al. Coccidioidomycosis outbreak among United States Navy SEALs training in a Coccidioides immitis-endemic area–Coalinga, California. J Infect Dis 2002;186(6): 865–8.
17. Schneider E, Hajjeh RA, Spiegel RA, et al. A coccidioidomycosis outbreak following the Northridge, Calif, earthquake. JAMA 1997; 277(11):904–8.
18. Tamerius JD, Comrie AC. Coccidioidomycosis incidence in Arizona predicted by seasonal precipitation. PLoS One 2011;6(6):e21009.
19. Comrie AC. Climate factors influencing coccidioidomycosis seasonality and outbreaks. Environ Health Perspect 2005;113(6):688–92.
20. Valdivia L, Nix D, Wright M, et al. Coccidioidomycosis as a common cause of community-acquired pneumonia. Emerg Infect Dis 2006; 12(6):958–62.

21. Stockamp NW, Thompson GR 3rd. Coccidioidomycosis. Infect Dis Clin North Am 2016;30(1):229–46.

22. Hector RF, Rutherford GW, Tsang CA, et al. The public health impact of coccidioidomycosis in Arizona and California. Int J Environ Res Public Health 2011;8(4):1150–73.

23. Chang DC, Anderson S, Wannemuehler K, et al. Testing for coccidioidomycosis among patients with community-acquired pneumonia. Emerg Infect Dis 2008;14(7):1053–9.

24. Desai SA, Minai OA, Gordon SM, et al. Coccidioidomycosis in non-endemic areas: a case series. Respir Med 2001;95(4):305–9.

25. Ogiso A, Ito M, Koyama M, et al. Pulmonary coccidioidomycosis in Japan: case report and review. Clin Infect Dis 1997;25(5):1260–1.

26. Lan F, Tong YZ, Huang H, et al. Primary pulmonary coccidioidomycosis in China. Respirology 2010; 15(4):722–5.

27. Wang XL, Wang S, An CL. Mini-Review of published reports on coccidioidomycosis in China. Mycopathologia 2015;180(5–6):299–303.

28. Centers for Disease Control and Prevention (CDC). Coccidioidomycosis in travelers returning from Mexico–Pennsylvania, 2000. MMWR Morb Mortal Wkly Rep 2000;49(44):1004–6.

29. Cairns L, Blythe D, Kao A, et al. Outbreak of coccidioidomycosis in Washington state residents returning from Mexico. Clin Infect Dis 2000;30(1):61–4.

30. D'Avino A, Di Giambenedetto S, Fabbiani M, et al. Coccidioidomycosis of cervical lymph nodes in an HIV-infected patient with immunologic reconstitution on potent HAART: a rare observation in a non-endemic area. Diagn Microbiol Infect Dis 2012; 72(2):185–7.

31. Stagliano D, Epstein J, Hickey P. Fomite-transmitted coccidioidomycosis in an immunocompromised child. Pediatr Infect Dis J 2007;26(5):454–6.

32. Albert BL, Sellers TF Jr, Coccidioidomycosis. From fomites. Report of a case and review of the literature. Arch Intern Med 1963;112:253–61.

33. Centers for Disease Control and Prevention (CDC). Coccidioidomycosis in workers at an archeologic site–Dinosaur National Monument, Utah, June-July 2001. MMWR Morb Mortal Wkly Rep 2001; 50(45):1005–8.

34. Marsden-Haug N, Hill H, Litvintseva AP, et al. Coccidioides immitis identified in soil outside of its known range - Washington, 2013. MMWR Morb Mortal Wkly Rep 2014;63(20):450.

35. Dzawachiszwili N, Landau JW, Newcomer VD, et al. The effect of Sea Water and Sodium Chloride on the growth of fungi pathogenic to man. J Invest Dermatol 1964;43:103–9.

36. Reidarson TH, Griner LA, Pappagianis D, et al. Coccidioidomycosis in a bottlenose dolphin. J Wildl Dis 1998;34(3):629–31.

37. Leake JA, Mosley DG, England B, et al. Risk factors for acute symptomatic coccidioidomycosis among elderly persons in Arizona, 1996-1997. J Infect Dis 2000;181(4):1435–40.

38. Sunenshine RH, Anderson S, Erhart L, et al. Public health surveillance for coccidioidomycosis in Arizona. Ann N Y Acad Sci 2007;1111:96–102.

39. Drutz DJ, Huppert M, Sun SH, et al. Human sex hormones stimulate the growth and maturation of Coccidioides immitis. Infect Immun 1981;32(2): 897–907.

40. Weinberg ED. Pregnancy-associated depression of cell-mediated immunity. Rev Infect Dis 1984; 6(6):814–31.

41. Bercovitch RS, Catanzaro A, Schwartz BS, et al. Coccidioidomycosis during pregnancy: a review and recommendations for management. Clin Infect Dis 2011;53(4):363–8.

42. Louie L, Ng S, Hajjeh R, et al. Influence of host genetics on the severity of coccidioidomycosis. Emerg Infect Dis 1999;5(5):672–80.

43. Laniado-Laborin R. Expanding understanding of epidemiology of coccidioidomycosis in the Western hemisphere. Ann N Y Acad Sci 2007;1111:19–34.

44. Santelli AC, Blair JE, Roust LR. Coccidioidomycosis in patients with diabetes mellitus. Am J Med 2006;119(11):964–9.

45. Mertz LE, Blair JE. Coccidioidomycosis in rheumatology patients: incidence and potential risk factors. Ann N Y Acad Sci 2007;1111:343–57.

46. Bergstrom L, Yocum DE, Ampel NM, et al. Increased risk of coccidioidomycosis in patients treated with tumor necrosis factor alpha antagonists. Arthritis Rheum 2004;50(6):1959–66.

47. Rutala PJ, Smith JW. Coccidioidomycosis in potentially compromised hosts: the effect of immunosuppressive therapy in dissemination. Am J Med Sci 1978;275(3):283–95.

48. Blair JE, Smilack JD, Caples SM. Coccidioidomycosis in patients with hematologic malignancies. Arch Intern Med 2005;165(1):113–7.

49. Ampel NM, Dols CL, Galgani JN. Coccidioidomycosis during human immunodeficiency virus infection: results of a prospective study in a coccidioidal endemic area. Am J Med 1993;94:235–40.

50. Masannat FY, Ampel NM. Coccidioidomycosis in patients with HIV-1 infection in the era of potent antiretroviral therapy. Clin Infect Dis 2010;50(1):1–7.

51. Logan JL, Blair JE, Galgani JN. Coccidioidomycosis complicating solid organ transplantation. Semin Respir Infect 2001;16(4):251–6.

52. Blair JE, Logan JL. Coccidioidomycosis in solid organ transplantation. Clin Infect Dis 2001;33(9): 1536–44.

53. Blair JE. Coccidioidomycosis in liver transplantation. Liver Transpl 2006;12(1):31–9.

54. Braddy CM, Heilman RL, Blair JE. Coccidioidomy-cosis after renal transplantation in an endemic area. Am J Transplant 2006;6(2):340–5.

55. Vikram HR, Dosanjh A, Blair JE. Coccidioidomy-cosis and lung transplantation. Transplantation 2011;92(7):717–21.

56. Blair JE. Coccidioidomycosis in patients who have undergone transplantation. Ann N Y Acad Sci 2007;1111:365–76.

57. Calhoun D, Galgiani JN, Zukoski C. Coccidioido-mycosis in recent renal or cardiac transplant recip-ients. in Coccidioidomycosis. Proceedings of the 4th International Conference on Coccidioidomy-cosis. San Diego, March 14–17, 1984.

58. Brugiere O, Forget E, Biondi G, et al. Coccidioido-mycosis in a lung transplant recipient acquired from the donor graft in France. Transplantation 2009;88(11):1319–20.

59. Dierberg KL, Marr KA, Subramanian A, et al. Donor-derived organ transplant transmission of coccidioi-domycosis. Transpl Infect Dis 2012;14(3):300–4.

60. Miller MB, Hendren R, Gilligan PH. Posttransplanta-tion disseminated coccidioidomycosis acquired from donor lungs. J Clin Microbiol 2004;42(5): 2347–9.

61. Tripathy U, Yung GL, Kriett JM, et al. Donor transfer of pulmonary coccidioidomycosis in lung trans-plantation. Ann Thorac Surg 2002;73(1):306–8.

62. Blodget E, Geiseler PJ, Larsen RA, et al. Donor-derived Coccidioides immitis fungemia in solid or-gan transplant recipients. Transpl Infect Dis 2012; 14(3):305–10.

63. Wright PW, Pappagianis D, Wilson M, et al. Donor-related coccidioidomycosis in organ transplant re-cipients. Clin Infect Dis 2003;37(9):1265–9.

64. Carvalho C, Ferreira I, Gaião S, et al. Cerebral coccidioidomycosis after renal transplantation in a non-endemic area. Transpl Infect Dis 2010; 12(2):151–4.

65. Twarog M, Thompson GR 3rd. Coccidioidomy-cosis: recent updates. Semin Respir Crit Care Med 2015;36(5):746–55.

66. Azadeh N, Chang YH, Kusne S, et al. The impact of early and brief corticosteroids on the clinical course of primary pulmonary coccidioidomycosis. J Infect 2013;67(2):148–55.

67. Jude CM, Nayak NB, Patel MK, et al. Pulmonary coccidioidomycosis: pictorial review of chest radio-graphic and CT findings. Radiographics 2014; 34(4):912–25.

68. Naidich DP, Bankier AA, MacMahon H, et al. Rec-ommendations for the management of subsolid pulmonary nodules detected at CT: a statement from the Fleischner Society. Radiology 2013; 266(1):304–17.

69. Osaki T, Morishita H, Maeda H, et al. Pulmonary coccidioidomycosis that formed a fungus ball with 8-years duration. Intern Med 2005;44(2): 141–4.

70. Rohatgi PK, Schmitt RG. Pulmonary coccidioidal mycetoma. Am J Med Sci 1984;287(3):27–30.

71. Merchant M, Romero AO, Libke RD, et al. Pleural effusion in hospitalized patients with Coccidioido-mycosis. Respir Med 2008;102(4):537–40.

72. Thompson GR, Sharma S, Bays DJ, et al. Coccidi-oidomycosis: adenosine deaminase levels, sero-logic parameters, culture results, and polymerase chain reaction testing in pleural fluid. Chest 2013; 143(3):776–81.

73. Shekhel TA, Ricciotti RW, Blair JE, et al. Surgical pathology of pleural coccidioidomycosis: a clinico-pathological study of 36 cases. Hum Pathol 2014; 45(5):961–9.

74. Feldman BS, Snyder LS. Primary pulmonary coccidioidomycosis. Semin Respir Infect 2001; 16(4):231–7.

75. Malo J, Raz Y, Snyder L, et al. Treatment of coccidioidomycosis-associated eosinophilic pneu-monia with corticosteroids. Southwest J Pulm Crit Care 2012;4:61–6.

76. Garrett AL, Chang YH, Ganley K, et al. Uphill both ways: fatigue and quality of life in valley fever. Med Mycol 2016;54(3):310–7.

77. Muir Bowers J, Mourani JP, Ampel NM. Fatigue in coccidioidomycosis. Quantification and correlation with clinical, immunological, and nutritional factors. Med Mycol 2006;44(7):585–90.

78. Chan O, Low SW, Urcis R, et al. Coccidioidomycosis with pericardial involvement: case report and litera-ture review. Am J Med 2016;129(3):e21–5.

79. Crum-Cianflone NF, Truett AA, Teneza-Mora N, et al. Unusual presentations of coccidioidomy-cosis: a case series and review of the literature. Medicine (Baltimore) 2006;85(5):263–77.

80. Mangold AR, DiCaudo DJ, Blair JE, et al. Chronic interstitial granulomatous dermatitis in coccidioido-mycosis. Br J Dermatol 2016;174(4):881–4.

81. Campbell M, Kusne S, Renfree KJ, et al. Coccidioi-dal Tenosynovitis of the hand and Wrist: report of 9 cases and review of the literature. Clin Infect Dis 2015;61(10):1514–20.

82. Johnson RH, Einstein HE. Coccidioidal meningitis. Clin Infect Dis 2006;42(1):103–7.

83. Mischel PS, Vinters HV. Coccidioidomycosis of the central nervous system: neuropathological and vasculopathic manifestations and clinical corre-lates. Clin Infect Dis 1995;20(2):400–5.

84. Rempe S, Sachdev MS, Bhakta R, et al. Cocci-dioides immitis fungemia: clinical features and sur-vival in 33 adult patients. Heart Lung 2007;36(1): 64–71.

85. Malo J, Luraschi-Monjagatta C, Wolk DM, et al. Up-date on the diagnosis of pulmonary coccidioidomy-cosis. Ann Am Thorac Soc 2014;11(2):243–53.

86. Blair JE, Coakley B, Santelli AC, et al. Serologic testing for symptomatic coccidioidomycosis in immunocompetent and immunosuppressed hosts. Mycopathologia 2006;162(5):317–24.

87. Pappagianis D, Zimmer BL. Serology of coccidioidomycosis. Clin Microbiol Rev 1990;3(3):247–68.

88. Blair JE, Mendoza N, Force S, et al. Clinical specificity of the enzyme immunoassay test for coccidioidomycosis varies according to the reason for its performance. Clin Vaccine Immunol 2013;20(1):95–8.

89. Kaufman L, Sekhon AS, Moledina N, et al. Comparative evaluation of commercial Premier EIA and microimmunodiffusion and complement fixation tests for Coccidioides immitis antibodies. J Clin Microbiol 1995;33(3):618–9.

90. Kuberski T, Herrig J, Pappagianis D. False-positive IgM serology in coccidioidomycosis. J Clin Microbiol 2010;48(6):2047–9.

91. Blair JE, Currier JT. Significance of isolated positive IgM serologic results by enzyme immunoassay for coccidioidomycosis. Mycopathologia 2008;166(2):77–82.

92. Thompson GR 3rd, Lunetta JM, Johnson SM, et al. Early treatment with fluconazole may abrogate the development of IgG antibodies in coccidioidomycosis. Clin Infect Dis 2011;53(6):e20–4.

93. Crum NF, Lederman ER, Stafford CM, et al. Coccidioidomycosis: a descriptive survey of a reemerging disease. Clinical characteristics and current controversies. Medicine (Baltimore) 2004;83(3):149–75.

94. Galgiani JN. Coccidioidomycosis. West J Med 1993;159(2):153–71.

95. Lombard CM, Tazelaar HD, Krasne DL. Pulmonary eosinophilia in coccidioidal infections. Chest 1987;91(5):734–6.

96. Hajek J, Mohan SK, Marras TK. Eosinophilic pneumonia in a traveller returning from Mexico. Can J Infect Dis Med Microbiol 2007;18(5):313–5.

97. Swartz J, Stoller JK. Acute eosinophilic pneumonia complicating Coccidioides immitis pneumonia: a case report and literature review. Respiration 2009;77(1):102–6.

98. Helig D, Giampoli EJ. Mycelial form of Coccidioides immitis diagnosed in bronchoalveolar lavage. Diagn Cytopathol 2007;35(8):535–6.

99. Puckett TF. Hyphae of Coccidioides immitis in tissues of the human host. Am Rev Tuberc 1954;70(2):320–7.

100. Munoz-Hernandez B, Martínez-Rivera MA, Palma Cortés G, et al. Mycelial forms of Coccidioides spp. in the parasitic phase associated to pulmonary coccidioidomycosis with type 2 diabetes mellitus. Eur J Clin Microbiol Infect Dis 2008;27(9):813–20.

101. Saubolle MA. Laboratory aspects in the diagnosis of coccidioidomycosis. Ann N Y Acad Sci 2007;1111:301–14.

102. Sarosi GA, Lawrence JP, Smith DK, et al. Rapid diagnostic evaluation of bronchial washings in patients with suspected coccidioidomycosis. Semin Respir Infect 2001;16(4):238–41.

103. Sandhu GS, Kline BC, Stockman L, et al. Molecular probes for diagnosis of fungal infections. J Clin Microbiol 1995;33(11):2913–9.

104. Padhye AA, Smith G, Standard PG, et al. Comparative evaluation of chemiluminescent DNA probe assays and exoantigen tests for rapid identification of Blastomyces dermatitidis and Coccidioides immitis. J Clin Microbiol 1994;32(4):867–70.

105. Hall L, Wohlfiel S, Roberts GD. Experience with the MicroSeq D2 large-subunit ribosomal DNA sequencing kit for identification of filamentous fungi encountered in the clinical laboratory. J Clin Microbiol 2004;42(2):622–6.

106. Tintelnot K, De Hoog GS, Antweiler E, et al. Taxonomic and diagnostic markers for identification of Coccidioides immitis and Coccidioides posadasii. Med Mycol 2007;45(5):385–93.

107. Wallace JM, Catanzaro A, Moser KM, et al. Flexible fiberoptic bronchoscopy for diagnosing pulmonary coccidioidomycosis. Am Rev Respir Dis 1981;123(3):286–90.

108. DiTomasso JP, Ampel NM, Sobonya RE, et al. Bronchoscopic diagnosis of pulmonary coccidioidomycosis. Comparison of cytology, culture, and transbronchial biopsy. Diagn Microbiol Infect Dis 1994;18(2):83–7.

109. Durkin M, Connolly P, Kuberski T, et al. Diagnosis of coccidioidomycosis with use of the Coccidioides antigen enzyme immunoassay. Clin Infect Dis 2008;47(8):e69–73.

110. Durkin M, Estok L, Hospenthal D, et al. Detection of Coccidioides antigenemia following dissociation of immune complexes. Clin Vaccine Immunol 2009;16(10):1453–6.

111. Thompson GR 3rd, Bays DJ, Johnson SM, et al. Serum (1->3)-beta-D-glucan measurement in coccidioidomycosis. J Clin Microbiol 2012;50(9):3060–2.

112. Zangeneh TT, Malo J, Luraschi-Monjagatta C, et al. Positive (1-3) B-d-glucan and cross reactivity of fungal assays in coccidioidomycosis. Med Mycol 2015;53(2):171–3.

113. Johnson R, Kernerman SM, Sawtelle BG, et al. A reformulated spherule-derived coccidioidin (Spherusol) to detect delayed-type hypersensitivity in coccidioidomycosis. Mycopathologia 2012;174(5–6):353–8.

114. Pappagianis D, Johnson SM. Revision and return of a coccidioidal skin test reagent. Mycopathologia 2012;174(5–6):351–2.

115. Ampel NM, Hector RF, Lindan CP, et al. An archived lot of coccidioidin induces specific coccidioidal delayed-type hypersensitivity and correlates with in vitro assays of coccidioidal cellular immune response. Mycopathologia 2006;161(2):67–72.

116. Nesbit LA, Knox KS, Nguyen CT, et al. Immunological characterization of bronchoalveolar lavage fluid in patients with acute pulmonary coccidioidomycosis. J Infect Dis 2013;208(5):857–63.

117. Binnicker MJ, Buckwalter SP, Eisberner JJ, et al. Detection of Coccidioides species in clinical specimens by real-time PCR. J Clin Microbiol 2007;45(1):173–8.

118. Vucicevic D, Blair JE, Binnicker MJ, et al. The utility of Coccidioides polymerase chain reaction testing in the clinical setting. Mycopathologia 2010;170(5):345–51.

119. Galgiani JN, Ampel NM, Blair JE, et al. 2016 Infectious Diseases Society of America (IDSA) clinical practice guideline for the treatment of coccidioidomycosis. Clin Infect Dis 2016;63(6):e112–46.

120. Ampel NM, Giblin A, Mourani JP, et al. Factors and outcomes associated with the decision to treat primary pulmonary coccidioidomycosis. Clin Infect Dis 2009;48(2):172–8.

121. Ampel NM. The treatment of coccidioidomycosis. Rev Inst Med Trop Sao Paulo 2015;57(Suppl 19):51–6.

122. Ashfaq A, Vikram HR, Blair JE, et al. Video-assisted thoracoscopic surgery for patients with pulmonary coccidioidomycosis. J Thorac Cardiovasc Surg 2014;148(4):1217–23.

123. Jaroszewski DE, Halabi WJ, Blair JE, et al. Surgery for pulmonary coccidioidomycosis: a 10-year experience. Ann Thorac Surg 2009;88(6):1765–72.

124. Baalachandran R, Trutter LR, Raz Y, et al. Successful use of extracorporeal membrane oxygenation in a patient with pulmonary coccidioidomycosis-related acute respiratory distress syndrome. Am J Respir Crit Care Med 2016;193:A7130.

125. Galgiani JN, Catanzaro A, Cloud GA, et al. Comparison of oral fluconazole and itraconazole for progressive, nonmeningeal coccidioidomycosis. A randomized, double-blind trial. Mycoses Study Group. Ann Intern Med 2000;133(9):676–86.

126. Galgiani JN, Catanzaro A, Cloud GA, et al. Fluconazole therapy for coccidioidal meningitis. The NIAID-Mycoses Study Group. Ann Intern Med 1993;119(1):28–35.

127. Dewsnup DH, Galgiani JN, Graybill JR, et al. Is it ever safe to stop azole therapy for Coccidioides immitis meningitis? Ann Intern Med 1996;124(3):305–10.

128. Kim MM, Vikram HR, Kusne S, et al. Treatment of refractory coccidioidomycosis with voriconazole or posaconazole. Clin Infect Dis 2011;53(11):1060–6.

129. Falci DR, Pasqualotto AC. Profile of isavuconazole and its potential in the treatment of severe invasive fungal infections. Infect Drug Resist 2013;6:163–74.

130. Valley Fever Center for Excellence Homepage. 2016. Available at: http://www.vfce.arizona.edu/. Accessed September 31, 2016.

131. Li RK, Ciblak MA, Nordoff N, et al. In Vitro activities of voriconazole, itraconazole, and amphotericin B against Blastomyces dermatitidis, Coccidioides immitis, and Histoplasma capsulatum. Antimicrobial Agents Chemother 2000;44(6):1734–6.

132. Mendoza N, Noel P, Blair JE. Diagnosis, treatment, and outcomes of coccidioidomycosis in allogeneic stem cell transplantation. Transpl Infect Dis 2015;17(3):380–8.

133. Ampel NM. Delayed-type hypersensitivity, in vitro T-cell responsiveness and risk of active coccidioidomycosis among HIV-infected patients living in the coccidioidal endemic area. Med Mycol 1999;37(4):245–50.

134. Taroumian S, Knowles SL, Lisse JR, et al. Management of coccidioidomycosis in patients receiving biologic response modifiers or disease-modifying antirheumatic drugs. Arthritis Care Res (Hoboken) 2012;64(12):1903–9.

135. Arunachalam A, Grewal H, Khirafan G, et al. Reactivation of indolent pulmonary coccidiodomycosis presenting as acute respiratory distress syndrome. Am J Respir Crit Care 2016;193:A1883.

136. Kotton CN, Marconi VC, Fishman JA, et al. Coccidioidal meningitis after liver transplantation in a nonendemic region: a case report. Transplantation 2006;81(1):132–4.

137. Vartivarian SE, Coudron PE, Markowitz SM. Disseminated coccidioidomycosis. Unusual manifestations in a cardiac transplantation patient. Am J Med 1987;83(5):949–52.

138. Cha JM, Jung S, Bahng HS, et al. Multi-organ failure caused by reactivated coccidioidomycosis without dissemination in a patient with renal transplantation. Respirology 2000;5(1):87–90.

139. Blair JE. Approach to the solid organ transplant patient with latent infection and disease caused by Coccidioides species. Curr Opin Infect Dis 2008;21(4):415–20.

140. Kahn A, Carey EJ, Blair JE. Universal fungal prophylaxis and risk of coccidioidomycosis in liver transplant recipients living in an endemic area. Liver Transpl 2015;21(3):353–61.

Clinical Manifestations and Treatment of Blastomycosis

Joseph A. McBride, MD[a,b], Gregory M. Gauthier, MD[a],*,
Bruce S. Klein, MD[a,b,c],*

KEYWORDS

- Blastomycosis • Dimorphic fungi • Pneumonia • Acute respiratory distress syndrome

KEY POINTS

- *Blastomyces dermatitidis* and *Blastomyces gilchristii* are the causal agents of blastomycosis.
- *Blastomyces* spp infect healthy and immunocompromised hosts.
- Pulmonary manifestations of blastomycosis range from subclinical infection to acute respiratory distress syndrome.
- Diagnosis of blastomycosis requires a high degree of clinical suspicion and involves the use of culture and nonculture diagnostic methods.
- Blastomycosis should be considered in patients who live in or visit regions where *Blastomyces* is endemic and have unresolving pneumonia despite antibiotic therapy, concomitant pulmonary and cutaneous infection, acute respiratory distress syndrome, or a compatible illness following recognizable risk factors for *Blastomyces* exposure.

INTRODUCTION

Blastomyces dermatitidis and *Blastomyces gilchristii* are the causal agents of blastomycosis. *Blastomyces* spp are thermally dimorphic fungi that grow as a filamentous mold in the environment and as a yeast in human tissues. Blastomycosis is endemic to North America, particularly states/provinces bordering the Mississippi, Ohio and St Lawrence Rivers, and the Great Lakes. The clinical manifestations of blastomycosis are broad, ranging from asymptomatic infection to acute respiratory distress syndrome (ARDS) and death. Extrapulmonary dissemination to the skin, bone, and central nervous system can occur. Although culture and non-culture diagnostic tests are available, a high index of clinical suspicion is essential for prompt diagnosis. Treatment guidelines published by the Infectious Disease Society of America and the American Thoracic Society recommend the use of polyene or azole antifungal agents, with selection influenced by disease severity, site of infection, immunosuppression, and pregnancy.

MYCOLOGY

Recent phylogenic analysis has divided *Blastomyces* into 2 species, *B dermatitidis* and *B gilchristii*.[1] *Blastomyces* spp belong to a group of fungi that includes *Histoplasma capsulatum*, *Coccidioides immitis* and *Coccidioides posadasii*, *Paracoccidioides brasiliensis* and *Paracoccidioides lutzii*,

Disclosure: The authors have nothing to disclose.
[a] Division of Infectious Disease, Department of Medicine, University of Wisconsin School of Medicine and Public Health, 600 Highland Avenue, Madison, WI 53792, USA; [b] Division of Infectious Disease, Department of Pediatrics, University of Wisconsin School of Medicine and Public Health, 1675 Highland Avenue, Madison, WI 53792, USA; [c] Department of Medical Microbiology and Immunology, University of Wisconsin School of Medicine and Public Health, 1550 Linden Drive, Madison, WI 53706, USA
* Corresponding author. Division of Infectious Disease, Department of Medicine, University of Wisconsin School of Medicine and Public Health, 600 Highland Avenue, Madison, WI 53792.
E-mail addresses: gmg@medicine.wisc.edu (G.M.G.); bsklein@wisc.edu (B.S.K.)

Sporothrix schenckii, and *Talaromyces marneffei* (formerly *Penicillium marneffei*). *Blastomyces* undergoes a reversible morphologic switch between hyphae at 22°C to 25°C and yeast at 37°C. *Blastomyces* yeast forms (8–20 μm diameter) are characterized by a broad-based bud (4–10 μm) and doubly refractile cell wall (**Fig. 1**).[2] Although this appearance is unique among dimorphic fungi, giant forms (28–40 μm diameter) have been described and can be confused with *Coccidioides* species.[3] The mycelial form is characterized by septate hyphae (1–2 μm diameter) that produce asexual spores (4–5 μm diameter).[2] In contrast with the yeast, hyphal morphology is not distinct and requires molecular confirmation or transition to yeast for identification.

GEOGRAPHIC DISTRIBUTION AND EPIDEMIOLOGY

Knowledge about the geographic distribution and epidemiologic risks is important for including blastomycosis in the differential diagnosis in patients with pulmonary, cutaneous, bone, and central nervous system (CNS) infections. In North America, *Blastomyces* is endemic to the midwestern, south-central, and southeastern regions of the United States and 4 Canadian provinces from Saskatchewan to Quebec (**Fig. 2**). In the endemic region, *Blastomyces* is not uniformly distributed; it inhabits an ecologic niche that is characterized by forested, sandy soils with an acidic pH, decaying vegetation or organic material, and rotting wood located near water sources.[4] Similar to *H*

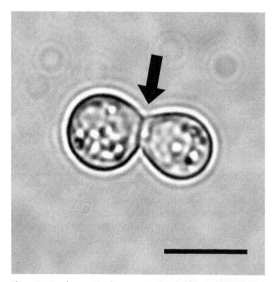

Fig. 1. *B dermatitidis* yeast. Broad-based budding yeast at 37°C. Arrow points to the broad-based bud between mother and daughter cells. Scale bar is 10 μm.

capsulatum and *Cryptococcus*, *Blastomyces* can grow in bird guano. Although most infections are sporadic, occupational and recreational activities that disrupt soil (eg, construction, exploration of beaver damns or underground forts, use of community compost piles, clearing brush or cutting trees, hunting, canoeing, boating, tubing, fishing) have all been associated with outbreaks of the disease (**Table 1**).[4,5]

Rare autochthonous cases of culture-proven blastomycosis have been reported outside of North America. Approximately 100 cases have been described in 18 African nations, whereas fewer than 10 confirmed autochthonous cases have been reported in India.[6,7] *Blastomyces* is not considered endemic to Central America, South America, Europe, Australia, or Asia outside India.

The epidemiology of blastomycosis in North America is based mainly on retrospective studies and passive surveillance. Within endemic zones, 6 American states (Arkansas, Louisiana, Michigan, Minnesota, Missouri, and Wisconsin) and 2 Canadian provinces (Manitoba and Ontario) require reporting of new cases. In North America, the annual incidence of blastomycosis ranges from 0.2 to 1.94 cases per 100,000 persons.[8–11] Several hyperendemic regions exist, including Kenora, Ontario (117.2 human cases per 100,000 population); Eagle River, Wisconsin (101.3 per 100,000); Vilas County, Wisconsin (40.4 per 100,000); Washington Parish, Louisiana (6.8 per 100,000); and central/south-central Mississippi (>5 per 100,000).[12–15] The true incidence of blastomycosis is likely greater than the reported numbers. Reliable skin and serologic tests are not available. Moreover, approximately 50% of infected persons have subclinical or asymptomatic illness.[4] Thus, epidemiologic data are limited to patients with clinically apparent infection that is diagnosed and reported. In the United States from 2007 to 2011 a total of 4688 patients in 46 states were hospitalized for blastomycosis.[16] Most of these patients were hospitalized in the state in which they resided; however, 8% of patients were admitted to hospitals outside of known endemic regions.[16]

Most blastomycosis cases occur in adults, with less than 13% occurring in the pediatric population.[5,17] Similar to histoplasmosis and coccidioidomycosis, blastomycosis epidemiologic studies of adults show a slight male predominance. *Blastomyces* is a primary fungal pathogen because it causes invasive disease in immunocompetent hosts; most patients with blastomycosis are immunocompetent. Patients who are immunocompromised by solid organ transplant (SOT), tumor necrosis factor-alpha (TNF-α) inhibitors, malignancy, or human immunodeficiency virus

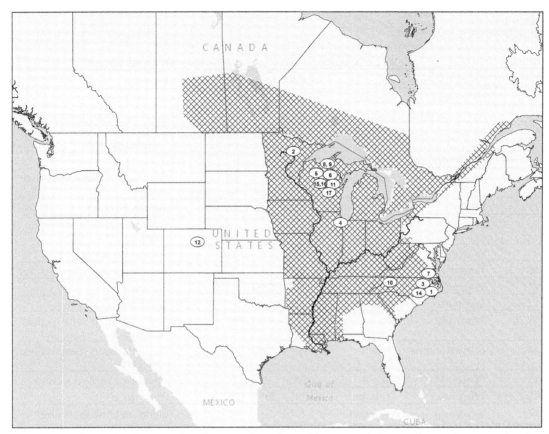

Fig. 2. Map of the distribution of endemic and epidemic blastomycosis in North America. Cross-hatching denotes geographic distribution of cases. Circled numbers denote location of epidemics referred to in **Table 1**. (© OpenStreetMap contributors.)

(HIV)/AIDS (acquired immunodeficiency syndrome) can develop more severe disease.[18–22] The higher incidence of blastomycosis in some ethnic groups, including aboriginal ethnicity in Canada and Hmong populations in Wisconsin, may signal genetic predisposition.[9,23]

PATHOGENESIS
The Phase Transition

The ability to convert from mold to yeast is an essential event in the pathogenesis of all dimorphic fungi, including *Blastomyces* spp. This morphologic shift or phase transition is primarily influenced by a change in temperature and is a complex process involving global changes in transcription, metabolism, cell signaling, cell wall composition, and plasma membrane lipid content.[24] In the soil (22°C–25°C), *B dermatitidis* and *B gilchristii* grow as mold that produces infectious conidia (spores). After disruption of soil, often through human activity, aerosolized conidia and mold fragments inhaled into the lungs of a human

host (37°C) convert to pathogenic yeast, which evades host immune defenses to cause infection. Moreover, conidia phagocytized by lung macrophages are able to survive and convert into yeast.[25] This intracellular lifestyle is not unique to *Blastomyces*; other dimorphic pathogens, including *H capsulatum*, *Coccidioides* spp, and *Paracoccidioides* spp, show similar intracellular preferences. For fungi such as *H capsulatum* and *Cryptococcus neoformans*, survival in macrophages promotes dissemination; however, it is unknown whether *B dermatitidis* uses this so-called Trojan horse method for extrapulmonary dissemination.[26]

The development of molecular tools to genetically manipulate the dimorphic fungi has enabled the discovery of genes critical for the phase transition to yeast and virulence, including *DRK1* (dimorphism-regulating kinase-1) and *BAD1* (*Blastomyces* adhesion-1; formerly WI-1). *DRK1* encodes a hybrid histidine kinase that is essential for the conversion of mold to yeast in *B dermatitidis*, *B gilchristii*, and *H capsulatum* in response to a

Table 1
Blastomycosis outbreaks[a,b]

Number	State	City or County	Years	# Infected	Outbreak Source
1	North Carolina	Pitt	1953–1954	11	Unknown
2	Minnesota	Bigfork	1972	12	Cabin construction
3	North Carolina	Enfield	1975	5	Harvest at peanut farm
4	Illinois	Westmont	1974–1975	5	Apartment complex construction
5	Wisconsin	Hayward	1979	8	Canoeing
6	Wisconsin	Eagle River	1984	48	Visiting an abandoned beaver lodge
7	Virginia	Southampton	1984	4	Raccoon hunting
8	Wisconsin	Portage and Waupaca	1985	14	Underground timber fort; fishing
9	Wisconsin	Vilas	1988	32	Hotel construction
10	Tennessee	Elizabethton	1989	3	Construction at rayon factory
11	Wisconsin	Oconto	1989–1990	8	Unknown
12	Colorado	Boulder	1998	2	Prairie dog relocation
13	Wisconsin	Indian reservation[c]	1998–2000	9	Likely related to construction/excavation
14	North Carolina	Duplin	2001–2002	8	Likely related to construction projects
15	Wisconsin	Merrill	2006	21	Community yard waste site
16	Wisconsin	Marathon	2009–2010	55	Unknown
17	Wisconsin	Waupaca	2015	90	Tubing on Little Wolf River

[a] Refs.[5,23] and www.dhs.wisconsin.gov/disease/blastomycosis.htm (accessed January 2016).
[b] See **Fig. 2**.
[c] The specific Indian reservation was not published and thus the location is not reflected in **Fig. 2**.

shift in temperature from 22°C to 37°C.[27] Deletion of *DRK1* results in *Blastomyces* and *Histoplasma* cells that fail to convert to yeast and grow as hyphae at 37°C. *DRK1* null mutants (*DRK1Δ*) also have altered distribution of cell wall carbohydrates, such as α-(1,3)-glucan and chitin, and fail to express *BAD1*, an essential virulence factor.[27] *Blastomyces* and *Histoplasma* cells with reduced transcription of *DRK-1* are avirulent in a murine model of pulmonary infection.[27] These findings offer genetic proof that the morphologic switch to yeast is essential for pathogenicity.

In the yeast phase, *B dermatitidis* expresses BAD1, a 120-kDA protein that facilitates adhesion and immune evasion.[28] BAD1 is secreted by *B dermatitidis* yeast into the extracellular milieu and binds back to the cell surface via interactions with chitin in the cell wall. BAD1 functions as an adhesin that attaches yeast cells to host tissue by binding heparin sulfate.[29] BAD1 enables immune evasion by repressing TNF-α production through transforming growth factor-β (TGF-β)–dependent and TGF-β–independent mechanisms.[30] TNF-α is an important cytokine that contributes to host defense against blastomyces infection. In mice, neutralization of TNF-α results in progressive pulmonary blastomycosis.[31] In addition to its effects on innate immunity, BAD1 alters adaptive immunity through inhibiting CD4+ T-lymphocyte activation, which in turn reduces production of interleukin-17 and interferon gamma.[29] In a murine model of pulmonary infection, *BAD1* null mutants (*BAD1Δ*) strains are avirulent.[28] Moreover, the lungs of mice infected with *BAD1Δ* strains appear grossly normal and contain few granulomas.[28] In addition to *BAD1*, genes upregulated during pulmonary infection have been identified by *in vivo* transcriptional profiling of *B dermatitidis* yeast.[32]

During phase transition to yeast, changes in cell wall carbohydrate composition may also contribute to virulence and immune evasion. During the transition from mold to yeast, the amount of cell wall α-(1,3)-glucan increases, whereas β-(1,3)-glucan decreases from 40% to 50% in mycelia to less than 5% in yeast.[33] The decreased β-(1,3)-glucan concentration in *Blastomyces* yeast cell walls has substantial diagnostic and therapeutic implications because it precludes the use of β-(1,3)-glucan assays for diagnosis and renders echinocandins ineffective.

The transition in the opposite direction, yeast to mycelia, is important for environmental survival, mating to promote genetic diversity, and transmission to mammalian hosts. Recent genetic analyses identified a GATA transcription factor encoded by *SREB* that mediates the conversion from yeast to mycelia after a reduction in temperature from 37°C to 22°C.[34] *SREB* null mutants (*SREBΔ*) have a defect in the morphologic shift that corresponds with a reduction in neutral lipid (ergosterol, triacylglycerol) biosynthesis and lipid droplet formation. In *B dermatitidis* and *H capsulatum*, *N*-acetylglucosamine transporters *NGT1* and *NGT2* accelerate the transition to mycelia at 22°C.[35]

HOST RESPONSE

Both the innate and adaptive immune responses are required to combat blastomyces infection, whereas humoral immunity is dispensable. Following inhalation of aerosolized conidia, alveolar macrophages and neutrophils phagocytize and kill conidia.[36] However, conidia that survive phagocytosis germinate to yeast, which is more challenging for the host immune system to kill. *B dermatitidis* yeast actively subverts host immune defenses by inhibiting host cell cytokine production, impairing CD4[+] T-lymphocyte activation, and suppressing nitric oxide production.[29,30,37] Moreover, *Blastomyces* yeasts are fairly resistant to reactive oxygen species produced by macrophages and neutrophils.[37] Following recovery from blastomycosis, hosts develop cell-mediate immunity that lasts at least 2 years,[38] and likely longer.

CLINICAL MANIFESTATIONS

The clinical manifestations of blastomycosis are heterogeneous and range from asymptomatic infection to pneumonia to acute respiratory distress syndrome (ARDS). Because of this clinical variability, blastomycosis has been described as "the great pretender."[39] The lung is the primary portal of entry for aerosolized conidia following disruption of soil. Traumatic inoculation of skin (eg, laboratory accidents) is rare but has been reported.[40] Onset of symptoms occurs 3 weeks to 3.5 months following inhalation of mycelial fragments or spores.[4,41] When symptomatic, approximately 25% to 40% of patients develop extrapulmonary dissemination.[42] Common sites for disseminated disease are the skin, bone, genitourinary tract, and CNS; however, *Blastomyces* can infect nearly every organ in the body.[5]

PULMONARY BLASTOMYCOSIS

Pulmonary infection is reported in more than 79% of patients with documented blastomycosis.[5,8–10] The spectrum of pulmonary infection is broad and varies from subclinical pneumonia to ARDS.[42,43] In both adult and pediatric populations, symptomatic pneumonia presents with fevers, chills, headache, productive or non-productive cough, dyspnea, chest pain, and malaise.[5,8,9,44] Acute pulmonary blastomycosis may be mild and can be mistaken for other lower respiratory tract infections, including bacterial community-acquired pneumonia (CAP); moreover, consolidation is the most common chest radiographic finding and is indistinguishable from CAP. Undiagnosed or untreated acute pulmonary blastomycosis can progress to ARDS or chronic pneumonia (**Figs. 3** and **4**). Symptoms and radiographic findings for chronic pulmonary blastomycosis are nonspecific and can mimic other diagnoses, such as lung neoplasm or tuberculosis.[39] Symptoms can include fever, persistent cough, hemoptysis, night sweats, anorexia, weight loss, and malaise.[5,8,9,44] Chest radiography can show nodules, masses, or cavitation (see **Fig. 4**). Because the clinical picture is

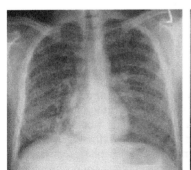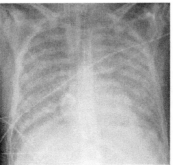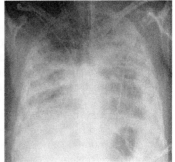

Fig. 3. Miliary blastomycosis and ARDS. Chest radiographs showing miliary blastomycosis that progressed to diffuse, dense consolidation in a patient with ARDS.

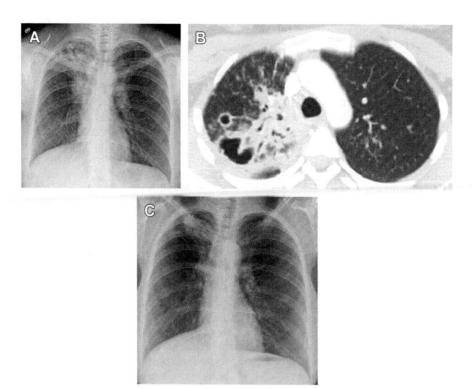

Fig. 4. Cavitary blastomycosis. Chest radiograph (*A*) and corresponding chest computed tomography image (*B*) of a patient with multiple cavities and consolidation in the right upper lung at the time of initial clinical presentation. (*C*) Chest radiograph after completion of antifungal therapy shows residual scarring and bronchiectasis.

nonspecific, blastomycosis is often not included in the differential diagnosis unless the patient has other findings such as skin lesions, fails to respond to antibacterial therapy, or has recognized risk factors for exposure to blastomycosis.[39] Thus, symptoms may be present for several months before diagnosis.

A subset of patients with acute pulmonary blastomycosis have a rapidly progressive infection resulting in respiratory failure or ARDS (see **Fig. 3**).[42,43] In retrospective analyses of patients from Mississippi and Tennessee, ARDS was encountered in 8.4% to 14.8% of hospitalized patients with pulmonary blastomycosis.[45,46] A delay in diagnosis of blastomycosis-induced ARDS is common with patients initially misdiagnosed with CAP that becomes fulminant in 5 to 7 days or progressive CAP that fails to respond to multiple courses of antibiotic therapy. Mortality caused by ARDS is high, often greater than 50%.[45–47] In most patients who die of blastomycosis-induced ARDS, the diagnosis was either not suspected or was considered after the patient was moribund.[44–46] Thus, early diagnosis of blastomycosis-induced ARDS is critical to decrease mortality.

EXTRAPULMONARY AND DISSEMINATED BLASTOMYCOSIS
Overview

Blastomyces can disseminate to any organ in the body. Evidence of dissemination occurs in approximately 25% to 40% of cases.[42] Aside from rare cases of direct inoculation through penetrating trauma, accidental needle stick, or laboratory exposure, extrapulmonary blastomycosis represents disseminated disease and should be treated accordingly.

Cutaneous Blastomycosis

The skin is the most common extrapulmonary site of infection and cutaneous involvement occurs in up to 40% to 80% of patients with disseminated disease.[48,49] Cutaneous disease often begins as papulopustular lesions that progress to ulcerative, verrucous, or crusted lesions (**Fig. 5**). Other manifestations include violaceous nodules, plaques, and abscesses.[48] Although erythema nodosum is common in patients with histoplasmosis or coccidioidomycosis, it is rarely described in blastomyces infection. Cutaneous lesions can expand in an asymmetric fashion creating ulcerations and

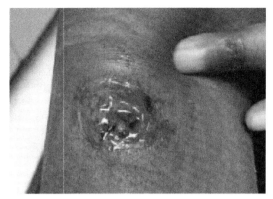

Fig. 5. Cutaneous ulcer caused by blastomycosis in a patient who received TNF-α inhibitor therapy.

necrosis that can lead to disfigurement, including permanent scarring.[50] Less commonly, cutaneous blastomycosis manifests as a draining sinus tract or ulcer from underlying osteomyelitis.[48] Skin lesions can occur anywhere on the body but are often found on exposed areas, including the head and extremities.[48] *Blastomycosis* is much less likely than *H capsulatum* or *Paracoccidioides* spp to involve the mucous membranes; however, intraoral, nasal, and pharyngeal lesions have rarely been described.[51] Although uncommon, cutaneous involvement of the eyelid is the most common ophthalmologic finding.[52] Endophthalmitis and orbital abscess are exceedingly rare.[52] Involvement of the periorbital skin can be complicated by ectropion, which can require surgical correction following successful treatment of infection.[50,52]

Osseous Blastomycosis

The bone is the second most common site for dissemination of *Blastomyces* and occurs in approximately 5% to 25% of patients.[8,44,46] Most patients with osteomyelitis have concomitant pulmonary blastomycosis. Osseous lesions are painful and can be associated with soft tissue abscess, draining sinus tracts, or cutaneous ulcers.[53] Osseous invasion by *Blastomyces* is characterized by lytic destruction, periosteal reaction or sclerotic margins on radiography, and granulomatous inflammation on histopathology.[53,54] Although any bone can be infected, the most common sites include the long bones, vertebrae, skull, and ribs.[44,53,54] Blastomycosis of the bone can mimic malignancy (eg, sarcoma, giant cell tumor, metastases) and Pott disease (*Mycobacterium tuberculosis*).[53,54] Through direct extension, infection can spread from bones to nearby joints and soft tissue, resulting in septic arthritis and abscess, respectively.[53,54] Progressive bone destruction can result in pathologic fracture (eg, vertebral body collapse).[54]

Genitourinary Blastomycosis

Case series published in the 1950s estimated the rate of genitourinary (GU) dissemination to be as high as 20% to 30%; however, modern case series report prostate involvement in less than 10% of patients.[8] In men, the most common sites of GU involvement are the prostate and epididymis. Symptoms of prostatitis include urinary obstruction, dysuria, and perineal or suprapubic discomfort.[55] Epididymitis presents with pain, scrotal swelling, testicular enlargement, and (rarely) a draining sinus. In women, dissemination to the GU system can cause tubo-ovarian abscess, endometritis, and salpingitis. This condition can be complicated by extension to the peritoneum and omentum with or without new-onset ascites.[56] A single case of sexual transmission has been described following intercourse between a man with *Blastomyces* prostatitis and his wife who had endometrial adenocarcinoma.[57]

Central Nervous System Blastomycosis

CNS blastomycosis is estimated to occur in less than 5% to 10% of immunocompetent patients.[58] Dissemination to the CNS results from either hematogenous seeding or direct invasion through untreated skull-based osteomyelitis and can manifest as meningitis, epidural abscess, or brain abscess.[58] Presenting symptoms can include headache, focal neurologic defects, confusion, visual disturbances, and seizures. In patients with meningitis, cerebrospinal fluid (CSF) analysis reveals a lymphocytic or neutrophilic pleocytosis with increased protein levels and hypoglycorrhachia.[58] *Blastomyces* grow about 45% of the time from CSF cultures; however, a positive CSF *Blastomyces* antigen test may facilitate diagnosis.[58] A wide range of CNS complications have been reported, including hydrocephalus, mass effect from edema, cerebral herniation, infarction, seizures, panhypopituitarism, weakness, and impaired ability to function at school.[5,58]

BLASTOMYCOSIS IN IMMUNOCOMPROMISED HOSTS
Human Immunodeficiency Virus/Acquired Immunodeficiency Syndrome

In contrast with histoplasmosis, blastomycosis is an uncommon infection in patients with HIV/AIDS. Most patients with HIV with blastomycosis have a CD4+ T-lymphocyte count less than 200 cells/mm³ and two-thirds have a history of prior opportunistic infections.[22] Patients with AIDS are more likely to have severe pulmonary disease (eg, ARDS, miliary disease) and up to 40% have dissemination to the CNS.[22] In one case series, approximately one-quarter of AIDS-related blastomycosis was postulated to be caused by reactivation of latent infection.[22] Before the era of modern antiretrovirals, mortality in patients with AIDS and blastomycosis exceeded 50%.[22]

Solid Organ Transplant

Blastomycosis is an uncommon infection in SOT recipients, with a cumulative incidence of 0.13% to 0.14% in SOT patients from an endemic region.[18,19] This rate is lower than the reported incidence of posttransplant histoplasmosis or coccidioidomycosis.[18,19] The onset of disease after transplant ranges from 12 days to 250 months.[18,19] This variability may reflect different disease pathogenesis including (1) primary infection; (2) reactivation of latent disease; (3) and conversion of recently acquired, pretransplant, asymptomatic infection to symptomatic disease.[18] In contrast with histoplasmosis and coccidioidomycosis, donor-derived blastomycosis has not been reported. Compared with immunocompetent hosts, SOT patients have similar rates of disseminated disease (33%–50%) but are at increased risk for severe pulmonary disease, including respiratory failure and ARDS.[18,19] Mortality for transplant-associated blastomycosis ranges from 33% to 38% but increases to 67% in patients with ARDS. Lifelong suppressive antifungal therapy is generally not required following appropriately treated blastomycosis.[18]

Anti–Tumor Necrosis Factor Alpha Therapy

TNF-α is a critical cytokine for host defense against blastomycosis. In murine models, antibody-mediated neutralization of TNF-α results in progressive pulmonary infection.[31] Clinical data on blastomycosis in the setting of TNF-α exposure are sparse and are limited to case reports.[20,59] Nevertheless, blastomycosis was listed in the 2008 warning issued by the US Food and Drug Administration regarding increased risk of fulminant infections with endemic mycosis in patients receiving TNF inhibitor therapy.[20]

BLASTOMYCOSIS IN PREGNANCY AND NEWBORNS

Blastomycosis in pregnancy and the newborn is rare and clinical information is limited to case reports.[60–63] Women can be infected in any trimester but the disease is most frequently diagnosed in the second or third trimester.[63] Case reports suggest

disseminated disease (62%) is more common than isolated pulmonary infection (38%).[63] Reliable data regarding the frequency of placental infection are lacking because examination by culture or histology has been conducted in only one-third of clinical cases; however, placental involvement has been reported.[60,63] Blastomycosis does not seem to increase risk for congenital malformations, but there is potential for transmission during the peripartum period. Neonatal pulmonary blastomycosis is rare and can be fatal.[61,62] The underlying pathogenesis of neonatal blastomycosis is not well defined and may involve transplacental transmission or aspiration of infected vaginal secretions.

DIAGNOSIS

The clinical presentation, physical examination, and the radiographic manifestations of blastomycosis are nonspecific; therefore, a high index of suspicion is essential for prompt diagnosis. Delays in diagnosis are common, even in endemic areas, because few patients are correctly diagnosed at initial presentation and delays in diagnosis exceeding 1 month occur in more than 40% of patients.[15,39,46] A detailed history to identify possible exposures and at-risk hosts can facilitate a diagnosis. In patients with pneumonia, medical histories should include place of residence, travel, outdoor activities (eg, fishing, canoeing, rafting), hobbies, recent home remodeling, exposure to road construction, and use of a wood-burning stove or community compost pile. Blastomycosis in a household pet, such as a dog, suggests a common source of exposure and can serve as a harbinger of human infection.[64] In patients with concomitant pulmonary and cutaneous disease, blastomycosis must be considered in the differential diagnosis.

Microscopic and Culture-Based Diagnostics

The most expeditious method to diagnose blastomycosis remains the examination of stained clinical specimens. Although *Blastomyces* is not well visualized with Gram or hematoxylin and eosin stains, sputum or tissue samples stained with 10% potassium hydroxide, calcofluor white, Gomori methenamine silver, or periodic acid–Schiff can facilitate visualization of the characteristic *Blastomyces* yeast.[49] The discovery of the characteristic yeast forms (8–20 μm) with broad-based budding and a doubly refractile cell wall can lead to a presumptive diagnosis of blastomycosis before the results of culture and non-culture tests are available. In one case series, the use of appropriately stained clinical specimens identified nearly 80% of culture-confirmed cases.[65] Despite the effectiveness of fungal-specific stains in diagnosis, this technique is often underused.[66] In tissue specimens, the presence of neutrophilic infiltration with noncaseating granulomas (ie, pyogranulomatous inflammation) can suggest blastomycosis and thorough microscopic examination for *Blastomyces* yeast should be performed.

Culture of *Blastomyces* provides a definitive diagnosis. In the setting of pulmonary blastomycosis, the yield of culture from invasive bronchoscopy is excellent. One study showed a 92% diagnostic yield for bronchoscopy.[66] Even noninvasive methods, including cultures from sputum, tracheal secretion, or gastric washings, yielded *Blastomyces* growth in 86% of samples.[66] Specialized media, including Sabouraud dextrose agar, potato dextrose agar, and brain-heart infusion media, are required for growth.[49] Incubator temperatures used in most clinical laboratories (25°C to 30°C) promote the growth of *Blastomyces* as a mold. Although highly specific, *Blastomyces* grows slowly in culture. Fungal colonies take an average of 5 to 14 days to be visualized; however, when burden of infection is low, growth can take longer.[49]

Non-culture Diagnostics

Classic antibody testing by complement fixation (CF) or immunodiffusion (ID) is not clinically useful for the diagnosis of blastomycosis because of poor sensitivity and specificity.[41] A newer enzyme immunoassay that uses microplates coated with BAD1 protein has enhanced sensitivity (87%) and specificity (94%–99%); however, it is not yet commercially available.[67] Because BAD1 is unique to *Blastomyces*, BAD1 assays can distinguish between histoplasmosis and blastomycosis.[67]

An antigen assay that detects a galactomannan component in the cell wall of *Blastomyces* has supplanted CF and ID, and can be used to test urine, serum, bronchoalveolar lavage fluid, and CSF specimens.[67–69] Sensitivity of antigenuria in patients with proven disease is 76.3% to 92.9% and specificity is 79.3%.[69–71] False-positives can occur in the setting of other fungal infections, such as histoplasmosis, paracoccidioidomycosis, and penicilliosis (talaromycosis).[67] The clinical impact of a false-positive test is often minimal because paracoccidioidomycosis and penicilliosis (talaromycosis) can be removed from the differential diagnosis if the patient has not traveled to Central and South America (paracoccidioidomycosis), or southeast Asia and China (talaromycosis). Moreover, the treatment of blastomycosis is similar to that of histoplasmosis. Serial urine antigen concentrations can be used to monitor response to treatment.[71] Following initiation of therapy, an increase in antigenuria can occur (median of 11 days), which is followed by progressive decline in antigen titer with successful therapy.[71] Initial posttreatment increase in titer may reflect increased urinary excretion of antigen caused by fungal cell death.[71]

RADIOGRAPHIC MANIFESTATIONS

There are no pathognomonic radiographic patterns for pulmonary blastomycosis. Radiographic findings are nonspecific and may mimic bacterial pneumonia, tuberculosis, or malignancy. Radiographic abnormalities may include diffuse airspace disease, consolidation, nodular masses, interstitial disease, cavitation disease, or miliary disease (see **Figs. 3** and **4**).[72] Consolidation is the most common radiographic findings and may be present in the absence of pulmonary symptoms.[72] Calcified lung lesions, hilar/mediastinal adenopathy, and pleural effusions are uncommon.[72] MRI is the preferred imaging modality for CNS disease and is frequently abnormal in patients with CNS blastomycosis.[58]

TREATMENT

Guidelines for the diagnosis and treatment of blastomycosis are published by the Infectious Disease Society of America and the American Thoracic Society (**Table 2**).[42,43] Treatment recommendations are based on the site and severity of infection, host immune status, and pregnancy. Antifungal treatment is recommended for all patients diagnosed with blastomycosis, including those with resolution of clinical symptoms before receiving therapy.[42,43] Before the initiation of therapy, baseline evaluation of hematologic, hepatic, and renal function should be obtained. Careful review of all medications is required to limit drug interactions commonly associated with azole antifungals. Itraconazole, voriconazole, posaconazole, and fluconazole can lengthen the QT interval, especially when administered with other medications that prolong the QT interval. In contrast, isavuconazole can shorten the QT interval and is contraindicated in patients with familial short QT syndrome. Itraconazole has a negative inotropic effect and the potential to exacerbate existing congestive heart failure and should be used with caution in patients with ventricular dysfunction.[73] Azole antifungals increase the serum concentration of HMG-CoA (3-hydroxy-3-methylglutaryl-coenzyme A) reductase inhibitors metabolized via cytochrome P450 3A4, which can increase the risk for statin-induced rhabdomyolysis. Pravastatin can

Table 2
Summary of clinical practice guidelines for antifungal therapy against blastomycosis

Site of Infection	Disease Severity	Initial Therapy	Step-Down Therapy
Pulmonary blastomycosis	Mild to moderate	Oral itraconazole 200 mg 3× daily for 3 d and then 1× or 2× daily for 6–12 mo[a]	Not applicable
	Moderately severe to severe	Lipid formulation of AmB 3–5 mg/kg daily or AmB deoxycholate 0.7–1 mg/kg daily for 1–2 wk or until improvement is noted	Oral itraconazole 200 mg 3× daily for 3 d and then 2× daily for 6–12 mo[a]
Disseminated or extrapulmonary blastomycosis	Mild to moderate	Oral itraconazole 200 mg 3× daily for 3 d and then 1× or 2× daily for 6–12 mo[a,b]	Not applicable
	Moderately severe to severe	Lipid formulation of AmB 3–5 mg/kg daily or AmB deoxycholate 0.7–1 mg/kg daily for 1–2 wk or until improvement is noted	Oral itraconazole 200 mg 3× daily for 3 d and then 2× daily for at least 12 mo[a,b]
Central nervous system disease	—	Lipid formulation AmB 5 mg/kg/d for 4–6 wk	Options include: 1. Oral fluconazole 800 mg daily 2. Oral itraconazole 200 mg 2× or 3× daily 3. Voriconazole (200–400 mg 2× daily) Treatment should continue for at least 12 mo and until resolution of CSF abnormalities
Immunocompromised patients	—	Lipid formulation of AmB 3–5 mg/kg daily or AmB deoxycholate 0.7–1 mg/kg daily for 1–2 wk or until improvement is noted	Oral itraconazole 200 mg 3× daily for 3 d and then 2× daily for at least 12 mo[a,c]
Pregnant women	All disease	Lipid formulation of AmB 3–5 mg/kg/d	Azoles should be avoided because of risks of teratogenicity and spontaneous abortion
Newborn	All disease	AmB deoxycholate 1.0 mg/kg/d	Not applicable
Children	Mild to moderate (nonmeningeal)	Oral itraconazole 10 mg/kg/d (maximum of 400 mg/d) for 6–12 mo[a]	Not applicable
	Severe	AmB deoxycholate 0.7–1.0 mg/kg daily or lipid AmB at 3–5 mg/kg daily until improvement	Oral itraconazole 10 mg/kg/d (maximum of 400 mg/d) for 12 mo[a]

Abbreviations: AmB, amphotericin B; CSF, cerebrospinal fluid.

[a] Therapeutic drug monitoring is required with goal serum levels (sum of itraconazole + hydroxy-itraconazole concentrations) of greater than or equal to 1 μg/mL.

[b] Osteoarticular blastomycosis should be treated with at least 12 months' total antifungal treatment.

[c] Lifelong suppressive therapy with oral itraconazole, 200 mg/d may need to be considered in select patients including those with immunosuppression that cannot be reversed and in those who experience relapse despite appropriate therapy.

safely be used with azoles because it is not metabolized by P450 3A4.[42] Other significant azole drug-drug interactions include immunosuppressive medications, dihydropyridine calcium channel blockers, sulfonylureas, and anticonvulsants. Because of adverse effects of azole exposure on pregnancy, including teratogenicity, all women of childbearing age should be screened for pregnancy.[74,75]

Amphotericin B

Polyene amphotericin B (AmB) formulations are recommended for the treatment of patients with severe pulmonary infection, disseminated disease, CNS involvement, and underlying immunosuppression (eg, HIV/AIDS, SOT). AmB is also the first-line agent for neonates and pregnant women.[42,43] AmB deoxycholate has a long track record of clinical success with high cure rates.[15,42] Despite well-proven efficacy, the use of AmB is associated with significant cumulative toxicity. Nephrotoxicity is the most common treatment-limiting toxicity and occurs in more than 30% of treated patients.[76] Other adverse effects include infusion reactions (eg, fever, rigors, hypoxia, nausea, vomiting, hypertension, hypotension) and electrolyte disturbances (hypokalemia, hypomagnesemia).[76] The risks of nephrotoxicity can be minimized by 0.9% normal saline infusions administered before and after AmB, and by avoidance of diuretics and nephrotoxic agents. Most patients require scheduled replacement potassium and magnesium to offset renal loss of these electrolytes. Frequent monitoring of electrolytes and creatinine is essential during AmB therapy (eg, at least 2–3 times per week). Lipid AmB preparations (eg, liposomal amphotericin, AmB lipid complex, and AmB colloidal dispersion) are preferred to AmB deoxycholate because these formulations have lower rates of nephrotoxicity. For CNS blastomycosis, liposomal amphotericin is the preferred polyene because it has the best penetration of the blood-brain barrier among the lipid formulations.[42]

Triazoles

In contrast with AmB, azole antifungal agents are fungistatic against *Blastomyces*. Itraconazole is the first-line agent for the treatment of mild to moderate, non-CNS blastomycosis, and for step-down therapy following induction treatment with AmB.[42,43] Oral itraconazole can be prescribed as a solution or a capsule; however, administration of these formulations is not equivalent. Therapeutic drug monitoring (TDM) is important to optimize itraconazole dosing because serum concentrations are influenced by formulation, dosage, and interpatient variability in drug metabolism. Serum concentrations are approximately 30% higher with the use of solution than with capsule formulation.[42] Itraconazole solution can be taken without regard to food and does not require gastric acidity for absorption. In contrast, itraconazole capsules must be taken with food and an acidic beverage to maximize absorption.[42,43] Therefore, in patients who are taking H_2-blockers or proton-pump inhibitors, itraconazole solution is the preferred formulation. Itraconazole levels should be obtained after 2 weeks of therapy when a steady-state concentration is reached. Because of a long half-life of approximately 24-hours, serum specimens for TDM can be obtained at any time, independent of when the itraconazole dose was administered. Total itraconazole level is calculated by adding itraconazole and hydroxy-itraconazole concentrations with a goal level between 1 and 5.5 µg/mL. Hydroxy-itraconazole, which is a metabolite of itraconazole, has antifungal activity. Serum levels of greater than or equal to 10.0 µg/mL are unnecessary and associated with drug toxicity.[42] Liver function tests should be obtained at baseline and at 2 and 4 weeks into therapy and then every 3 months thereafter.[42]

Newer triazoles, including voriconazole, posaconazole, and isavuconazole, have activity against *B dermatitidis*.[77–79] Voriconazole should be taken in the absence of food to optimize absorption. The goal serum trough concentration for voriconazole is between 1 and 5.5 µg/mL.[80] The absorption of posaconazole solution is maximized by high-fat meals, whereas posaconazole delayed-release tablets are not affected by food or gastric acid inhibitors. The target posaconazole level is not well defined but most experts recommend levels greater than 0.5 to 1 µg/mL.[80] Isavuconazole capsules can be administered without regard to food or stomach acidity and TDM is not needed. Parental formations are available for voriconazole, posaconazole, and isavuconazole. Voriconazole and posaconazole have been successfully used to treat blastomycosis, including the use of voriconazole for CNS infection.[77,78]

Steroids and Acute Respiratory Distress Syndrome

Despite appropriate antifungal therapy, the mortality of blastomycosis-induced ARDS remains high.[45–47] Case reports have suggested the potential for adjunctive steroids to improve survival; however, a recent retrospective analysis of 43 patients (1992–2014) with ARDS caused by blastomycosis did not show reduced mortality in patients who received steroids.[81–83] Nevertheless, additional research is needed regarding the dose, duration, and efficacy of adjuvant steroids in ARDS.

MORTALITY

Large case series from Wisconsin and Manitoba report a case fatality rate between 4.3% and 6.3%.[16,17] Mortality has been associated with a shorter duration of symptoms, likely suggesting more fulminant presentation and a compromised immune status of the host. Blastomycosis-induced ARDS is associated with high mortality even in patients receiving appropriate antifungal treatment.[18,45–47,83] The mortality of blastomycosis in patients with AIDS in the absence of immune reconstitution is nearly 40% and most deaths occur within 3 weeks of diagnosis.[22] Similarly, the mortality of patients immunosuppressed by SOT is 33% to 38% and increases in the setting of respiratory failure.[18,19]

SUMMARY

Blastomycosis is often a diagnostic and therapeutic challenge. Even in endemic areas, the nonspecific clinical manifestations of blastomycosis frequently lead to a delay in diagnosis. For physicians within areas of *Blastomyces* endemicity, certain clinical characteristics should trigger suspicion, including (1) unresolving pneumonia despite appropriate CAP management, (2) simultaneous pulmonary/cutaneous infection, (3) ARDS, and (4) illness following recognizable risk factors for *Blastomyces* exposure. The knowledge that *Blastomyces* spp can infect, and disseminate, in both the immunocompromised and the immunocompetent is essential. An understanding of phase transition reminds clinicians that β-(1,3)-glucan assays and echinocandin antifungals have no role in diagnosis or therapy for blastomycosis. Ultimately, an awareness of common issues confronting clinicians using polyene and azole antifungals decreases the risks associated with treatment.

REFERENCES

1. Brown EM, McTaggart LR, Zhang SX, et al. Phylogenetic analysis reveals a cryptic species *Blastomyces gilchristii*, sp. nov. within the human pathogenic fungus *Blastomyces dermatitidis*. PLoS One 2013;8(3): e59237.
2. Wolf PL, Russel B, Shimoda A, editors. Practical clinical microbiology and mycology: techniques and interpretations. Section x: identification of dimorphic fungi causing systemic mycosis. New York: John Wiley; 1975. p. 486–8.
3. Wu SJ, Valyi-Nagy T, Engelhard HH, et al. Secondary intracerebral blastomycosis with giant yeast forms. Mycopathologia 2005;160(3):253–7.
4. Klein BS, Vergeront JM, Weeks RJ, et al. Isolation of *Blastomyces dermatitidis* in soil associated with a large outbreak of blastomycosis in Wisconsin. N Engl J Med 1986;314(9):529–34.
5. Gauthier G, Klein BS. Blastomycosis. Chapter 198. In: Cherry JD, Harrison GJ, editors. Feigin and Cherry's textbook of pediatric infectious disease. 7th Edition. Philadelphia: Elsevier Saunders; 2014. p. 2723–43.
6. Baily GG, Robertson VJ, Neill P, et al. Blastomycosis in Africa: clinical features, diagnosis, and treatment. Rev Infect Dis 1991;13(5):1005–8.
7. Randhawa HS, Chowdhary A, Kathuria S, et al. Blastomycosis in India; report of an imported case and current status. Med Mycol 2013;51(2):185–92.
8. Carlos WG, Rose AS, Wheat LJ, et al. Blastomycosis in Indiana: digging up more cases. Chest 2010; 138(6):1377–82.
9. Crampton TL, Light RB, Berg GM, et al. Epidemiology and clinical spectrum of blastomycosis diagnosed at Manitoba hospitals. Clin Infect Dis 2002; 34(10):1310–6.
10. Centers for Disease Control and Prevention (CDC). Blastomycosis – Wisconsin, 1986-1995. MMWR Morb Mortal Wkly Rep 1996;45(28):601–3.
11. Furcolow ML, Chick EW, Busey JP, et al. Prevalence and incidence studies of human and canine blastomycosis. 1. Cases in the United Stated, 1885-1968. Am Rev Respir Dis 1970;102(1):60–7.
12. Baumgardner DJ, Buggy BP, Mattson BJ, et al. Epidemiology of blastomycosis in a region of high endemicity in north central Wisconsin. Clin Infect Dis 1992;15(4):629–35.
13. Dwight PJ, Naus M, Sarsfield P, et al. An outbreak of human blastomycosis: the epidemiology of blastomycosis in the Kenora catchment region of Ontario, Canada. Can Commun Dis Rep 2000;26(10):82–91.
14. Lowry PW, Kelso KY, McFarland LM. Blastomycosis in Washington Parish, Louisiana 1976-1985. Am J Epidemiol 1989;130(1):151–9.
15. Chapman SW, Lin AC, Hendricks KA, et al. Endemic blastomycosis in Mississippi: epidemiologic and clinical studies. Semin Respir Infect 1997;12(3): 219–28.
16. Seitz AE, Younes N, Steiner CA, et al. Incidence and trends of blastomycosis- associated hospitalizations in the United States. PLoS One 2014;9(8):e105466.
17. Morris S, Brophy J, Richardson SE, et al. Blastomycosis in Ontario, 1994-2003. Emerg Infect Dis 2006; 12:274–9.
18. Gauthier GM, Safdar N, Klein BS, et al. Blastomycosis in solid organ transplant recipients. Transpl Infect Dis 2007;9(4):310–7.
19. Grim SA, Proria L, Miller R, et al. A multicenter study of histoplasmosis and blastomycosis after solid organ transplantation. Transpl Infect Dis 2012;14(1): 17–23.

20. Smith JA, Kauffman CA. Endemic fungal infections in patients receiving tumour necrosis factor-alpha inhibitor therapy. Drugs 2009;69(11):1403–15.

21. Pappas PG. Blastomycosis in the immunocompromised patient. Semin Respir Infect 1997;12(3): 243–51.

22. Pappas PG, Pottage JC, Powderly WG, et al. Blastomycosis in patients with the acquired immunodeficiency syndrome. Ann Intern Med 1992;116(10): 847–53.

23. Roy M, Benedict K, Deak E, et al. A large community outbreak of blastomycosis in Wisconsin with geographic and ethnic clustering. Clin Infect Dis 2013; 57(5):655–62.

24. Gauthier GM, Klein BS. Insights into fungal morphogenesis and immune evasion: fungal conidia, when situated in mammalian lungs, may switch from mold to pathogenic yeasts or spore-forming spherules. Microbe Wash DC 2008;3:416–23.

25. Sterkel AK, Mettelman R, Wüthrich M, et al. The unappreciated intracellular lifestyle of Blastomyces dermatitidis. J Immunol 2015;194(4):1796–805.

26. Charlier C, Nielsen K, Daou S, et al. Evidence of a role for monocytes in dissemination and brain invasion by Cryptococcus neoformans. Infect Immun 2009;77(1):120–7.

27. Nemecek JC, Wüthrich M, Klein BS. Global control of dimorphism and virulence in fungi. Science 2006;312(5773):583–8.

28. Brandhorst TT, Wüthrich M, Warner T, et al. Targeted gene disruption reveals an adhesion indispensable for pathogenicity of Blastomyces dermatitidis. J Exp Med 1999;189(8):1207–16.

29. Brandhorst TT, Roy R, Wüthrich M, et al. Structure and function of a fungal adhesion that binds heparin and mimics thrombospondin-1 by blocking T cell activation and effector function. PLoS Pathog 2013; 9(7):e1003464.

30. Finkel-Jimenez B, Wüthrich M, Klein BS. BAD1, an essential virulence factor of Blastomyces dermatitidis, suppress hosts TNF-α production through TGF-β-dependent and -independent mechanisms. J Immunol 2002;168(11):5746–55.

31. Finkel-Jimenez B, Wüthrich M, Brandhorst T, et al. The WI-1 adhesin blocks phagocyte TNF-α production, imparting pathogenicity on Blastomyces dermatitidis. J Immunol 2001;166(4):2665–73.

32. Muñoz JF, Gauthier GM, Desjardins CA, et al. The dynamic genome and transcriptome of the human fungal pathogen Blastomyces and close relative Emmonsia. PLoS Pathog 2015;11(10): e1005493.

33. Kanetsuna F, Carbonell LM. Cell wall composition of the yeast-like and mycelial forms of Blastomyces dermatitidis. J Bacteriol 1971;106(3):946–8.

34. Marty AJ, Broman AT, Zarnowski R, et al. Fungal morphology, iron homeostasis, and lipid metabolism regulated by a GATA transcription factor in Blastomyces dermatitidis. PLoS Pathog 2015;11(6): 31004959.

35. Gilmore SA, Naseem S, Konopka JB, et al. N-acetylglucosamine (G1cNAc) triggers a rapid temperature-responsive morphogenetic program in thermally dimorphic fungi. PLoS Genet 2013;9:e1003799.

36. Sugar AM, Picard M, Wagner R, et al. Interactions between human bronchoalveolar macrophages and Blastomyces dermatitidis conidia: demonstration of fungicidal and fungistatic effects. J Infect Dis 1995;171(6):1559–62.

37. Rocco NM, Carmen JC, Klein BS. Blastomyces dermatitidis yeast cells inhibit nitric oxide production by alveolar macrophage inducible nitric oxide synthase. Infect Immun 2001;79(6):2385–95.

38. Klein BS, Bradsher RW, Vergeront JM, et al. Development of long-term specific cellular immunity after acute Blastomyces dermatitidis infection: assessments following a large point source outbreak in Wisconsin. J Infect Dis 1990;151(1):97–101.

39. Lemos LB, Baliga M, Guo M. Blastomycosis: the great pretender can also be an opportunist. Initial clinical diagnosis and underlying disease in 123 patients. Ann Diagn Pathol 2002;6(3):194–203.

40. Larson DM, Eckman MR, Alber RL, et al. Primary cutaneous (inoculation) blastomycosis: an occupational hazard to pathologist. Am J Clin Pathol 1983; 79(2):253–5.

41. Klein BS, Vergeront JM, Kaufman L, et al. Serologic tests for blastomycosis: assessments during a large point-source outbreak in Wisconsin. J Infect Dis 1987;155(2):262–8.

42. Chapman SW, Dismukes WE, Proia LA, et al, Infectious Diseases Society of America. Clinical practice guidelines for the management of blastomycosis: 2008 updated by the Infectious Disease Society of America. Clin Infect Dis 2008;46(12): 1801–11.

43. Limper AH, Knox KS, Sarosi GA, et al. An official American Thoracic Society statement: treatment of fungal infections in adult pulmonary and critical care patients. Am J Respir Crit Care Med 2011; 183:96–128.

44. Fanella S, Skinner S, Trepnman E, et al. Blastomycosis in children and adolescents: a 30-year experience from Manitoba. Med Mycol 2011;49(6): 627–32.

45. Lemos LB, Baliga M, Guo M. Acute respiratory distress syndrome and blastomycosis: presentation of nine cases and review of the literature. Ann Diagn Pathol 2001;5(1):1–9.

46. Vasquez JE, Mehta JB, Agrawal R, et al. Blastomycosis in northeast Tennessee. Chest 1998;114(2): 436–43.

47. Meyer KC, McManus EJ, Maki DG. Overwhelming pulmonary blastomycosis associated with the adult

respiratory distress syndrome. N Engl J Med 1993; 329(17):1231–6.

48. Smith JA, Riddell JIV, Kauffman CA. Cutaneous manifestations of endemic mycoses. Curr Infect Dis Rep 2013;15(5):440–9.

49. Saccente M, Woods GL. Clinical and laboratory update on blastomycosis. Clin Microbiol Rev 2010; 23(2):367–81.

50. Saucier J, Gauthier G. Photo quiz. Verrucous lesions and ectropion in an immunocompetent individual. Clin Infect Dis 2012;55(10):1390–1, 1426–8.

51. Reder PA, Neel HB. Blastomycosis in otolaryngology: review of a large series. Laryngoscope 1993;103(1 Pt 1):53–8.

52. Pariseau B, Lucarelli MJ, Appen RE. A concise history of ophthalmic blastomycosis. Ophthalmology 2007;114(11):e27–32.

53. Jain R, Sing K, Lamzabi I, et al. Blastomycosis of the bone: a clinicopathologic study. Am J Clin Pathol 2014;142(5):609–16.

54. Saccente M, Abernathy RS, Pappas PG, et al. Vertebral blastomycosis with paravertebral abscess: report of eight cases and review of the literature. Clin Infect Dis 1998;26(2):413–8.

55. Seo R, Oyasu R, Schaeffer A. Blastomycosis of the epididymis and prostate. Urology 1997;50(6): 980–2.

56. Barocas JA, Gauthier GM. Peritonitis caused by *Blastomyces dermatitidis* in a kidney transplant recipient: case report and literature review. Transpl Infect Dis 2014;16(4):634–41.

57. Farber E, Leahy M, Meadows T. Endometrial blastomycosis acquired by sexual contact. Obstet Gynecol 1968;32(2):195–9.

58. Bariola JR, Perry P, Pappas PG, et al. Blastomycosis of the central nervous system: a multicenter review of diagnosis and treatment in the modern era. Clin Infect Dis 2010;50(6): 797–804.

59. Smith RJ, Boos MD, Burnham JM, et al. Atypical cutaneous blastomycosis in a child with juvenile idiopathic arthritis on infliximab. Pediatrics 2015; 136(5):e1386–9.

60. MacDonald D, Alguire PC. Adult respiratory distress syndrome due to blastomycosis during pregnancy. Chest 1990;98(6):1527–8.

61. Maxson S, Miller SF, Tryka AF, et al. Perinatal blastomycosis: a review. Pediatr Infect Dis J 1992;11(9): 760–3.

62. Watts EA, Gard PD, Tuthill SW. First reported case of intrauterine transmission of blastomycosis. Pediatr Infect Dis J 1983;2(4):308–10.

63. Lemos LB, Soofi M, Amir E. Blastomycosis and pregnancy. Ann Diagn Pathol 2002;6(4):211–5.

64. Sarosi GA, Eckman MR, Davies SF, et al. Canine blastomycosis as a harbinger of human disease. Ann Intern Med 1979;91(5):733–5.

65. Patel AJ, Gattuso P, Reddy VB. Diagnosis of blastomycosis in surgical pathology and cytopathology: correlation with microbiologic culture. Am J Surg Pathol 2010;34(2):256–61.

66. Martynowicz MA, Prakash UB. Pulmonary blastomycosis: an appraisal of diagnostic techniques. Chest 2002;121(3):768–73.

67. Richer SM, Smedema ML, Durkin MM, et al. Development of a highly sensitive and specific blastomycosis antibody enzyme immunoassay using *Blastomyces dermatitidis* surface protein BAD-1. Clin Vaccine Immunol 2014;21(2):143–6.

68. Durkin M, Witt J, Lemonte A, et al. Antigen assay with the potential to aid in diagnosis of blastomycosis. J Clin Microbiol 2004;42:4873–5.

69. Bariola JR, Hage CA, Durkin M, et al. Detection of *Blastomyces dermatitidis* antigen in patients with newly diagnosed blastomycosis. Diagn Microbiol Infect Dis 2011;69(2):143–6.

70. Connolly P, Hage CA, Bariola JR, et al. *Blastomyces dermatitidis* antigen detection by quantitative enzyme immunoassay. Clin Vaccine Immunol 2012; 19(1):53–6.

71. Frost HM, Novicki TJ. *Blastomyces* antigen detection for diagnosis and management of blastomycosis. J Clin Microbiol 2015;53(11):3660–2.

72. Fang W, Washington L, Kumar N. Imaging manifestations of blastomycosis: a pulmonary infection with potential dissemination. Radiographics 2007;27(3): 641–55.

73. Ahmad SR, Singer SJ, Leissa BG. Congestive heart failure associated with itraconazole. Lancet 2001; 357(9270):1766–77.

74. De Santis M, Di Gianantonio E, Cesari E, et al. First-trimester itraconazole exposure and pregnancy outcome: a prospective cohort study of women contacting teratology information services in Italy. Drug Saf 2009;32(3):239–44.

75. Pursley TJ, Blomquist IK, Abraham J, et al. Fluconazole-induced congenital anomalies in three infants. Clin Infect Dis 1996;22(2):336–40.

76. Girois SB, Chapuis F, Decullier E, et al. Adverse effects of antifungal therapies in invasive fungal infections: review and meta-analysis. Eur J Clin Microbiol Infect Dis 2005;24(2):119–30.

77. Ta M, Flowers SA, Rogers PD. The role of voriconazole in the treatment of central nervous system blastomycosis. Ann Pharmacother 2009;43(10): 1696–700.

78. Proia LA, Harnisch DO. Successful use of posaconazole for treatment of blastomycosis. Antimicrob Agents Chemother 2012;56(7):4029.

79. Gonzalez GM. In vitro activities of isavuconazole against opportunistic filamentous and dimorphic fungi. Med Mycol 2009;47(1):71–6.

80. Andes D, Pascual A, Marchetti O. Antifungal therapeutic drug monitoring: established and emerging

indications. Antimicrob Agents Chemother 2009; 53(1):24–34.

81. Lahm T, Neese S, Thornburg AT, et al. Corticosteroids for blastomycosis-induced ARDS: a report of two patients and review of the literature. Chest 2008;133(6):1478–80.

82. Plamondon M, Lamontagne F, Allard C, et al. Corticosteroids as adjunctive therapy in severe blastomycosis-induced acute respiratory distress syndrome in an immunosuppressed patient. Clin Infect Dis 2010;51(1):e1–3.

83. Schwartz IS, Embil JM, Sharma A, et al. Management and outcome of acute respiratory distress syndrome caused by blastomycosis: a retrospective case series. Medicine 2016; 95(18):e3538.

Cryptococcal Lung Infections

Kate Skolnik, MD[a], Shaunna Huston, PhD[b], Christopher H. Mody, MD[c,d],*

KEYWORDS

- Cryptococcus • Cryptococcosis • Fungal lung infection • Endemic mycoses • Treatment

KEY POINTS

- *Cryptococcus* infections have high morbidity and mortality rates worldwide, particularly in the context of immune suppression and central nervous system involvement.
- *Cryptococcus neoformans* can be found globally and predominantly affects the immune-suppressed individual, whereas *Cryptococcus gattii* is endemic to certain regions and often affects immune-competent individuals.
- Most individuals with cryptococcal pulmonary infection present with symptoms; however, they may be mild and nonspecific, making timely diagnosis challenging.
- Pulmonary nodules or focal consolidation is the most common radiographic finding with *Cryptococcus*.
- Azoles (specifically fluconazole) and amphotericin B (in severe disease) are key cryptococcal therapies. There is no role for echinocandins.

INTRODUCTION

Cryptococcus remains one of the leading causes of acquired immunodeficiency syndrome (AIDS)-related deaths, and is among the most common fungal pathogens worldwide.[1] *Cryptococcus* demands global attention because of the high mortality, unique geographic distribution, and its propensity to cause severe and rapidly progressive disease in both healthy and immunosuppressed individuals.[1,2] *Cryptococcus neoformans*, which mainly infects immunosuppressed individuals, and *Cryptococcus gattii*, which has a high propensity to infect healthy individuals, are the 2 major species of *Cryptococcus* that are associated with

mortality.[1] Arguably, the greatest virulence factor for both species is the cryptococcal polysaccharide capsule, which helps evade immune detection.[3] The organism often leads to respiratory infection but can also disseminate to other organs, in particular to the meninges causing meningoencephalitis, which is associated with poor clinical outcomes.[2,4] Current diagnostics are based on detection of antigen and culture techniques, and treatment recommendations are tailored based on fungal susceptibility, location, and severity of disease. Research is advancing technologies to enable more effective and efficient diagnostics for early detection along with improved prophylactic and therapeutic regimes.

Disclosure Statement: The authors have nothing to disclose.
[a] Division of Respirology, Department of Internal Medicine, Rockyview General Hospital, University of Calgary, Respirology Offices, 7007 14th Street Southwest, Calgary, Alberta T2V 1P9, Canada; [b] Department of Physiology and Pharmacology, Health Research Innovation Centre, University of Calgary, Room 4AA08, 3330 Hospital Drive Northwest, Calgary, Alberta T2N 4N1, Canada; [c] Department of Microbiology and Infectious Diseases, Health Research Innovation Centre, University of Calgary, Room 4AA14, 3330 Hospital Drive Northwest, Calgary, Alberta T2N 4N1, Canada; [d] Department of Internal Medicine, Health Research Innovation Centre, University of Calgary, Room 4AA14, 3330 Hospital Drive Northwest, Calgary, Alberta T2N 4N1, Canada
* Corresponding author. Health Research Innovation Centre, Room 4AA14, 3330 Hospital Drive Northwest, Calgary, Alberta T2N 4N1, Canada.
E-mail address: cmody@ucalgary.ca

chestmed.theclinics.com

EPIDEMIOLOGY

General Cryptococcal Epidemiology

Among the 37 species of *Cryptococcus*, only a few are human pathogens.[5] *C neoformans* is characterized as an opportunistic pathogen because it commonly causes infections in individuals with impaired immunity. *C neoformans* causes more than 1 million infections in AIDS patients annually, and, unfortunately, most of these patients will die within a few months of diagnosis.[2] By contrast, *C gattii* has a more distinct geographic range and is more likely to affect healthy individuals leading to its characterization as an endemic mycosis.[6,7] *C gattii* is classically located in tropical and subtropical areas of the world such as Australia and Papua New Guinea, but more recently it has emerged as an endemic mycosis on the west coast of Canada and the United States.[7] Rarely, *Cryptococcus laurentii* causes infection in individuals with compromised immunity[8–10] and even less often in patients who are immune competent.[11,12] Immunosuppression is a significant risk factor, and the prevalence of cryptococcal infection significantly increased during the emergence of AIDS.[13] Currently, in developed countries with effective antiretroviral therapies, the prevalence of opportunistic cryptococcal infections has decreased, but *Cryptococcus* continues to affect those with other defects in cell-mediated immunity. Infections also occur in healthy individuals, especially if exposed in endemic areas.[14,15]

Although *Cryptococcus* causes both endemic and opportunistic mycosis, transmission of *Cryptococcus* occurs directly from the environment rather than from human to human.[16–18] Although *Cryptococcus* can cause infection in animals such as cats, dogs, ferrets, cockatiels, parrots, llamas, horses, and marine mammals,[19,20] direct transmission from these species is exceptionally rare. The primary environmental sources of *C gattii* are trees, such as eucalyptus, Douglas-fir, red cedar, and Garry oak, among others,[16,17,21] but it can also be found in the soil, water, and air in endemic regions.[22] *C gattii* has been isolated from the environment mainly in Australia, New Zealand, Papa New Guinea, Central America, parts of South America, and the Pacific Northwest of North America including Vancouver Island.[18,21,23–25] Interestingly, *C gattii* has also been identified in the Mediterranean basin on various trees, including olive and eucalyptus, which marks the first detection of the species in Europe.[26] In contrast, *C neoformans* is found worldwide, with the primary source being pigeon excrement, although certain subtypes are more common in particular regions of the world.[16,18] *C neoformans* has also been linked to other bird species such as magpies and cockatiels.[27,28] Additionally, there seems to be a seasonality to *C gattii* infections in some regions, which has not been noted with *C neoformans*.[29]

Cryptococcal Subtypes

It is important to differentiate between subtypes of *C neoformans* and *C gattii* for clinical purposes. *C neoformans* is divided into 2 major groups known as *C neoformans* var *grubii* (serotype A) and *C neoformans* var *neoformans* (serotype D).[30] Additionally, a hybrid serotype, AD, has also been identified as a clinically significant subtype.[30] *C neoformans* and *C gattii* have also more recently been subdivided into 4 molecular types, termed *VNI, VNII, VNIII, VNIV* and *VGI, VGII, VGIII, VGIV*, respectively, which may lead to further species distinctions.[30,31] *C neoformans* var *grubii* and *C neoformans* var *neoformans* have important differences in their genomes and replication methods,[30] which have clinical implications, as certain serotypes and molecular types may be more likely to respond to treatment.[31]

STRUCTURE AND LIFE CYCLE

Cryptococci are eukaryotic organisms that belong to the phylum Basidiomycota of filamentous fungi.[32] The cryptococcal cell is enveloped by a cell membrane, cell wall, and a characteristic polysaccharide capsule.[4] The capsule is unique to *Cryptococcus* and sets it apart from other pathogenic fungi.[33] It is composed of glucuronoxylomannan (GXM), which is the predominant polysaccharide, GalXM (galactoxylomannan), and mannoproteins.[34,35] Structural differences in GXM allow for the identification of *Cryptococcus* based on serotype.[36] The fungal cell wall consists of chitin and β-glucans (which provide structural integrity), pores (which allow for the movement of important molecules and transport vesicles), melanin (which protects the cell from oxidative stress), and proteins that serve a variety of cellular functions.[37–39] Cryptococcal cells can be identified by light microscopy but require special stains such as mucicarmine or Periodic-acid Schiff to identify the capsule or silver stains to identify the cell wall.[40] *Cryptococcus* is also readily identified with India ink staining, in which exclusion of the stain in the perimeter of the fungal cell is indicative of the fungal capsule (Fig. 1).[41,42]

Cryptococcus species are able to reproduce asexually through simple budding, and sexually, through the mating of α- and a-mating types.[43,44] Asexual reproduction is more common and occurs in the human host.[43,45] Sexual reproduction

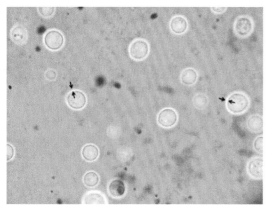

Fig. 1. Cryptococcus species as visualized by India ink staining. Arrows indicate the fungal cell capsule.

provides greater genetic diversity and, with this, the potential for increased virulence.[46] Both mating strategies have the potential to increase genetic diversity.[45,46] The reproductive strategy is also influenced by Cryptococcus variety. For example, less than half of C neoformans var grubii are fertile, whereas most C neoformans var neoformans are capable of sexual reproduction.[30,47] Interestingly, the highly virulent C gattii subtype VGIIa, which is responsible for the outbreak on Vancouver Island, seems to have emerged specifically from same-sex reproduction, suggesting that different types of reproduction may provide environmental adaptation and virulence.[45]

PATHOGENESIS

The primary risk factor for C gattii infection is exposure from environmental sources in endemic regions. It is unclear why most C gattii infections occur in healthy individuals.[48] By contrast, C neoformans infection is more common in immunosuppressed patients, in particular, those with defective cell-mediated immunity such as those with human immunodeficiency virus (HIV), idiopathic CD4 lymphopenia, organ transplant, hematologic malignancies or those receiving immune-suppressive medications (including systemic steroids, biologic agents, chemotherapy, and other cytotoxic therapies).[16,49] Although it is much less common, individuals with a milder degree of immune suppression (such as splenectomy, cirrhosis, diabetes mellitus, systemic lupus erythematosus, and pregnancy) have an increased risk of getting C neoformans infections.[50–53]

Independent of the type of cryptococcal infection or the primary organ involved, the fungus typically enters the body through the lungs.[54] After entering, the organism undergoes changes to a phenotype that facilitates invasive infection of the host.[54] Although C neoformans takes advantage of natural weak points in the immune system, C gattii is postulated to have additional unique virulence factors that allow it to evade the immune system.[3,55–57]

C neoformans infections may also occur owing to the reactivation of latent infection, similar to tuberculosis.[57–60] In one study, antibodies to Cryptococcus were found in most individuals in the borough of the Bronx, New York, independent of prior exposure or HIV status, suggesting that exposure is surprisingly common.[61] Additionally, years after emigrants from Africa moved to France, infections developed with organisms of an African phenotype rather than a French phenotype, suggesting that organisms were dormant in these hosts for years.[58] There is evidence that anticryptococcal antibodies (and Cryptococcus) can persist in the body for years without symptom development.[58,61] However, when impairment in immunity occurs, as with solid-organ transplantation or AIDS, dormant Cryptococcus may reactivate and develop into an active fungal infection.[58,60] By contrast, C gattii infections seem to occur de novo,[62] although it must be noted that clinical disease may occur months or years after exposure.[63,64]

VIRULENCE FACTORS

The distinctive polysaccharide capsule of Cryptococcus spp. acts as a key virulence factor.[4,37] The polysaccharide capsule prevents phagocytosis, allowing the organism to bypass the host innate immune response.[65] In addition, GXM is known to directly interfere with T lymphocyte function,[66] whereas GalXM has been shown to induce cytokine dysregulation and T lymphocyte apoptosis,[67] and both GXM and GalXM are capable of stimulating macrophage apoptosis.[68]

In addition to the polysaccharide capsule, Cryptococcus has several virulence factors that act as antioxidants, neutralizing host innate immune molecules and preventing oxidative damage to the cell.[69] These antioxidants include mannitol,[70] superoxide dismutase,[71] thioredoxin reductase,[72] and pigments such as melanin.[69] Melanin also binds to antibiotics, which may confer antifungal resistance.[73] Additional virulence factors target the host by various mechanisms including destabilization of the cell membrane (as with β1 phospholipase),[74] degradation of host proteins (as with metalloproteinases),[75] and altering pH (via urease).[76] The α-mating type of C gattii is also a virulence factor.[77] C gattii likely has additional virulence factors that allow it to cause invasive infection in hosts with intact immune systems;

however, the exact nature of these factors is yet to be discovered.

CLINICAL OUTCOMES OF CRYPTOCOCCAL PULMONARY INFECTION
Clinical Manifestations of Cryptococcal Pulmonary Infection

Cryptococcal infection can produce a range of manifestations from minimal symptoms to severe life-threatening disease.[78] *Cryptococcus* most often leads to pulmonary[75,76] and central nervous system (CNS) disease,[79,80] the latter being a major source of morbidity and mortality. However, *Cryptococcus* can also present as infection in the bone,[78] skin,[81] eyes,[82] and prostate[83,84] and may even cause disseminated disease and cryptococcemia.[85,86] These findings may occur in isolation or in association with pulmonary *Cryptococcus* infection. Interestingly, these presentations can occur in both immune-suppressed and immune-competent individuals, although cryptococcemia is rare in those with intact immunity.

An individual's underlying risk factors may affect the manifestations of cryptococcal disease. For example, those with pre-existing lung disease are more likely to have significant pulmonary infection,[78] whereas those with HIV or organ transplant and healthy subjects are more likely to have CNS infection.[78,87–89] Lung involvement occurs in 28% to 64% of HIV-negative individuals infected with *Cryptococcus*[52,90] compared with less than 5% of those co-infected with *Cryptococcus* and HIV.[90] By contrast, *C gattii* tends to cause more pulmonary disease and is generally seen in immune-competent individuals.[91] Furthermore, the prevalence of pulmonary cryptococcal infection may be underestimated, as individuals can have asymptomatic pulmonary nodules that never come to medical attention.[92]

Cryptococcal pulmonary infection can cause vague symptoms and a wide spectrum of disease severity including minimal or no symptoms in a subset of individuals.[93] Consequently, early diagnosis may be challenging, and cryptococcal disease may be overlooked in the setting of subtle symptoms. Most patients with cryptococcal lung infection are clinically symptomatic.[94–96] When present, pulmonary symptoms can include dry cough, dyspnea, chest tightness, and fever, with cough and fever being the most common (**Table 1**).[4,48,95] Mediastinal or hilar lymphadenopathy may occur in both immune-competent and immune-suppressed individuals, which may be a solitary finding or associated with other pulmonary manifestations.[97,98] Those with lymphadenopathy

---

Table 1
Potential manifestations of pulmonary cryptococcal infection

Symptoms	Radiographic Findings
• None	• Single or multiple pulmonary nodules[a]
• Fever[a]	
• Dry cough[a]	• Consolidation (lobar or segmental)[a]
• Dyspnea	
• Chest pain/ discomfort	• Nodular interstitial pattern
• Malaise	• Reticular interstitial pattern
	• Ground glass opacities
	• Mass
	• Mediastinal/hilar lymphadenopathy
	• Pleural effusions

[a] Most common.

---

may present with symptoms secondary to compression of adjacent structures if the adenopathy is severe. Cryptococcoma, a granulomatous mass harboring the fungus, may be mistaken for lung cancer on imaging[94,99–102] and has been described more frequently in infections caused by *C gattii* in immune-competent patients[99,100] but can also occur with *C neoformans*.[52] Rarely, endobronchial infection can occur.[101,102] In some cases, severe pulmonary disease leading to respiratory failure can be seen, and acute respiratory distress syndrome has occurred in immune-compromised individuals with pulmonary cryptococcosis.[103,104] A miliary tuberculosislike presentation with *Cryptococcus* in an AIDS patient has also been reported but is exceedingly rare.[105,106] Importantly, although immune-compromised individuals, such as those with HIV, are less likely to manifest with pulmonary symptoms, when present, the manifestations can be very severe.

Radiographic Findings of Cryptococcal Pulmonary Infection

Radiographic findings can include pulmonary nodules (single or multiple), lobar or segmental consolidation, nodular or reticulonodular interstitial pattern, ground glass opacities, masses, hilar/mediastinal lymphadenopathy, and even pleural effusions.[52,85,93,94,97,98,105] Cryptococcal pleural effusions are typically limited to severely immune-suppressed individuals, as is seen with AIDS or ideopathic CD4 lymphopenia (**Fig. 2**). Reticular or reticulonodular interstitial changes are the most frequent radiographic presentation in HIV, whereas dense nodules, consolidation, or interstitial changes seem to be the most common findings in the immune-competent population.[52,85,107,108]

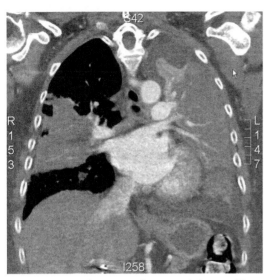

Fig. 2. Computed tomography scan of drowned lung in an adult with idiopathic CD4 lymphopenia secondary to invasive cryptococcal pneumonia and associated pleural effusion.

Overall, about half of all cryptococcal infections present with chest radiograph findings, with some variability depending on cryptococcal subtype and host immune status (see **Table 1**). In one study of predominantly C neoformans–affected individuals, 66% of those without HIV had an abnormal chest radiograph, compared with 40% of those with HIV.[96] In those with HIV and pulmonary C neoformans infection, infiltrates or several small nodules were most commonly seen.[96] Cryptococcal pulmonary involvement was confirmed in only 58% and 14%, respectively.[96] In comparison, a Colombian study focusing on C gattii (with a minority of individuals having concurrent HIV) found abnormal chest radiographs in 15% of individuals with known C gattii and only half of them had pulmonary involvement.[109] However, these numbers are likely an underestimate, as only 40% of subjects underwent chest imaging. A separate study of HIV-negative individuals had findings that fell between those of the aforementioned studies, with 36% having pulmonary involvement.[78] Computed tomography scanning would likely improve the sensitivity for detecting cryptococcal-related changes and should be pursued when radiographs are not helpful, but clinical suspicion for Cryptococcus persists.

DIAGNOSIS

Testing for Cryptococcus should be considered in anyone with risk factors or exposure history and persistent pulmonary symptoms or radiographic findings despite treatment of common bacterial pathogens. Diagnosis of cryptococcal pulmonary infections usually requires a combination of microbiologic and radiographic investigations. Although microbiologic tests are the key to diagnosis, pulmonary imaging may bring subclinical infection to the clinicians' attention and suggest Cryptococcus as part of a differential diagnosis (see **Table 1**). As part of the diagnostic process, there should be an assessment for possible extrapulmonary complications of disease; in particular, neurologic involvement should be considered and investigated.[49]

Cryptococcus can be identified by various methods, including fungal culture, special stains, and immunohistochemical tests that identify cryptococcal antigen.[6,110] Fungal culture may be obtained by plating respiratory samples on selective media. Cryptococcus grows best in temperatures between 30°C and 35°C,[111] and environmental concentrations decrease with hotter weather.[112] Cryptococcus can be identified by exclusion of India ink stain in the immediate cell perimeter; however, this method cannot differentiate between viable and dead fungal cells (see **Fig. 1**).[6] Alternatively, the diagnosis may be made by detection of cryptococcal polysaccharide antigen in body fluids by various immunologic techniques.[113,114] In respiratory secretions, the latex agglutination assay has a sensitivity between 93% and 100% and specificity of 93% to 98%,[113] whereas enzyme-linked immunosorbent assay has a sensitivity of 99% and specificity of 97% for Cryptococcus.[114] These results are similar to assays performed on cerebrospinal fluid samples.[115,116] However, the latex agglutination assay was found to be slightly more sensitive than enzyme-linked immunosorbent assay for blood and cerebrospinal fluid samples from a larger study.[116] The lateral flow assay is the newest test for cryptococcal antigen with good yield and has been adopted at most centers because it is easier to use.[115,117] An important downfall of these assays is suboptimal sensitivity in detecting C gattii. In one study, 40% of C gattii were missed despite the application of all 3 tests.[118] Nevertheless, lateral flow assay seems to have the best sensitivity for C gattii and has largely replaced other methods.[119] Furthermore, although the enzyme-linked immunosorbent assay, latex agglutination assay, and lateral flow assay are generally highly sensitive and specific, none of the tests can differentiate viable from dead fungal cells.[6] In addition, DNA amplification has largely replaced canavanine-glycine-bromothymol blue selective media for further identification and confirmation of the presence of C gattii.[120] If the aforementioned tests are nondiagnostic, but clinical suspicion for *Cryptococcus* remains high because of exposure history, further diagnostic testing may be required. In some situations, a video-assisted thoracoscopic biopsy or a surgical wedge resection may be considered if a pulmonary nodule is growing and cannot be accessed by bronchoscopy or percutaneous biopsy.[93] Surgical intervention may be important in individuals with risk factors for lung cancer or immune suppression. These biopsy and surgical specimens should be sent for fungal cultures in addition to histopathology.

TREATMENT
Treatment Indications

Antifungal treatment may not be required for everyone with *Cryptococcus* that is isolated from the lungs. In some individuals, *Cryptococcus* may simply be colonizing the airways, and patients remain asymptomatic. Occasionally, cryptococcal pulmonary nodules may also not require treatment if involvement is minimal and patients have no symptoms.[48] However, immune-suppressed individuals with pulmonary *Cryptococcus* should be offered antifungal therapy.[48,121] Therapy is particularly important in those with impaired cell-mediated immunity, such as those receiving immunosuppressive therapy after organ transplant, those with hematologic malignancies, those receiving chemotherapy or biologic agents, and those with long-term prednisone use. There is also a lower threshold to treat asymptomatic individuals with mild immune impairment, such as diabetes or severe renal failure. In addition, immune-competent individuals with mild to severe symptomatic pulmonary cryptococcal infection should be treated.[48,121] One must be mindful that some immune-competent individuals may have impaired immunity in the future; therefore, it is essential that those with previously identified *Cryptococcus* be followed up carefully for signs of reactivation and active infection.

Treatment of Cryptococcus neoformans Pulmonary Disease

Recommended treatment regimens for cryptococcal pulmonary infection are summarized in **Table 2**. Immune-suppressed individuals (specifically, those infected with HIV or have had organ transplant) with mild cryptococcal pulmonary disease or asymptomatic colonization (*Cryptococcus* isolated from respiratory specimens in the absence of symptoms or radiographic findings) can be treated with fluconazole alone. However, CNS or disseminated disease must be first ruled out.[48,121] The standard dose of fluconazole is

400 mg once daily for 6 to 12 months (longer duration preferred).[48,121] In the setting of severe cryptococcal lung infection or milder lung disease with concurrent disseminated or CNS infection, more aggressive therapy is warranted.[48,121] In these cases, the induction treatment consists of intravenous amphotericin B deoxycholate (AmB; 0.7–1 mg/kg/d) with intravenous or oral flucytosine (100 mg/kg/d) for 2 weeks followed by fluconazole, 400 mg once daily (OD) for a minimum of 8 weeks.[48,121–124] Alternative induction regimens that can be considered in the absence of flucytosine (if it is not available or not tolerated) include a longer duration of AmB or increasing the dose and duration of fluconazole (see **Table 2**).[48,121] Liposomal AmB should be used in place of the usual deoxycholate formulation in those at risk of renal dysfunction, which is often the case for transplant patients. Of note, fluconazole has superior efficacy against *Cryptococcus* compared with other azoles. Doses as high as 1200 mg daily have been used with minimal toxicity, and it has excellent CNS penetration.[48,121] Consequently, alternate azoles are reserved for resistant isolates or rare patients with fluconazole intolerance.[121] After induction, maintenance therapy (or secondary prophylaxis) should be continued with fluconazole, 200 mg/d, in organ transplants or other forms of severe immunosuppression for 6 to 12 months.[121] In contrast, secondary prophylaxis should be continued until a CD4 count of 200 or greater is sustained for at least 3 months in HIV patients on antiretroviral therapy.[48,121] In those with HIV, antiretroviral therapy should commence 5 weeks after initiation of cryptococcal treatment to reduce the risk of immune reconstitution inflammatory syndrome, which can be particularly severe and detrimental with CNS cryptococcal infection.[121,122,125]

The evidence behind what has now become standard therapy is derived from a few key studies. A landmark treatment trial for cryptococcal meningitis in AIDS patients found that combined AmB (0.7 mg/kg/d) and flucytosine (100 mg/kg/d) for 2 weeks had a higher likelihood of achieving negative cryptococcal cultures compared with AmB alone.[123] Furthermore, patients who were placed on fluconazole for the following 8 weeks had a statistically significant lower fungal burden than those on itraconazole (regardless of flucytosine use).[123] Additional studies have validated these findings[124,126] and also demonstrated lower risk of relapse with flucytosine use,[126] although there was no corresponding difference in mortality.[127]

In immunocompetent individuals with mild-to-moderate pulmonary disease (based on combination of symptoms and radiographic findings) the

Table 2
Summary of treatment regimens for pulmonary cryptococcal infection

Form of Disease	Treatment	Comments
Immune suppressed[d] + mild/moderate lung infection	Fluconazole[a] 400 mg po OD for 6–12 mo	Secondary prophylaxis required; fluconazole 200 mg po OD
Immunosuppressed (HIV+ and CD4<100/mm^3) + positive cryptococcal serum antigen	Fluconazole 800 mg/d for 2 weeks, followed by 400 mg/d for 8 weeks	Secondary prophylaxis required
Immune suppressed + severe lung infection and/or extrapulmonary infection	AmB 0.7–1.0 mg/kg/d IV + flucytosine[b] 100 mg/kg/d for 2 wk followed by fluconazole 400 mg po OD for 8 wk Alternatives 1. Liposomal Amphotericin B (3–6 mg/kg IV daily) or amphotericin B lipid complex (5 mg/kg IV daily)+ flucytosine[b] 100 mg/kg/d for 2 wk in those with renal failure or chronic kidney disease followed by fluconazole 400 mg po OD for 8 wk 2. AmB 0.7–1.0 mg/kg/d IV + flucytosine 100 mg/kg/d for 6–10 wk 3. AmB 0.7–1.0 mg/kg/d IV for 6–10 wk 4. AmB 0.7–1.0 mg/kg/d IV and fluconazole 800 mg OD for 2 wk then fluconazole 800 mg OD for 8 wk 5. Fluconazole 1200 mg OD + flucytosine 100 mg/kg OD for 6 wk 6. Fluconazole 1200–2000 mg OD for 10–12 wk	Secondary prophylaxis required; fluconazole 200 mg po OD
Immune competent + mild/moderate lung infection	Fluconazole[a] 400 mg po OD for 6 mo Alternatives 1. Itraconazole 200 mg po bid for 6 mo 2. Voriconazole 200 mg po bid for 6 mo 3. Posaconazole delayed release (DR) 300 mg po bid once then 300 mg OD for 6 mo (guided by drug levels) 4. Fluconazole 400 mg po bid for 6 mo[c]	No secondary prophylaxis
Immune competent + severe lung infection and/or extrapulmonary infection	AmB 0.7–1.0 mg/kg/d IV ± flucytosine 100 mg/kg/d for 2 wk followed by fluconazole 400 mg po OD for 8 wk Alternatives Same as *C neoformans* treatment in severe lung or disseminated disease in the immune suppressed	No secondary prophylaxis
C gattii + mild/moderate lung infection	Same as *C neoformans* treatment in mild lung disease in immune suppressed but may require longer duration of therapy	No secondary prophylaxis
C gattii + severe lung infection and/or extrapulmonary infection	Same as *C neoformans* treatment in severe lung or disseminated disease in immune suppressed but may require longer duration of therapy	No secondary prophylaxis

Abbreviations: bid, twice a day; IV, intravenous; po, orally.

[a] Fluconazole may be replaced with one of the following if it is unavailable or contraindicated: itraconazole, 200 mg po bid; voriconazole, 200 mg po bid; or posaconazole delayed release (DR) 300 mg po bid once then 300 mg OD for 6 mo (guided by drug levels) (but fluconazole is preferred as first line).

[b] Flucytosine is given in 4 divided doses.

[c] If not responding to standard dosing fluconazole.

[d] Immune-suppressed individuals include those with HIV, organ transplant, hematologic malignancy, and on immune suppressing medications. Treatment regimen may require extension if inadequate response with standard duration.

Data from Limper AH, Knox KS, Sarosi GA, et al. An official American Thoracic Society statement: treatment of fungal infections in adult pulmonary and critical care patients. Am J Respir Crit Care Med 2011;183(1):96–128; and Perfect JR, Dismukes WE, Dromer F, et al. Clinical practice guidelines for the management of cryptococcal disease: 2010 update by the Infectious Diseases Society of America. Clin Infect Dis 2010;50(3):291–322.

mainstay of therapy is daily fluconazole for 6 months (see **Table 2**).[48,121] Treatment for severe pulmonary cryptococcal disease or milder lung disease with disseminated or extrapulmonary infection is similar to immunocompromised patients, where parenteral AmB should be used for at least the first 2 weeks of treatment, and flucytosine is strongly recommended (see **Table 2**).[48,121] The remainder of treatment may be completed using 8 to 10 weeks of a daily azole or 6 to 10 additional weeks of AmB.[48,121] As with immune-suppressed patients, maintenance therapy is advised.

Treatment of Cryptococcus gattii Pulmonary Disease

The treatment for mild *C gattii* pulmonary disease, such as a single pulmonary cryptococcoma (nodule) is the same as for *C neoformans*.[121] However, for severe *C gattii* pulmonary infection, a longer induction regimen is recommended (4–6 weeks of AmB and flucytosine) and longer maintenance therapy (up to 18 months of fluconazole therapy). The longer regimen is thought to be necessary because *C gattii* tends to form multiple or large cryptococcomas, which may be more difficult to penetrate with antifungal agents.[121] There is also a recommendation against the use of interferon therapy in *C gattii* lung infections but greater use of thoracic surgery compared with *C neoformans*.[121]

Treatment Challenges and Complications

Clinicians must maintain a high index of suspicion for CNS infection regardless of the patient's immune status, as symptoms may be subtle. Consequently, a lumbar puncture is usually performed in immunosuppressed individuals and in many immunocompetent individuals with cryptococcal lung infection, unless the extent of disease is limited, such as a nodule with negative serum cryptococcal antigen.[120] Surgical intervention may also be required if there are complications caused by compression of vital structures or persistent focal infection despite optimal medical therapy, which tends to occur more frequently with *C gattii*.

Occasionally, severe cryptococcal infection can be associated with a profound inflammatory response and potentially life threatening acute respiratory distress syndrome. In these circumstances, a short (approximately 1 week) course of oral corticosteroids is suggested, despite minimal evidence to support this practice.[48,121] Notably, dexamethasone was recently found to have no benefit in patients with cryptococcal

meningitis.[128] Adjunctive interferon-γ may also be considered in those with severe *C neoformans* infection.[48,121] Finally, it is important to monitor complications from therapy in the form of renal toxicity (with AmB) or hepatotoxicity (with azoles, including high dose fluconazole).

Treatment Failure and Resistant Cryptococcal Infection

The therapeutic goal is resolution of clinical symptoms and radiographic findings with eradication of viable organisms. Residual radiographic abnormalities may be present despite microbiologic cure and persistent positive cryptococcal antigen. However, this should not necessarily be deemed a treatment failure if the patient exhibits resolution of clinical symptoms. Reasons for treatment failure may include drug intolerance, drug resistance, inaccessibility to key drugs (as with flucytosine in developing countries), suboptimal drug concentrations, and surgical complications.

Of particular concern, *Cryptococcus* strains resistant to key antifungals have emerged in recent years and require adjustment of standard therapeutic regimens. In the setting of fluconazole resistance or intolerance, an alternative azole[121] can be trialed. Itraconazole is one option, although it sacrifices the superior CNS penetration and lower toxicity of fluconazole.[121] Similar outcomes have been observed with voriconazole and AmB/high-dose fluconazole induction for cryptococcal meningitis.[129] In the setting of AmB resistance/intolerance, flucytosine and high-dose fluconazole (800 mg/d to 1200 mg/d) have been used for induction.[121] Flucytosine-resistant strains may be managed with AmB and high-dose fluconazole. Antifungal susceptibility testing should be considered treatment failure or when relapse occurs in the patient. Drug level monitoring (specifically azoles) may also be helpful in cases slow to respond to treatment.

Prophylaxis

Primary cryptococcal prophylaxis should be initiated in those with HIV and continued until the CD4 count is 200 or greater for at least 3 months.[48,121] In contrast, guidelines do not routinely recommend primary cryptococcal prophylaxis in transplant patients; however, screening for cryptococcal antigen may be considered in areas with a high incidence of cryptococcal infection and with primary prophylaxis in those who are positive for cryptococcal antigen.[121] Nevertheless, most lung transplant centers have some form of antifungal prophylaxis directly after transplant (although not necessarily cryptococcal specific).[130] Secondary cryptococcal prophylaxis with daily fluconazole should be initiated at the time of completion of induction therapy as discussed above.[48,121]

PROGNOSIS

Despite improved diagnostic techniques and treatment options, cryptococcal mortality remains high even in developed countries (25% to 35%), with a range between 7% and 65%.[52,73,85,89,90,131,132] Mortality with invasive cryptococcal infections is substantial regardless of immune status, type of organ involvement, or species (C neoformans vs C gattii).[52,85,90] However, certain modifying factors seem to increase mortality risk, such as CNS involvement[2,132] and cryptococcemia.[132,133] The presence of organ failure or hematologic malignancy has variable effects on cryptococcal mortality.[132,133] Interestingly, investigators found that there was no statistically significant difference in deaths between HIV-positive and HIV-negative patients with C neoformans infection in one study.[48]

NEW DEVELOPMENTS AND FUTURE DIRECTIONS

Research priorities in Cryptococcus include developing antifungal treatment regimens with lower toxicity and better efficacy. Recent advances include the development of novel conjugates or delivery methods for AmB to improve drug delivery and efficacy, and lower toxicity. A preparation has been described that combines AmB with polyethylene glycol, which resulted in a compound that had comparable in vitro efficacy against C neoformans but 2 times less toxicity than AmB.[134] A novel delivery method through encapsulated AmB in a biodegradable fibrin microsphere has been described.[135] This AmB-fibrin microsphere not only led to sustained drug release but was also significantly more efficacious at reducing cryptococcal burden and survival in mice compared with AmB alone.[135]

Additionally, adjuncts have been developed to augment standard anticryptococcal therapy. Because iron is required for microbial growth, inhibition of iron uptake has been examined in Cryptococcus.[136] Lai and colleagues[136] found that several iron chelators such as lactoferrin significantly improved AmB efficacy in vitro. However, some chelators interfered with azole therapy indicating that further work will be needed.[136] Novel compounds, such as quercetin and rutin, have also been investigated as adjuncts to AmB.[137] Both agents improved in vitro AmB efficacy, but only quercetin reduced AmB-related cell toxicity.

There continues to be much interest in developing a cryptococcal vaccine. Approaches include cryptococcal proteins, polysaccharide, and whole avirulent or genetically modified organisms.[138–140] Eliciting antibody-mediated immunity and cell-mediated immunity has shown promise and we await clinical trials.[141,142]

Finally, novel antifungal agents and cryptococcal molecular targets are also under investigation.[143,144] Interestingly, sertraline had comparable efficacy to fluconazole against Cryptococcus in vitro and in murine models.[143] Highly effective non–flucytosine-containing regimens are also of interest, as this drug is not available in many countries. The combination of terbinafine with fluconazole is one such example with excellent in vitro activity against C neoformans compared with other regimens.[31]

Invasive cryptococcal infections contribute to a high global burden of morbidity and mortality. Although diagnosis and therapy has improved over the years, there is still much work to be done to optimize Cryptococcus management and improve mortality. Ongoing research is essential to tackle these important problems.

REFERENCES

1. Vallabhaneni S, Mody RK, Walker T, et al. The global burden of fungal diseases. Infect Dis Clin North Am 2016;30(1):1–11.
2. Park BJ, Wannemuehler KA, Marston BJ, et al. Estimation of the current global burden of cryptococcal meningitis among persons living with HIV/AIDS. AIDS 2009;23(4):525–30.
3. Huston SM, Ngamskulrungroj P, Xiang RF, et al. Cryptococcus gattii capsule blocks Surface Recognition required for dendritic cell maturation independent of internalization and antigen processing. J Immunol 2016;196(3):1259–71.
4. Li SS, Mody CH. Cryptococcus. Proc Am Thorac Soc 2010;7(3):186–96.
5. Findley K, Rodriguez-Carres M, Metin B, et al. Phylogeny and phenotypic characterization of pathogenic Cryptococcus species and closely related saprobic taxa in the Tremellales. Eukaryot Cell 2009;8(3):353–61.
6. Huston SM, Mody CH. Cryptococcosis: an emerging respiratory mycosis. Clin Chest Med 2009;30(2):253–64, vi.
7. Galanis E, Macdougall L, Kidd S, et al. Epidemiology of Cryptococcus gattii, British Columbia, Canada, 1999-2007. Emerg Infect Dis 2010;16(2):251–7.
8. Mittal N, Vatsa S, Minz A. Fatal meningitis by Cryptococcus laurentii in a post-partum woman: a manifestation of immune reconstitution inflammatory

syndrome. Indian J Med Microbiol 2015;33(4): 590–3.

9. Neves RP, Lima Neto RG, Leite MC, et al. *Cryptococcus laurentii* fungaemia in a cervical cancer patient. Braz J Infect Dis 2015;19(6):660–3.

10. Conti F, Spinelli FR, Colafrancesco S, et al. Acute longitudinal myelitis following *Cryptococcus laurentii* pneumonia in a patient with systemic lupus erythematosus. Lupus 2015;24(1):94–7.

11. Banerjee P, Haider M, Trehan V, et al. *Cryptococcus laurentii* fungemia. Indian J Med Microbiol 2013;31(1):75–7.

12. Molina-Leyva A, Ruiz-Carrascosa JC, Leyva-Garcia A, et al. Cutaneous *Cryptococcus laurentii* infection in an immunocompetent child. Int J Infect Dis 2013;17(12):e1232–3.

13. Coker RJ. Cryptococcal infection in AIDS. Int J STD AIDS 1992;3(3):168–72.

14. Dromer F, Mathoulin S, Dupont B, et al. Comparison of the efficacy of amphotericin B and fluconazole in the treatment of cryptococcosis in human immunodeficiency virus-negative patients: retrospective analysis of 83 cases. French Cryptococcosis Study Group. Clin Infect Dis 1996;22(Suppl 2):S154–60.

15. Maziarz EK, Perfect JR. Cryptococcosis. Infect Dis Clin North Am 2016;30(1):179–206.

16. Gugnani HC, Mitchell TG, Litvintseva AP, et al. Isolation of *Cryptococcus gattii* and *Cryptococcus neoformans* var. grubii from the flowers and bark of Eucalyptus trees in India. Med Mycol 2005;43(6): 565–9.

17. Escandon P, Quintero E, Granados D, et al. Isolation of *Cryptococcus gattii* serotype B from detritus of Eucalyptus trees in Colombia. Biomedica 2005; 25(3):390–7.

18. Pfeiffer T, Ellis D. Environmental isolation of *Cryptococcus neoformans* gattii from California. J Infect Dis 1991;163(4):929–30.

19. Stephen C, Lester S, Black W, et al. Multispecies outbreak of cryptococcosis on southern Vancouver Island, British Columbia. Can Vet J 2002;43(10): 792–4.

20. MacDougall L, Kidd SE, Galanis E, et al. Spread of *Cryptococcus gattii* in British Columbia, Canada, and detection in the Pacific Northwest, USA. Emerg Infect Dis 2007;13(1):42–50.

21. Pfeiffer TJ, Ellis DH. Environmental isolation of *Cryptococcus neoformans* var. gattii from Eucalyptus tereticornis. J Med Vet Mycol 1992;30(5):407–8.

22. Mak S, Klinkenberg B, Bartlett K, et al. Ecological niche modeling of *Cryptococcus gattii* in British Columbia, Canada. Environ Health Perspect 2010;118:653–8.

23. Campbell LT, Currie BJ, Krockenberger M, et al. Clonality and recombination in genetically differentiated subgroups of Cryptococcus gattii. Eukaryot Cell 2005;4(8):1403–9.

24. Firacative C, Roe CC, Malik R, et al. MLST and whole-genome-based population analysis of *Cryptococcus gattii* VGIII links clinical, veterinary and environmental strains, and reveals divergent serotype specific sub-populations and distant ancestors. PLoS Negl Trop Dis 2016;10(8):e0004861.

25. Bartlett KH, Cheng PY, Duncan C, et al. A decade of experience: *Cryptococcus gattii* in British Columbia. Mycopathologia 2012;173(5–6):311–9.

26. Cogliati M, D'Amicis R, Zani A, et al. Environmental distribution of *Cryptococcus neoformans* and *C. gattii* around the Mediterranean basin. FEMS Yeast Res 2016;16(4) [pii:fow086].

27. Lagrou K, Van Eldere J, Keuleers S, et al. Zoonotic transmission of *Cryptococcus neoformans* from a magpie to an immunocompetent patient. J Intern Med 2005;257(4):385–8.

28. Shrestha RK, Stoller JK, Honari G, et al. Pneumonia due to Cryptococcus neoformans in a patient receiving infliximab: possible zoonotic transmission from a pet cockatiel. Respir Care 2004;49(6): 606–8.

29. Chen YC, Chang SC, Shih CC, et al. Clinical features and in vitro susceptibilities of two varieties of *Cryptococcus neoformans* in Taiwan. Diagn Microbiol Infect Dis 2000;36(3):175–83.

30. Desnos-Ollivier M, Patel S, Raoux-Barbot D, et al. Cryptococcosis serotypes impact outcome and provide evidence of *Cryptococcus neoformans* Speciation. MBio 2015;6(3):e00311.

31. Reichert-Lima F, Busso-Lopes AF, Lyra L, et al. Evaluation of antifungal combination against *Cryptococcus* spp. Mycoses 2016;59(9):585–93.

32. Kidd SE, Chow Y, Mak S, et al. Characterization of environmental sources of the human and animal pathogen *Cryptococcus gattii* in British Columbia, Canada, and the Pacific Northwest of the United States. Appl Environ Microbiol 2007;73(5): 1433–43.

33. Perfect JR, Casadevall A. Cryptococcosis. Infect Dis Clin North Am 2002;16(4):837–74, v–vi.

34. Bose I, Reese AJ, Ory JJ, et al. A yeast under cover: the capsule of *Cryptococcus neoformans*. Eukaryot Cell 2003;2(4):655–63.

35. Doering TL. How sweet it is! Cell wall biogenesis and polysaccharide capsule formation in *Cryptococcus neoformans*. Annu Rev Microbiol 2009; 63:223–47.

36. Kwon-Chung KJ, Varma A. Do major species concepts support one, two or more species within *Cryptococcus neoformans*? FEMS Yeast Res 2006;6(4):574–87.

37. Wang Y, Aisen P, Casadevall A. *Cryptococcus neoformans* melanin and virulence: mechanism of action. Infect Immun 1995;63(8):3131–6.

38. Adams DJ. Fungal cell wall chitinases and glucanases. Microbiology 2004;150(Pt 7):2029–35.

39. Longo LV, Nakayasu ES, Pires JH, et al. Characterization of lipids and proteins associated to the cell wall of the acapsular mutant *Cryptococcus neoformans* Cap 67. J Eukaryot Microbiol 2015;62(5):591–604.

40. Makino Y, Nishiyama O, Sano H, et al. Cavitary pulmonary cryptococcosis with an *Aspergillus* fungus ball. Intern Med 2014;53(23):2737–9.

41. Mora DJ, Fortunato LR, Andrade-Silva LE, et al. Cytokine profiles at admission can be related to outcome in AIDS patients with cryptococcal meningitis. PLoS One 2015;10(3):e0120297.

42. Cohen J. Comparison of the sensitivity of three methods for the rapid identification of *Cryptococcus neoformans*. J Clin Pathol 1984;37:332–4.

43. Wickes BL, Mayorga ME, Edman U, et al. Dimorphism and haploid fruiting in *Cryptococcus neoformans*: association with the alpha-mating type. Proc Natl Acad Sci U S A 1996;93(14):7327–31.

44. McClelland CM, Chang YC, Varma A, et al. Uniqueness of the mating system in *Cryptococcus neoformans*. Trends Microbiol 2004;12(5):208–12.

45. Fraser JA, Heitman J. Sex, MAT, and the evolution of fungal virulence. In: Heitman J, Filler GF, Edwards JEJ, et al, editors. Molecular principles of fungal pathogenesis. Washington, DC: ASM Press; 2006. p. 13–33.

46. Sun S, Heitman J. From two to one: unipolar sexual reproduction. Fungal Biol Rev 2015;29(3–4):118–25.

47. Wang X, Darwiche S, Heitman J. Sex-induced silencing operates during opposite sex and unisexual reproduction in *Cryptococcus neoformans*. Genetics 2013;193(4):1163–74.

48. Limper AH, Knox KS, Sarosi GA, et al. An official American Thoracic Society statement: treatment of fungal infections in adult pulmonary and critical care patients. Am J Respir Crit Care Med 2011;183(1):96–128.

49. Pagano L, Fianchi L, Leone G. Fungal pneumonia due to molds in patients with hematological malignancies. J Chemother 2006;18(4):339–52.

50. Qazzafi Z, Thiruchunapalli D, Birkenhead D, et al. Invasive *Cryptococcus neoformans* infection in an asplenic patient. J Infect 2007;55(6):566–8.

51. Singh N, Husain S, De Vera M, et al. *Cryptococcus neoformans* infection in patients with cirrhosis, including liver transplant candidates. Medicine (Baltimore) 2004;83(3):188–92.

52. Kiertiburanakul S, Wirojtananugoon S, Pracharktam R, et al. Cryptococcosis in human immunodeficiency virus-negative patients. Int J Infect Dis 2006;10(1):72–8.

53. Nath R, Laskar B, Ahmed J, et al. *Cryptococcus neoformans* var. grubii Infection in HIV-Seronegative Patients from Northeast India: report of two cases with review of literature. Mycopathologia 2016;181(3–4):315–21.

54. Kronstad JW, Attarian R, Cadieux B, et al. Expanding fungal pathogenesis: *Cryptococcus* breaks out of the opportunistic box. Nat Rev Microbiol 2011;9(3):193–203.

55. Cheng PY, Sham A, Kronstad JW. *Cryptococcus gattii* isolates from the British Columbia cryptococcosis outbreak induce less protective inflammation in a murine model of infection than *Cryptococcus neoformans*. Infect Immun 2009;77(10):4284–94.

56. Huston SM, Li SS, Stack D, et al. *Cryptococcus gattii* is killed by dendritic cells, but evades adaptive immunity by failing to induce dendritic cell maturation. J Immunol 2013;191(1):249–61.

57. Ngamskulrungroj P, Chang Y, Roh J, et al. Differences in nitrogen metabolism between *Cryptococcus neoformans* and *C. gattii*, the two etiologic agents of cryptococcosis. PLoS One 2012;7(3):e34258.

58. Garcia-Hermoso D, Janbon G, Dromer F. Epidemiological evidence for dormant *Cryptococcus neoformans* infection. J Clin Microbiol 1999;37(10):3204–9.

59. Dromer F, Ronin O, Dupont B. Isolation of *Cryptococcus neoformans* var. gattii from an Asian patient in France: evidence for dormant infection in healthy subjects. J Med Vet Mycol 1992;30(5):395–7.

60. Saha DC, Goldman DL, Shao X, et al. Serologic evidence for reactivation of cryptococcosis in solid-organ transplant recipients. Clin Vaccine Immunol 2007;14(12):1550–4.

61. Chen LC, Goldman DL, Doering TL, et al. Antibody response to *Cryptococcus neoformans* proteins in rodents and humans. Infect Immun 1999;67(5):2218–24.

62. Lindberg J, Hagen F, Laursen A, et al. *Cryptococcus gattii* risk for tourists visiting Vancouver Island, Canada. Emerg Infect Dis 2007;13(1):178–9.

63. Levy PY, Habib G, Reynaud-Gaubert M, et al. Pericardial effusion due to *Cryptococcus neoformans* in a patient with cystic fibrosis following lung transplantation. Int J Infect Dis 2008;12(4):452.

64. Johannson KA, Huston SM, Mody CH, et al. *Cryptococcus gattii* pneumonia. CMAJ 2012;184(12):1387–90.

65. Del Poeta M. Role of phagocytosis in the virulence of *Cryptococcus neoformans*. Eukaryot Cell 2004;3(5):1067–75.

66. Syme RM, Spurrell JC, Amankwah EK, et al. Primary dendritic cells phagocytose *Cryptococcus neoformans* via mannose receptors and Fcgamma receptor II for presentation to T lymphocytes. Infect Immun 2002;70(11):5972–81.

67. Pericolini E, Cenci E, Monari C, et al. *Cryptococcus neoformans* capsular polysaccharide component galactoxylomannan induces apoptosis of human T-cells through activation of caspase-8. Cell Microbiol 2006;8(2):267–75.

68. Villena SN, Pinheiro RO, Pinheiro CS, et al. Capsular polysaccharides galactoxylomannan and glucuronoxylomannan from *Cryptococcus neoformans* induce macrophage apoptosis mediated by Fas ligand. Cell Microbiol 2008;10(6):1274–85.

69. Kwon-Chung KJ, Rhodes JC. Encapsulation and melanin formation as indicators of virulence in *Cryptococcus neoformans*. Infect Immun 1986; 51(1):218–23.

70. Suvarna K, Bartiss A, Wong B. Mannitol-1-phosphate dehydrogenase from *Cryptococcus neoformans* is a zinc-containing long-chain alcohol/polyol dehydrogenase. Microbiology 2000; 146(Pt 10):2705–13.

71. Jacobson ES, Jenkins ND, Todd JM. Relationship between superoxide dismutase and melanin in a pathogenic fungus. Infect Immun 1994;62(9): 4085–6.

72. Wong B, Perfect JR, Beggs S, et al. Production of the hexitol D-mannitol by *Cryptococcus neoformans* in vitro and in rabbits with experimental meningitis. Infect Immun 1990;58(6): 1664–70.

73. Nosanchuk JD, Casadevall A. The contribution of melanin to microbial pathogenesis. Cell Microbiol 2003;5(4):203–23.

74. Ghannoum MA. Potential role of phospholipases in virulence and fungal pathogenesis. Clin Microbiol Rev 2000;13(1):122–43.

75. Supasorn O, Sringkarin N, Srimanote P, et al. Matrix metalloproteinases contribute to the regulation of chemokine expression and pulmonary inflammation in *Cryptococcus* infection. Clin Exp Immunol 2016;183(3):431–40.

76. Cox GM, Mukherjee J, Cole GT, et al. Urease as a virulence factor in experimental cryptococcosis. Infect Immun 2000;68(2):443–8.

77. Phadke SS, Feretzaki M, Clancey SA, et al. Unisexual reproduction of *Cryptococcus gattii*. PLoS One 2014;9(10):e111089.

78. Pappas PG, Perfect JR, Cloud GA, et al. Cryptococcosis in human immunodeficiency virus-negative patients in the era of effective azole therapy. Clin Infect Dis 2001;33(5):690–9.

79. Cabello Ubeda A, Fortes Alen J, Gadea I, et al. Cryptococcal meningoencephalitis. Epidemiology and mortality risk factors in pre- and post-HAART era. Med Clin (Barc) 2016;146(9):397–401 [in Spanish].

80. Guevara-Campos J, Gonzalez-Guevara L, Urbez-Cano J, et al. *Cryptococcus neoformans* meningoencephalitis in immunocompetent schoolchildren. Invest Clin 2009;50(2):231–9.

81. Hoang JK, Burruss J. Localized cutaneous *Cryptococcus albidus* infection in a 14-year-old boy on etanercept therapy. Pediatr Dermatol 2007;24(3): 285–8.

82. Sheu SJ, Chen YC, Kuo NW, et al. Endogenous cryptococcal endophthalmitis. Ophthalmology 1998;105(2):377–81.

83. Shah VB, Patil PA, Agrawa V, et al. Primary cryptococcal prostatitis–rare occurrence. J Assoc Physicians India 2012;60:57–9.

84. de Lima MA, dos Santos JA, Lazo J, et al. *Cryptococcus* infection limited to the prostate in an AIDS patient with disseminated mycobacteriosis. A necropsy report. Rev Soc Bras Med Trop 1997;30(6): 501–5.

85. Jean SS, Fang CT, Shau WY, et al. Cryptococcaemia: clinical features and prognostic factors. QJM 2002;95(8):511–8.

86. Rachadi H, Senouci K, Lyagoubi M, et al. Multiple facial nodules revealing disseminated cryptococcosis in an immunocompetent patient. Ann Dermatol Venereol 2016;143(4):289–94.

87. Nasri H, Kabbani S, Bou Alwan M, et al. Retrospective study of cryptococcal meningitis with elevated minimum inhibitory concentration to fluconazole in immunocompromised patients. Open Forum Infect Dis 2016;3(2):ofw076.

88. McCarthy KM, Morgan J, Wannemuehler KA, et al. Population-based surveillance for cryptococcosis in an antiretroviral-naive South African province with a high HIV seroprevalence. AIDS 2006; 20(17):2199–206.

89. Lomes NR, Melhem MS, Szeszs MW, et al. Cryptococcosis in non-HIV/non-transplant patients: a Brazilian case series. Med Mycol 2016;54(7): 669–76.

90. Jongwutiwes U, Sungkanuparph S, Kiertiburanakul S. Comparison of clinical features and survival between cryptococcosis in human immunodeficiency virus (HIV)-positive and HIV-negative patients. Jpn J Infect Dis 2008;61(2):111–5.

91. Phillips P, Galanis E, MacDougall L, et al. Longitudinal clinical findings and outcome among patients with *Cryptococcus gattii* infection in British Columbia. Clin Infect Dis 2015;60(9):1368–86.

92. Sweeney DA, Caserta MT, Korones DN, et al. A ten-year-old boy with a pulmonary nodule secondary to *Cryptococcus neoformans*: case report and review of the literature. Pediatr Infect Dis J 2003; 22(12):1089–93.

93. Jang DW, Jeong I, Kim SJ, et al. Pulmonary cryptococcosis that mimicked rheumatoid nodule in rheumatoid arthritis lesion. Tuberc Respir Dis (Seoul) 2014;77(6):266–70.

94. Haddad N, Cavallaro MC, Lopes MP, et al. Pulmonary cryptococcoma: a rare and challenging diagnosis in immunocompetent patients. Autops Case Rep 2015;5(2):35–40.

95. Nadrous HF, Antonios VS, Terrell CL, et al. Pulmonary cryptococcosis in nonimmunocompromised-patients. Chest 2003;124(6):2143–7.

96. Chan M, Lye D, Win MK, et al. Clinical and microbiological characteristics of cryptococcosis in Singapore: predominance of *Cryptococcus neoformans* compared with *Cryptococcus gattii*. Int J Infect Dis 2014;26:110–5.

97. Wong M, Loong F, Khong PL, et al. Mediastinal cryptococcosis masquerading as therapy-refractory lymphoma. Ann Hematol 2011;90(5): 601–2.

98. Vawda F, Maharajh J, Naidoo K. Massive cryptococcal lymphadenopathy in an immunocompetent pregnant patient. Br J Radiol 2008;81(962):e53–6.

99. Oliveira Fde M, Severo CB, Guazzelli LS, et al. *Cryptococcus gattii* fungemia: report of a case with lung and brain lesions mimicking radiological features of malignancy. Rev Inst Med Trop Sao Paulo 2007;49(4):263–5.

100. Prasad KT, Sehgal IS, Shivaprakash MR, et al. Uncommon mycosis in a patient with diabetes. BMJ Case Rep 2016;2016 [pii:bcr2016214453].

101. Zhou Q, Hu B, Shao C, et al. A case report of pulmonary cryptococcosis presenting as endobronchial obstruction. J Thorac Dis 2013;5(4):E170–3.

102. Nakashima K, Akamatsu H, Endo M, et al. Endobronchial cryptococcosis induced by *Cryptococcus gattii* mimicking metastatic lung cancer. Respirol Case Rep 2014;2(3):108–10.

103. Gunda DW, Bakshi FA, Rambau P, et al. Pulmonary cryptococcosis presenting as acute severe respiratory distress in a newly diagnosed HIV patient in Tanzania: a case report. Clin Case Rep 2015; 3(9):749–52.

104. Orsini J, Blaak C, Tam E, et al. Disseminated cryptococcal infection resulting in acute respiratory distress syndrome (ARDS) as the initial clinical presentation of AIDS. Intern Med 2016;55(8):995–8.

105. Rigby AL, Glanville AR. Miliary pulmonary cryptococcosis in an HIV-positive patient. Am J Respir Crit Care Med 2012;186(2):200–1.

106. Shimoda M, Saraya T, Tsujimoto N, et al. Fatal disseminated cryptococcosis resembling miliary tuberculosis in a patient with HIV infection. Intern Med 2014;53(15):1641–4.

107. Friedman EP, Miller RF, Severn A, et al. Cryptococcal pneumonia in patients with the acquired immunodeficiency syndrome. Clin Radiol 1995; 50(11):756–60.

108. Balloul E, Couderc LJ, Molina JM, et al. Pulmonary cryptococcosis during HIV infection. 15 cases. Rev Mal Respir 1997;14(5):365–70.

109. Lizarazo J, Escandon P, Agudelo CI, et al. Retrospective study of the epidemiology and clinical manifestations of *Cryptococcus gattii* infections in Colombia from 1997-2011. PLoS Negl Trop Dis 2014;8(11):e3272.

110. McTaggart L, Richardson SE, Seah C, et al. Rapid identification of Cryptococcus neoformans var. grubii, C. neoformans var. neoformans, and C. gattii by use of rapid biochemical tests, differential media, and DNA sequencing. Journal of Clinical Microbiology 2011;49(7):2522–7.

111. Johnston SA, Voelz K, May RC. *Cryptococcus neoformans* Thermotolerance to avian body temperature is sufficient for extracellular growth but not intracellular survival in macrophages. Sci Rep 2016;6:20977.

112. Uejio CK, Mak S, Manangan A, et al. Climatic influences on *Cryptococcus gattii* populations, Vancouver Island, Canada, 2002-2004. Emerg Infect Dis 2015;21(11):1989–96.

113. Baughman RP, Rhodes JC, Dohn MN, et al. Detection of cryptococcal antigen in bronchoalveolar lavage fluid: a prospective study of diagnostic utility. Am Rev Respir Dis 1992;145(5):1226–9.

114. Gade W, Hinnefeld SW, Babcock LS, et al. Comparison of the PREMIER cryptococcal antigen enzyme immunoassay and the latex agglutination assay for detection of cryptococcal antigens. J Clin Microbiol 1991;29(8):1616–9.

115. Ji S, Ni L, Zhang J, et al. Value of three capsular antigen detection methods in diagnosis and efficacy assessment in patients with cryptococcal meningoencephalitis. Zhonghua Yi Xue Za Zhi 2015;95(46): 3733–6.

116. Panackal AA, Dekker JP, Proschan M, et al. Enzyme immunoassay versus latex agglutination cryptococcal antigen assays in adults with non-HIV-related cryptococcosis. J Clin Microbiol 2014; 52(12):4356–8.

117. Mamuye AT, Bornstein E, Temesgen O, et al. Point-of care testing for cryptococcal disease among hospitalized human immunodeficiency virus-infected adults in Ethiopia. Am J Trop Med Hyg 2016;95(4):786–92.

118. Tintelnot K, Hagen F, Han CO, et al. Pitfalls in serological diagnosis of *Cryptococcus gattii* infections. Med Mycol 2015;53(8):874–9.

119. Vidal JE, Boulware DR. Lateral flow assay for cryptococcal antigen: an important advance to improve the continuum of HIV care and reduce cryptococcal meningitis-related mortality. Rev Inst Med Trop Sao Paulo 2015;57(Suppl 19):38–45.

120. Klein KR, Hall L, Deml SM, et al. Identification of *Cryptococcus gattii* by use of L-canavanine glycine bromothymol blue medium and DNA sequencing. J Clin Microbiol 2009;47(11):3669–72.

121. Perfect JR, Dismukes WE, Dromer F, et al. Clinical practice guidelines for the management of cryptococcal disease: 2010 update by the infectious diseases society of America. Clin Infect Dis 2010; 50(3):291–322.

122. Boulware DR, Meya DB, Muzoora C, et al. Timing of antiretroviral therapy after diagnosis of cryptococcal meningitis. N Engl J Med 2014;370:2487–98.

123. van der Horst CM, Saag MS, Cloud GA, et al. Treatment of cryptococcal meningitis associated with the acquired immunodeficiency syndrome. N Engl J Med 1997;337:15–21.

124. Brouwer AE, Rajanuwong A, Chierakul W, et al. Combination antifungal therapies for HIV associated cryptococcal meningitis: a randomised trial. Lancet 2004;363(9423):1764–7.

125. Jarvis JN, Bicanic T, Loyse A, et al. Determinants of mortality in a combined cohort of 501 patients with HIV-associated Cryptococcal meningitis: implications for improving outcomes. Clin Infect Dis 2014,58(5):736–45.

126. Dromer F, Bernede-Bauduin C, Guillemot D, et al. Major role for amphotericin B-flucytosine combination in severe cryptococcosis. PLoS One 2008;3(8): e2870.

127. Bicanic T, Wood R, Meintjes G, et al. High-dose amphotericin B with flucytosine for the treatment of cryptococcal meningitis in HIV-infected patients: a randomized trial. Clin Infect Dis 2008;47(1): 123–30.

128. Beardsley J, Wolbers M, Kibengo FM, et al. Adjunctive dexamethasone in HIV-associated cryptococcal meningitis. N Engl J Med 2016; 374(6):542–54.

129. Loyse A, Wilson D, Meintjes G, et al. Comparison of the early fungicidal activity of high-dose fluconazole, voriconazole, and flucytosine as second-line drugs given in combination with amphotericin B for the treatment of HIV associated cryptococcal meningitis. Clin Infect Dis 2012;54(1):121–8.

130. Avery RK. Antifungal prophylaxis in lung transplantation. Semin Respir Crit Care Med 2011;32(6): 717–26.

131. Aye C, Henderson A, Yu H, et al. Cryptococcosis-the impact of delay to diagnosis. Clin Microbiol Infect 2016;22(7):632–5.

132. Pappas PG. Cryptococcal infections in non-HIV-infected patients. Trans Am Clin Climatol Assoc 2013;124:61–79.

133. Brizendine KD, Baddley JW, Pappas PG. Predictors of mortality and differences in clinical features among patients with Cryptococcosis according to immune status. PLoS One 2013;8(3):e60431.

134. Tan TR, Hoi KM, Zhang P, et al. Characterization of a polyethylene glycol amphotericin B conjugate loaded with free amb for improved antifungal efficacy. PLoS One 2016;11(3):e0152112.

135. Khan AA, Jabeen M, Alanazi AM, et al. Antifungal efficacy of amphotericin B encapsulated fibrin microsphere for treating Cryptococcus neoformans infection in Swiss albino mice. Braz J Infect Dis 2016;20(4):342–8.

136. Lai YW, Campbell LT, Wilkins MR, et al. Synergy and antagonism between iron chelators and antifungal drugs in Cryptococcus. Int J Antimicrob Agents 2016;48(4):388–94.

137. Oliveira VM, Carraro E, Auler ME, et al. Quercetin and rutin as potential agents antifungal against Cryptococcus spp. Braz J Biol 2016;76(4):1029–34.

138. Wormley FL Jr, Perfect JR, Steele C, et al. Protection against cryptococcosis by using a murine gamma interferon-producing Cryptococcus neoformans strain. Infect Immun 2007;75(3):1453–62.

139. Chaturvedi AK, Hameed RS, Wozniak KL, et al. Vaccine-mediated immune responses to experimental pulmonary Cryptococcus gattii infection in mice. PLoS One 2014;9(8):e104316.

140. Specht CA, Lee CK, Huang H, et al. Protection against Experimental Cryptococcosis following vaccination with glucan particles containing Cryptococcus alkaline extracts. MBio 2015;6(6): e01905–15.

141. Casadevall A, Pirofski LA. Immunoglobulins in defense, pathogenesis, and therapy of fungal diseases. Cell Host Microbe 2012;11(5):447–56.

142. Leopold Wager CM, Wormley FL Jr. Is development of a vaccine against Cryptococcus neoformans feasible? PLoS Pathog 2015;11(6): e1004843.

143. Trevino-Rangel Rde J, Villanueva-Lozano H, Hernandez-Rodriguez P, et al. Activity of sertraline against Cryptococcus neoformans: in vitro and in vivo assays. Med Mycol 2016;54(3):280–6.

144. Park YD, Sun W, Salas A, et al. Identification of multiple cryptococcal fungicidal drug targets by combined gene dosing and drug affinity responsive targetstability screening. MBio 2016;7(4): e01073–116.

Approach to Fungal Infections in Human Immunodeficiency Virus–Infected Individuals
Pneumocystis and Beyond

Richard J. Wang, MD[a],
Robert F. Miller, MBBS, CBiol, FRSB, FRCP[b,c],
Laurence Huang, MD[a,*]

KEYWORDS

- Human immunodeficiency virus • Opportunistic infection • Pneumonia • Mycoses • *Pneumocystis*

KEY POINTS

- Among patients with human immunodeficiency virus (HIV) infection, major fungal pathogens include *Pneumocystis jirovecii*, *Cryptococcus neoformans*, *Aspergillus* species, *Histoplasma capsulatum*, *Coccidioides* species, *Blastomyces dermatitidis*, *Paracoccidioides brasiliensis*, *Talaromyces marneffei*, and *Emmonsia* species.
- Clinical manifestations of fungal infection in HIV–infected patients frequently depend on the degree of immunosuppression and the CD4+ helper T cell count.
- Establishing definitive diagnosis is important because treatments differ.
- Primary and secondary prophylaxis depends on CD4+ helper T cell counts and geographic location and local prevalence of disease.

The recognition of an outbreak of *Pneumocystis* pneumonia (PCP) in 1981 was a fraught moment in the history of medicine.[1] It heralded the coming human immunodeficiency virus (HIV) pandemic, a disease heretofore unknown to humankind. Opportunistic fungal pathogens, *Pneumocystis jirovecii* in particular, have contributed significantly to the morbidity and mortality of HIV-infected patients. Fortunately, the development of and increasing access to effective combination antiretroviral therapy (ART) have reduced the incidence of opportunistic infections in HIV-infected patients worldwide. Nevertheless, fungi remain an important cause of disease, especially for patients with undiagnosed HIV infection and for patients without access to, or who fail to adhere to, ART.

In immunocompetent hosts, an array of immune mechanisms averts disease caused by fungi. Potential fungal pathogens are detected by pattern recognition receptors of innate immune cells.[2] These in turn produce cytokines, including interleukin-12, that result in activation of CD4+ helper T (T$_H$) cells. Production of interferon-γ by T$_H$1 cells then triggers cell-mediated, adaptive,

Disclosure Statement: None.
[a] Department of Medicine, University of California, San Francisco, 505 Parnassus Avenue, San Francisco, CA 94143, USA; [b] Research Department of Infection and Population Health, Institute of Global Health, University College London, Gower Street, London WC1E 6BT, UK; [c] Faculty of Infectious and Tropical Diseases, Department of Clinical Research, London School of Hygiene and Tropical Medicine, Keppel Street, Bloomsbury, London WC1E 7HT, UK
* Corresponding author.
E-mail address: laurence.huang@ucsf.edu

Clin Chest Med 38 (2017) 465–477
http://dx.doi.org/10.1016/j.ccm.2017.04.008
0272-5231/17/© 2017 Elsevier Inc. All rights reserved.

cytotoxic immunity. The downstream effects of interferon-γ production include recruitment of leukocytes to the site of infection and enhanced macrophage phagocytosis and killing, typically resulting in elimination of the invading fungi.[3]

The hallmark of HIV is infection of CD4$^+$ T$_H$ cells and, to a lesser degree, other CD4$^+$ cells including macrophages. Left untreated, HIV disrupts the function of CD4$^+$ T$_H$ cells and, ultimately, depletes them. The consequences of HIV-mediated immune dysregulation are wide ranging and include decreased production of interferon-γ,[4] impaired macrophage phagocytosis,[5] impaired neutrophil chemotaxis,[6] impaired neutrophil oxidative killing,[7] B-cell exhaustion, and decreased B-cell antigen responsiveness.[8] These defects in immunity conspire against the host and result in susceptibility to opportunistic fungal infections.

Because the clinical presentation and radiographic findings of opportunistic fungal infections are frequently nonspecific, diagnosis relies on maintaining a high index of suspicion. The intensity and duration of immunosuppression in HIV-infected patients is a major risk factor. The likelihood of some infections, like PCP, is inversely related to a patient's CD4$^+$ T$_H$ cell count; for other infections, like coccidioidomycosis, the clinical manifestations differ among patients with lower CD4$^+$ T$_H$ cell counts than for immunocompetent patients. Diagnosis typically relies on identification of the fungus by microscopy or culture, except in select instances in which antigen or serum antibody testing can be definitive.

This review discusses the clinical presentation, radiographic findings, diagnosis, and management of selected respiratory fungal infections in patients with HIV. Particular attention is extended to *Pneumocystis* pneumonia, which, in some geographic locales even today, remains the most common acquired immunodeficiency syndrome (AIDS)-defining opportunistic infection.[9]

PNEUMOCYSTIS PNEUMONIA
Pneumocystis jirovecii

Pneumocystis is a genus of host obligate ascomycete fungus. There are numerous species of *Pneumocystis*, each of which is specific to a particular mammalian host species. *P jirovecii* infects and colonizes humans. It is host obligate, it cannot be cultured or grown outside of the human body, and there is as yet no reliable evidence for an environmental reservoir for this organism other than the human host.[10–12]

In immunocompetent humans, *Pneumocystis* does not cause any clear clinical syndrome.

Serologic studies indicate that humans are exposed to *Pneumocystis* as infants or young children.[13] *Pneumocystis* is unlikely to cause anything more than mild, self-limiting respiratory symptoms.[14,15] Animal models indicate that *Pneumocystis* is spread from host to host via airborne transmission, and *P jirovecii* is likely spread among human hosts in the same fashion.[16] Most healthy adults do not have detectable *Pneumocystis* in respiratory specimens, but it is possible for immunocompetent adults, especially those with chronic obstructive pulmonary disease or cystic fibrosis, to harbor an asymptomatic colonization with *Pneumocystis*. The consequences of chronic colonization may be progressive impairment of lung function over time.[17]

By contrast, in immunocompromised hosts, *Pneumocystis* causes a devastating and frequently fatal pneumonia. The risk of *Pneumocystis* pneumonia increases with the degree of immunosuppression, and lower CD4$^+$ T$_H$ cell counts predict risk of PCP. Among patients with HIV, 95% of cases of PCP occur in patients with a CD4$^+$ T$_H$ cell count less than 200 cells/μL; at a CD4$^+$ T$_H$ cell count of 50 cells/μL, the risk of PCP is higher than at 100 cells/μL or 200 cells/μL.[18–20]

What is the Clinical Presentation of Pneumocystis Pneumonia?

The clinical presentation of PCP is nonspecific and cannot reliably be distinguished from other infectious pulmonary processes. Typical symptoms include fever, dyspnea, and a cough that can be either nonproductive or productive of scant sputum but is rarely purulent. Although the disease can be fulminant, PCP in patients with HIV frequently presents with an indolent course. Patients may experience weeks of slowly progressive symptoms, including a sensation of chest discomfort or chest tightness and exercise intolerance.[21] This is different from the presentation of PCP in medically immunosuppressed patients without HIV infection, which is more frequently acute and may rapidly progress to respiratory failure within days.[22] Physical examination is also nonspecific. Chest auscultation may reveal end-inspiratory crackles but is frequently normal.[21] Severe disease may be characterized by signs of acute respiratory failure. Hypoxemia is characteristic and can be mild (partial pressure of arterial oxygen when breathing room air greater than 70 mm Hg and alveolar-arterial O$_2$ difference <35 mm Hg), moderate (alveolar-arterial O$_2$ difference 35–45 mm Hg), or severe (alveolar-arterial O$_2$ difference >45 mm Hg).[23]

What Tests Can Be Used for Diagnosing Pneumocystis Pneumonia?

There is no serologic test that is specific for PCP. Lactate dehydrogenase is a nonspecific biomarker of cell turnover and cellular damage, and serum levels are frequently elevated in patients with PCP but are also elevated in the setting of other diseases including pneumonia caused by bacteria, mycobacteria, and other fungi.[24,25] The marker (1-3) β-D-glucan is a component of the fungal cell wall and can be detected in the serum of patients with PCP but also does not distinguish between PCP and other fungal pneumonias.[26] These tests can be useful to support a clinical suspicion for PCP but on their own are not specific enough for definitive diagnosis in most cases.

Chest imaging has an important role in the diagnosis of PCP. The classic appearance of a chest radiograph for a patient with PCP is diffuse, bilateral, interstitial type (commonly described as reticular, granular, or ground glass) opacities (**Fig. 1**).[27] However, the chest radiograph in a patient with early disease may be normal; with late or severe disease, the chest radiograph may show frank alveolar consolidation. Unusual but not inconsistent features of PCP on chest radiography include focal asymmetric interstitial or alveolar opacities, nodules, pneumatoceles, cavities, and pneumothoraces.[28] Computed high-resolution tomography (HRCT) of the chest is a highly sensitive test for PCP with a high negative predictive value. The classic appearance of PCP on an HRCT scan is bilateral and frequently patchy but sometimes diffuse and homogenous, ground glass opacities (**Fig. 2**).[29] Importantly, in a symptomatic patient with a normal chest radiograph, the absence of ground glass opacities on HRCT

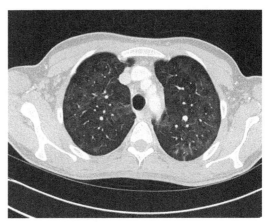

Fig. 2. Axial HRCT of the upper chest of an HIV-infected patient with PCP. There are bilateral patchy ground glass infiltrates, with subpleural sparing. (*Courtesy of* Robert F. Miller, MBBS, CBiol, FRSB, FRCP, London; with permission.)

significantly diminishes the probability of PCP. However, ground glass opacities on HRCT are not specific for PCP and can be seen in other cardiopulmonary pathologic conditions including viral pneumonia, pulmonary edema, and diffuse alveolar hemorrhage.[30] As with chest radiography, an HRCT scan of the chest in advanced disease may show consolidation, nodules, or pneumatoceles.

Because clinical presentation, serologic tests, and chest imaging are not definitive for PCP, PCP is typically diagnosed by investigation of respiratory specimens. Appropriate specimens include induced sputum or bronchoalveolar lavage (BAL) fluid. *Pneumocystis* is rarely identified in spontaneously expectorated sputum. Diagnostic yield is higher with induced sputum, that is, sputum provoked by inhalation of an aerosol of hypertonic saline solution, and sensitivity is 74% to 83%.[31] However, a negative result for *Pneumocystis* in induced sputum should be followed by bronchoscopy. In the hands of an experienced cytopathologist, the sensitivity and specificity of BAL fluid obtained during fiberoptic bronchoscopy approaches 100% for diagnosis of PCP.[32]

There is no method for culturing *Pneumocystis*, so the principal diagnostic test is cytopathologic examination. Diagnosis is established by the microscopic visualization of trophic or cystic forms of *Pneumocystis*. A variety of histologic stains can be used to identify *Pneumocystis* by light microscopy. The Diff-Quick and Wright-Giemsa stains identify the nuclei of *Pneumocystis* organisms of all developmental stages. Grocott-Gomori methenamine silver, toluidine blue O, and cresyl violet stain the wall of the cystic form but not that

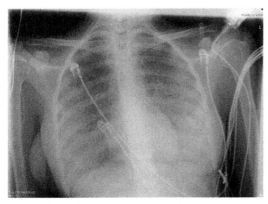

Fig. 1. Chest radiograph of a patient with newly diagnosed HIV infection presenting with severe PCP. There is diffuse bilateral interstitial shadowing, more marked on the left. (*Courtesy of* Robert F. Miller, MBBS, CBiol, FRSB, FRCP, London; with permission.)

of the trophic form. Other stains, such as the chemifluorescence calcofluor white (that binds to β-polymers of Pneumocystis and other fungi) and Papanicolaou (which detects the foamy eosinophilic exudate that surrounds Pneumocystis), can be used. The use of direct fluorescent antibody stains for Pneumocystis, which bind to both trophic and cystic forms, can increase sensitivity further.[31]

Molecular detection of Pneumocystis DNA by polymerase chain reaction (PCR) is offered by some laboratories for use on respiratory specimens. Although PCR testing is highly sensitive, it has only moderate specificity for diagnosis of PCP. PCR testing detects the presence of Pneumocystis DNA not only in those patients with pneumonia caused by Pneumocystis, but also in patients who are merely colonized and who have symptoms that can be attributed to another confirmed diagnosis or have no symptoms at all. A negative PCR test result, however, significantly decreases the likelihood that a patient has PCP.[33,34]

Diagnosis of PCP can be made by transbronchial biopsy through a fiberoptic bronchoscope or by video-assisted thoracoscopic biopsy. Histopathologically, PCP is characterized by a pattern of diffuse alveolar damage, a vacuolated and foamy exudate that fills alveolar airspaces, a lymphocytic interstitial infiltrate, and hyperplasia of type 2 pneumocytes. Because of the high diagnostic yield of bronchoscopy with BAL, biopsy is seldom necessary to confirm or rule out the diagnosis of PCP.

What are Treatment Options for Pneumocystis Pneumonia?

If there is clinical suspicion for PCP in an HIV-infected patient, it is reasonable to initiate empiric therapy while awaiting the results of diagnostic tests. Treatment need not be deferred, as the yield for diagnosis of PCP from BAL fluid is unchanged for up to 14 days after starting treatment.[23]

The first choice of treatment is trimethoprim-sulfamethoxazole (TMP-SMX). The 1:5 fixed-dose combination of TMP 15 to 20 mg/kg/d and SMX 75 to 100 mg/kg/d is given in 3 to 4 divided doses. It can be administered orally or intravenously (IV). Although oral bioavailability is excellent, IV therapy is often preferred initially for cases of moderate to severe PCP.[35] The total recommended dose duration is 21 days; shorter courses have resulted in higher rates of treatment failure.[22] Use of TMP-SMX may be limited by adverse reactions, including rash, fever, transaminitis, nephritis, hyperkalemia, and cytopenias.

There are alternative treatment options if TMP-SMX is not tolerated or if treatment fails. IV pentamidine given at 4 mg/kg once daily has equivalent efficacy to IV TMP-SMX but greater toxicity.[35,36] Adverse reactions include infusion site phlebitis, severe hypotension during infusion, prolonged QT, torsades de pointes, pancreatitis, hypoglycemia, transaminitis, nausea and vomiting, nephrotoxicity, hypocalcemia, hypomagnesemia, hyponatremia, and leukopenia. Given the variety and severity of these toxicities, IV pentamidine is typically reserved for patients with severe, life-threatening PCP who cannot tolerate or are unresponsive to TMP-SMX.

Other alternative therapies include clindamycin with primaquine. Clindamycin can be administered intravenously, 900 mg 3 times daily, or orally, 600 mg 3 times daily. Primaquine is only available in an oral formulation and is given 30 mg once daily.[35] Clindamycin with primaquine has equivalent efficacy to TMP-SMX for initial treatment of mild to moderate PCP, and there is evidence to suggest that it is more effective than IV pentamidine as a salvage therapy, although there are no randomized controlled trials comparing them.[37]

Oral dapsone, 100 mg daily, with TMP, 15 mg/kg/d in 3 divided doses, is as effective as oral TMP-SMX for mild or moderate PCP but is ineffective for severe PCP. Atovaquone suspension, 750 mg orally twice daily, is inferior therapy compared with TMP-SMX for mild or moderate PCP and is ineffective for severe PCP.[35]

Adjunctive corticosteroids decrease the need for intensive care unit admission, mechanical ventilation, and mortality in HIV-infected patients with moderate to severe PCP (partial pressure of arterial oxygen when breathing room air less than 70 mm Hg or alveolar-arterial O_2 difference >35 mm Hg).[38,39] Ideally, steroids should be started at the time that Pneumocystis-specific treatment is initiated and definitely within the first 72 hours of treatment. The recommended dosing schedule is 40 mg of prednisone (or an equipotent dose of IV methylprednisolone) twice daily for 5 days, then 40 mg once daily for 5 days, and 20 mg once daily for the remaining 11 days of treatment.[35]

With treatment, the overall mortality rate from PCP in HIV-infected patients is about 10%. With appropriate treatment, early clinical deterioration is common, attributed to a host inflammatory response provoked by antibiotic-induced lysis of Pneumocystis organisms. If there is no improvement or further clinical decline after at least 5 days of treatment, treatment failure is a possibility, and it would be reasonable to consider switching to an alternative therapy, although other causes of clinical deterioration, such as iatrogenic hypervolemia, pneumothorax, and methemoglobinemia would need to be excluded.

When is Prophylaxis Appropriate and with what Regimen?

The National Institutes of Health, Centers for Disease Control, and Infectious Diseases Society of America consensus guidelines recommend PCP prophylaxis for patients with $CD4^+$ T_H cell counts less than 200 cells/μL. TMP-SMX is the preferred agent. Traditionally, 1 double-strength tablet (160 mg TMP and 800 mg SMX) once daily has been the regimen of choice, but 1 single-strength tablet (80 mg TMP and 400 mg SMX) once daily is also effective. Alternatively, one double-strength tablet can be taken 3 times weekly. If TMP-SMX cannot be used because of adverse effects, alternative options for prophylaxis include aerosolized pentamidine, 300 mg once monthly; dapsone, 100 mg once daily; dapsone, 50 mg once daily with pyrimethamine, 50 mg once weekly; and atovaquone, 1500 mg oral suspension once daily. These regimens are less effective than prophylaxis with TMP-SMX. PCP prophylaxis can be discontinued if the $CD4^+$ T_H cell count increases to greater than 200 cells/μL for at least 3 months as a result of ART. Although PCP can occur when $CD4^+$ T_H counts are greater than 200 cells/μL, the benefit of ongoing PCP chemoprophylaxis is diminished and may be outweighed by the risk of drug toxicity.[35]

CRYPTOCOCCUS

Cryptococcus is a genus of encapsulated yeast that is ubiquitous in human-populated environments and can be isolated from bird excrement, rotting fruit, and soil.[40] Some species, such as *Cryptococcus gattii*, are known to cause disease in immunocompetent hosts. The species that most frequently affects HIV-infected patients is *Cryptococcus neoformans*. Although it is known to occasionally cause asymptomatic colonization in immunocompetent hosts with structural lung disease, *C neoformans* is almost exclusively an opportunistic pathogen. A $CD4^+$ T_H cell count less than 100 cells/μL is a risk factor for cryptococcosis.[41]

C neoformans gains access to the human host through inhalation of fungal basidiospores. Host immunosuppression allows *C neoformans* to disseminate throughout the body. In HIV-infected patients, cryptococcal meningitis is the most common manifestation. In disseminated disease, multiple organs including the skin, bone, eye, prostate, and lung can be affected. Although the respiratory system is the portal of entry, isolated cryptococcal pneumonia without other organ involvement is less common than disseminated disease.[42] Symptoms of cryptococcal pneumonia are nonspecific and include cough, dyspnea, sputum production, chest pain, and pleurisy. Findings on chest radiography are varied, and include unilateral or bilateral interstitial opacities, focal consolidation, solitary or multiple pulmonary nodules, cavitation, hilar adenopathy, and pleural effusion (**Fig. 3**).[43] Because of the severity of immunosuppression that permits invasive cryptococcosis, simultaneous co-infection with other pulmonary pathogens is common.

The cryptococcal antigen (CrAg) test, which detects the presence of capsular polysaccharides, is important for investigating cryptococcal infection. The test can be performed on serum, cerebrospinal fluid, BAL fluid, or pleural fluid. The serum CrAg test is highly sensitive for both cryptococcemia and cryptococcal meningitis; a negative serum CrAg result markedly decreases the likelihood of cryptococcal meningitis. The serum CrAg test is often positive in cases of cryptococcal pneumonia, although it can be negative in cases of isolated cryptococcal pneumonia without dissemination.[43,44] The CrAg test can also be performed on BAL fluid, although caution is warranted; in one study, the sensitivity of the test was 71% and the positive predictive value was 0.59.[45]

Definitive diagnosis of cryptococcal pneumonia is typically made by cytopathologic examination of a respiratory specimen, histopathologic examination of a biopsy specimen, or culture of either. The yield of expectorated sputum is low; in one series, sputum microscopy detected only one of 11

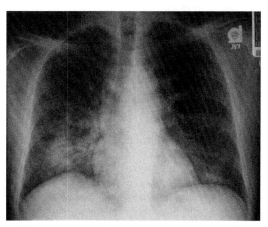

Fig. 3. Chest radiograph of an HIV-infected patient with isolated cryptococcal pneumonia. There is a focal consolidation in the right lower lobe with areas of cavitation. (*Courtesy of* Laurence Huang, MD, San Francisco, USA; with permission.)

patients with cryptococcal pneumonia.[46] BAL fluid is significantly better with a diagnostic yield of 82%.[44,46] The use of PCR for the detection of *Cryptococcus* DNA in respiratory specimens is offered by some laboratories and seems promising, but the clinical utility remains to be determined.[47]

There are no randomized, controlled clinical trials for HIV-infected patients with isolated cryptococcal pneumonia or disseminated cryptococcosis with pulmonary involvement. Treatment recommendations are extrapolated from trials of treatment of cryptococcal meningitis. For isolated pulmonary disease with mild symptoms, treatment with oral fluconazole, 400 mg daily for 12 months, is recommended. For severe pulmonary disease or disseminated disease, the standard initial (induction) treatment regimen is IV amphotericin B and oral flucytosine for at least 2 weeks. If clinical improvement is noted, treatment can be changed to consolidation therapy with oral fluconazole, 400 mg daily for at least an additional 8 weeks, followed by maintenance therapy with oral fluconazole, 200 mg daily for at least 1 year, to prevent relapse. Extrapolating from data on patients who have recovered from cryptococcal meningitis, secondary prophylaxis can be stopped if $CD4^+$ T_H counts are greater than 200 cells/μL and the HIV viral load is undetectable for 3 months on ART.[35]

Current guidelines do not support primary prophylaxis of cryptococcal disease regardless of $CD4^+$ T_H count. However, routine screening for asymptomatic cryptococcal antigenemia is recommended by some experts for patients with a new diagnosis of HIV and a $CD4^+$ T_H count less than 100 cells/μL. If the serum CrAg test result is positive, CSF evaluation is required to assess for meningitis. Asymptomatic cryptococcal antigenemia is treated with fluconazole, 400 mg oral daily for 12 months.[35]

ASPERGILLUS

Aspergillus is a genus of mold that is ubiquitous in the environment and can be isolated from soil worldwide.[48] Various species are known to cause human disease, but the most frequent pathogen is *Aspergillus fumigatus*. Human exposure to *Aspergillus* spp. occurs by inhalation of airborne conidia. In immunocompetent hosts with normal lung architecture, it is rare for *Aspergillus* to cause disease. In immunocompromised patients or patients with structural lung abnormalities, *Aspergillus* is associated with several distinct chest syndromes: aspergilloma, allergic bronchopulmonary aspergillosis, tracheobronchial aspergillosis, chronic necrotizing aspergillosis, and invasive pulmonary aspergillosis (IPA). Different syndromes have unique risk factors. For aspergilloma, structural lung disease, like bullae in chronic obstructive pulmonary disease, is a major predisposing condition. Allergic bronchopulmonary aspergillosis has a predilection for patients with cystic fibrosis and severe asthma. IPA, the most severe and most dangerous manifestation of *Aspergillus* infection, affects immunocompromised hosts, particularly patients with absent or abnormal phagocyte function. The classic risk factors for IPA are corticosteroid use and granulocytopenia from hematologic malignancy or its therapies.[49,50]

All *Aspergillus* syndromes have been described in patients with HIV infection but compared with the occurrence of other opportunistic pathogens, *Aspergillus* infection is uncommon. Although IPA was initially included as an AIDS-defining opportunistic infection by the Centers for Disease Control, it was removed in 1984 when it was found that the incidence of IPA in patients with HIV infection was 0.1%; incidence is lower still today because of widespread use of effective ART.[51] Even in patients with very low $CD4^+$ T_H counts, IPA is unusual in the absence of additional risk factors such as neutropenia.

The clinical presentations of the various forms of *Aspergillus*-related disease in HIV-infected patients are not distinct from those of HIV-uninfected patients and are described elsewhere in this issue. For invasive aspergillosis, patients with and without HIV can present with fever, cough, dyspnea, pleurisy, and sometimes hemoptysis. Imaging findings vary and can include consolidation, cavities, nodules, and pleural effusions. Definitive diagnosis requires demonstration of tissue invasion on biopsy and isolation of the organism by culture. In patients for whom biopsy is infeasible or fails to demonstrate invasive disease but in whom IPA is still suspected, initiating empiric treatment of probable IPA is reasonable. Voriconazole is the preferred therapy; alternative treatments include amphotericin, caspofungin, or posaconazole.[52] Given its low incidence even in advanced HIV disease, prophylaxis is not recommended.[35]

ENDEMIC FUNGI

Around the world, there are pathogenic fungi that have limited geographic distribution. These include *Histoplasma capsulatum*, *Coccidioides* species, *Blastomyces dermatitidis*, *Paracoccidioides brasiliensis*, *Talaromyces* (formerly *Penicillium*) *marneffei*, and *Emmonsia* species. These fungi are dimorphic. In the environment, they grow as molds. The predominant method of human infection is through inhalation of spores from contaminated soils. Once deposited in the human respiratory tract, the fungi change and grow as yeasts. All are known to cause disease in immunocompetent hosts. Typically, the severity of disease is related to the size of the inoculum and to the state of host immunity. In patients who are immunocompromised, particularly with respect to cell-mediated immunity, infections are more severe, more likely to disseminate beyond the respiratory system, and more frequently fatal.

H capsulatum is found throughout the Americas, Africa, and Asia. It is endemic to the Ohio and Mississippi River Valleys in the United States and in regions of Mexico, Venezuela, Brazil, Ecuador, Paraguay, Argentina, and Uruguay. In Asia, it is endemic to parts of China, India, Thailand, and South Korea. Information is more limited from Africa, but cases have been reported from South Africa, Zimbabwe, Uganda, and Tanzania.[53] In immunocompetent hosts, histoplasmosis is typically a mild self-limited respiratory illness characterized by fevers, chills, headache, myalgias, nonproductive cough, and chest pain that resolves over weeks. Immunocompromised patients, including HIV-infected patients with CD4$^+$ T$_H$ cell counts less than 150 cells/μL, are at risk for disseminated histoplasmosis.[54–57] In addition to cough and dyspnea, disseminated disease presents with constitutional symptoms including fever and weight loss and evidence of other organ involvement including lymphadenopathy, hepatosplenomegaly, skin lesions, meningitis, and infiltration of bone marrow. The tempo of illness can vary from indolent to fulminant. Patterns on chest radiography associated with histoplasmosis include a diffuse interstitial pattern or a miliary nodular pattern (**Fig. 4**). Less common but also compatible are focal alveolar opacities or a normal chest radiograph. The *Histoplasma* antigen test can be helpful for diagnosis; in HIV-infected patients with disseminated disease, the sensitivity of the urine *Histoplasma* antigen test approaches 100%, although the test may also be positive in some patients with other endemic mycoses including blastomycosis, coccidioidomycosis, paracoccidioidomycosis, and penicilliosis (talaromycosis).[58] Antigen testing in BAL fluid can be diagnostic, especially for relatively immunocompetent patients with isolated pulmonary disease who may not have antigenuria or antigenemia.[59] In disseminated disease, fungal cultures are frequently positive from blood, bone marrow, lymph node, and skin. Preferred treatment of disseminated histoplasmosis is IV

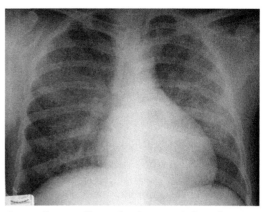

Fig. 4. Chest radiograph of an HIV-infected patient with disseminated histoplasmosis shows diffuse interstitial opacities. (*Courtesy of* Laurence Huang, MD, San Francisco, USA; with permission.)

liposomal amphotericin B for at least 2 weeks or until evidence of clinical improvement followed by oral itraconazole for at least 12 months.[35] Immunocompetent patients with mild pulmonary disease can be treated with itraconazole for at least 12 weeks.[60] Serial *Histoplasma* urine or serum antigen levels can be used to monitor therapeutic response. Primary prophylaxis for histoplasmosis is not recommended except for patients with CD4$^+$ T$_H$ cell counts less than 150 cells/μL and who live in an area with hyperendemic rates of histoplasmosis (>10 cases per 100 patient-years).[35]

Coccidioidomycosis is caused by 2 species of *Coccidioides*, *Coccidioides immitis* and *Coccidioides posadasii*. They are endemic to semiarid regions of North and South America, including parts of California, Arizona, New Mexico, Texas, Mexico, and Argentina. In immunocompetent hosts, including HIV-infected patients with CD4$^+$ T$_H$ cell counts greater than 250 cells/μL, the spectrum of disease ranges from asymptomatic exposure to an influenzalike illness characterized by fever, cough, fatigue, headache, and myalgia (colloquially called *valley fever*) to frank pneumonia. In immunocompromised hosts, including HIV-infected patients with CD4$^+$ T$_H$ cell counts less than 150 cells/μL, *Coccidioides* spp. can disseminate causing meningitis, lymphadenitis, hepatitis, and skin lesions.[61,62] Disseminated disease frequently presents with systemic symptoms including night sweats and weight loss. Radiographic findings include diffuse nodular opacities, focal consolidation, solitary pulmonary nodules, and cavitary lesions (**Fig. 5**). Definitive diagnosis is established by culture from infected tissues or cytopathologic or histopathologic identification of pathognomonic giant spherules in sputum, BAL fluid, or biopsy

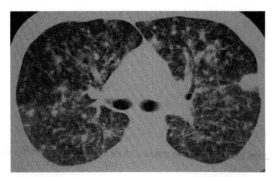

Fig. 5. Axial HRCT of the chest of an HIV-infected patient with coccidioidomycosis. There are numerous nodules in a military pattern. (*Courtesy of* Laurence Huang, MD, San Francisco, USA; with permission.)

specimens. Serologic tests are useful adjunctive tests. Detection of *Coccidioides*-specific antibodies by complement fixation, enzyme immunosorbent assay, or immunodiffusion can support a diagnosis of coccidioidomycosis and can also be used to monitor response to treatment. Preferred treatment of severe or disseminated coccidioidomycosis is amphotericin B.[35] When clinical improvement is noted, switching from amphotericin B to fluconazole or itraconazole for a minimum of another 12 months is appropriate.[60] HIV-infected patients who have recovered from coccidioidomycosis can be considered for secondary prophylaxis with fluconazole or itraconazole if CD4+ T_H cell counts remain less than 250 cells/μL. Current guidelines do not support primary prophylaxis of coccidioidomycosis regardless of CD4+ T_H count. However, annual screening for *Coccidioides* exposure with an antibody test is recommended for patients with a CD4+ T_H count less than 250 cells/μL and who live in an endemic region. Coccidioidal seroconversion is treated with daily oral fluconazole.[35]

B dermatitidis is found primarily in North America along the Ohio, Mississippi, and St. Lawrence Rivers. Blastomycosis is less common than either histoplasmosis or coccidioidomycosis. In immunocompetent hosts, the manifestations of blastomycosis range from asymptomatic infection to pneumonia to disseminated disease affecting the skin, bone, genitourinary tract, and central nervous system. The frequency of severe or disseminated disease is higher in immunocompromised hosts, including HIV-infected patients with CD4+ T_H cell counts less than 200 cells/μL.[63] Radiographic findings include diffuse interstitial opacities, a military nodular pattern, focal or diffuse airspace consolidation, solitary or multiple pulmonary nodules, mass lesions, or cavitary lesions.[64] Definitive diagnosis is established by culture of infected

tissues or respiratory samples, including BAL fluid. In the absence of a positive culture, histopathologic or cytopathologic identification of *Blastomyces* yeast forms can support a diagnosis of blastomycosis. For severe life-threatening disease, amphotericin B is the preferred treatment until there is evidence of clinical improvement, followed by itraconazole for 6 to 12 months. For mild to moderate severity disease, initial treatment with itraconazole is recommended for a duration of 6 to 12 months.[60] Secondary prophylaxis with itraconazole is recommended for HIV-infected patients with CD4+ T_H cell counts that remain less than 200 cells/μL. Current guidelines do not support primary prophylaxis for blastomycosis regardless of CD4+ T_H cell counts.[60]

P brasiliensis is found throughout much of South and Central America, but it is most common in parts of Brazil, Colombia, and Venezuela. Most infections are asymptomatic. Symptomatic disease is expected to manifest in 1% to 2% of infected persons. There are 2 patterns of disease manifestation. Acute or juvenile paracoccidioidomycosis occurs exclusively in children and young adults less than 30 years of age, and is characterized by fever, weight loss, lymphadenopathy, hepatosplenomegaly, and cytopenias as a result of disseminated disease within the reticuloendothelial system; the illness evolves and progresses over weeks to months. Chronic or reactivation paracoccidioidomycosis develops more slowly, over months, and can involve the lungs, mucosa, skin, lymph nodes, adrenal glands, bones, and central nervous system.[65] In HIV-infected patients, paracoccidioidomycosis tends to be disseminated, more severe, and more rapidly progressive.[66–69] Chest radiograph findings vary and can include diffuse bilateral reticular opacities, nodular opacities, airspace consolidation, cavitation, mediastinal adenopathy, and pleural effusion.[69,70] Definitive diagnosis is typically established by identification of *Paracoccidioides* yeast forms on microscopy of clinical specimens, including sputum, BAL fluid, pleural effusion, lymph node aspirate, or tissue biopsy.[67] Culture of the fungus is possible but can take several weeks so is clinically less useful. Detection of specific serum antibodies by immunodiffusion is also diagnostic, and reported sensitivity is 90%.[71] For severe life-threatening disease, amphotericin B is the preferred treatment until there is evidence of clinical improvement, followed by itraconazole for 6 to 12 months. For mild to moderate disease, initial treatment with itraconazole is recommended for 6 to 12 months.[60] There are no specific recommendations for primary prophylaxis against

Paracoccidioides in HIV-infected patients, although PCP prophylaxis with trimethoprim-sulfamethoxazole may confer some protection as *Paracoccidioides* is susceptible to sulfonamides.[35]

The causative agent for penicilliosis, previously known as *Penicillium marneffei*, was determined to be substantially genetically different from other members of the *Penicillium* genus and so was renamed *Talaromyces marneffei* in 2011.[72] It is endemic to parts of Asia including Vietnam, Thailand, Cambodia, Laos, Malaysia, Myanmar, Singapore, India, China, Hong Kong, and Taiwan.[73–76] Although penicilliosis can affect immunocompetent patients, it is predominantly an opportunistic infection, and symptoms are attributable to disseminated infection.[77] Clinical manifestations of penicilliosis are myriad and include cough, fever, dyspnea, chest pain, lymphadenopathy, anemia, hepatosplenomegaly, abdominal pain, diarrhea, skin and mucosal lesions, arthritis, and osteomyelitis.[76] Chest radiographic findings can mimic those of PCP and include interstitial opacities, airspace consolidation, pleural effusion, and cavitary lesions.[77] Definitive diagnosis is made by culture from blood or BAL, skin biopsy, bone marrow biopsy, or lymph node aspirate or biopsy. Presumptive diagnosis can be made by microscopic examination of clinical specimens, including BAL fluid. The preferred treatment is liposomal amphotericin B for at least 2 weeks until clinical improvement followed by oral itraconazole for 10 weeks.[78] For HIV-infected patients, it is reasonable to provide secondary prophylaxis with itraconazole for at least an additional 6 months and until $CD4^+$ T_H cell counts increase to greater than 100 cells/μL.[79] Primary prophylaxis is indicated for HIV-infected patients with a $CD4^+$ T_H count less than 100 cells/μL and who reside or travel to endemic regions.[35]

At least 4 species of *Emmonsia* are known to be pathogenic in humans. Three species are named: *Emmonsia parva*, *Emmonsia crescens*, and *Emmonsia pasteuriana*. *E parva* and *E crescens* cause adiaspiromycosis, a pulmonary infection that is common in rodents but has been known to affect immunocompetent humans. A striking feature of adiaspiromycosis is the identification of giant conidia, or adiaspores, on microscopy, which neither replicate nor disseminate but provoke a granulomatous response from the host. *E pasteuriana* does not cause adiaspiromycosis but, in case reports from Italy, Spain, China, and India, is described to cause disseminated fungal disease in patients with cell-mediated immunodeficiency from HIV infection, medical immunosuppression, or

both.[80–85] In 2013, a new species of an as yet unnamed *Emmonsia* species of fungus was described in HIV-infected patients in South Africa.[86] In a case series of 54 patients, 51 were HIV infected, 1 was medically immunosuppressed after renal transplantation, and 2 had no apparent cause for immunodeficiency.[87] Genetically, the novel pathogen is more similar to *E pasteuriana*, and, unlike *E parva* and *E crescens*, it does not create adiaspores. For HIV-infected patients in this case series, the median $CD4^+$ T_H count was 16 cells/μL; in 12 of the 51 HIV-infected patients, symptomatic disease was likely provoked by immune reconstitution after initiation of ART. Overall, 88% of the patients had lower respiratory disease as evidenced by chest radiograph abnormalities including diffuse or focal opacities, lobar atelectasis, hilar adenopathy, or an intrathoracic mass. Ninety-six percent of patients had cutaneous lesions, ranging from papules, plaques, nodules, and ulcers, mimicking Kaposi's sarcoma, varicella, cutaneous tuberculosis, or syphilis. Other clinical features included fever, weight loss, night sweats, and lymphadenopathy. Given the frequency of skin involvement, the most common diagnostic procedure was skin biopsy, which found yeast on histologic examination in 92% and was culture positive in 72%. Organisms were also identified in respiratory tissue, bone marrow, brain tissue, liver tissue, and blood. In total, 48% of patients died, half of them before diagnosis was established. Most patients were treated with amphotericin B followed by maintenance triazole therapy. However, much remains unknown about this new pathogen, including whether it causes asymptomatic and self-limited infection in immunocompetent hosts and its true geographic range. The final species name for this pathogen remains to be determined.

SUMMARY

Many fungi cause pulmonary disease in HIV-infected patients. Major pathogens include *P jirovecii*, *C neoformans*, *Aspergillus* species, *H capsulatum*, *Coccidioides* species, *B dermatitidis*, *P brasiliensis*, *T marneffei*, and *Emmonsia* species. Because symptoms are frequently nonspecific, a high index of suspicion for fungal infection is required for diagnosis. Clinical manifestations of fungal infection in HIV-infected patients frequently depend on the degree of immunosuppression and the CD_4^+ T_H cell count. Establishing definitive diagnosis is important because treatments differ. Primary and secondary prophylaxis depends on $CD4^+$ T_H cell counts and geographic location and local prevalence of disease.

REFERENCES

1. Gottlieb MS, Schanker HM, Fan PT, et al. Pneumocystis pneumonia–Los Angeles. MMWR Morb Mortal Wkly Rep 1981;30(21):250–2.

2. Romani L. Immunity to fungal infections. Nat Rev Immunol 2011;11(4):275–88.

3. Schroder K, Hertzog PJ, Ravasi T, et al. Interferon-gamma: an overview of signals, mechanisms and functions. J Leukoc Biol 2004;75(2):163–89.

4. Huson AM, Hoogendijk AJ, de Vos AF, et al. The impact of HIV infection on blood leukocyte responsiveness to bacterial stimulation in asymptomatic patients and patients with bloodstream infection. J Int AIDS Soc 2016;19(1):20759.

5. Koziel H, Eichbaum Q, Kruskal BA, et al. Reduced binding and phagocytosis of Pneumocystis carinii by alveolar macrophages from persons infected with HIV-1 correlates with mannose receptor down-regulation. J Clin Invest 1998;102(7):1332–44.

6. Nielsen H, Kharazami A, Faber V. Blood monocyte and neutrophil functions in the acquired immune deficiency syndrome. Scand J Immunol 2006; 24(3):291–6.

7. Murphy PM, Clifford Lane H, Fauci AS, et al. Impairment of neutrophil bactericidal capacity in patients with AIDS. J Infect Dis 1988;158(3):627–9.

8. Moir S, Fauci AS. B cells in HIV infection and disease. Nat Rev Immunol 2009;9(4):235–45.

9. Djawe K, Buchacz K, Hsu L, et al. Mortality risk after AIDS-defining opportunistic illness among HIV-Infected persons—San Francisco, 1981-2012. J Infect Dis 2015;212(9):1366–75.

10. Bartlett MS, Vermund SH, Jacobs R, et al. Detection of Pneumocystis carinii DNA in air samples: likely environmental risk to susceptible persons. J Clin Microbiol 1997;35(10):2511–3.

11. Skalski JH, Kottom TJ, Limper AH, et al. Pathobiology of Pneumocystis pneumonia: life cycle, cell wall and cell signal transduction. FEMS Yeast Res 2015;15(6):1.

12. Gigliotti F, Wright TW. Pneumocystis: where does it live? PLoS Pathog 2012;8(11):e1003025.

13. Vargas SL, Hughes WT, Santolaya ME, et al. Search for primary infection by Pneumocystis carinii in a cohort of normal, healthy infants. Clin Infect Dis 2001;32(6):855–61.

14. Wakefield AE, Stewart TJ, Moxon ER, et al. Infection with Pneumocystis carinii is prevalent in healthy Gambian children. Trans R Soc Trop Med Hyg 1990;84(6):800–2.

15. Respaldiza N, Medrano FJ, Medrano AC, et al. High seroprevalence of Pneumocystis infection in Spanish children. Clin Microbiol Infect 2004;10(11):1029–31.

16. Morris A, Norris KA. Colonization by Pneumocystis jirovecii and its role in disease. Clin Microbiol Rev 2012;25(2):297–317.

17. Morris A, Sciurba FC, Lebedeva IP, et al. Association of chronic obstructive pulmonary disease severity and Pneumocystis colonization. Am J Respir Crit Care Med 2004;170(4):408–13.

18. Walzer PD, Evans HER, Copas AJ, et al. Early predictors of mortality from Pneumocystis jirovecii pneumonia in HIV-infected patients: 1985-2006. Clin Infect Dis 2008;46(4):625–33.

19. Stansell JD, Osmond DH, Charlebois E, et al. Predictors of Pneumocystis carinii pneumonia in HIV-infected persons. Am J Respir Crit Care Med 1997;155(1):60–6.

20. Kaplan JE, Hanson DL, Navin TR, et al. Risk factors for primary Pneumocystis carinii pneumonia in human immunodeficiency virus-infected adolescents and adults in the United States: reassessment of indications for chemoprophylaxis. J Infect Dis 1998; 178(4):1126–32.

21. Kales CP, Murren JR, Torres RA, et al. Early predictors of in-hospital mortality for Pneumocystis carinii pneumonia in the acquired immunodeficiency syndrome. Arch Intern Med 1987;147(8):1413–7.

22. Kovacs JA, Hiemenz JW, Macher AM, et al. Pneumocystis carinii pneumonia: a comparison between patients with the acquired immunodeficiency syndrome and patients with other immunodeficiencies. Ann Intern Med 1984;100(5):663–71.

23. Miller RF, Huang L, Walzer PD. Pneumocystis pneumonia associated with human immunodeficiency virus. Clin Chest Med 2013;34(2):229–41.

24. Tasaka S, Hasegawa N, Kobayashi S, et al. Serum indicators for the diagnosis of Pneumocystis pneumonia. Chest 2007;131(4):1173–80.

25. Quist J, Hill AR. Serum lactate dehydrogenase (LDH) in Pneumocystis carinii pneumonia, tuberculosis, and bacterial pneumonia. Chest 1995;108(2):415–8.

26. Sax PE, Komarow L, Finkelman MA, et al. Blood (1-3)-beta-D-Glucan as a diagnostic test for HIV-related Pneumocystis jirovecii pneumonia. Clin Infect Dis 2011;53(2):197–202.

27. DeLorenzo LJ, Huang CT, Maguire GP, et al. Roentgenographic patterns of Pneumocystis carinii pneumonia in 104 patients with AIDS. Chest 1987;91(3):323–7.

28. Kennedy CA, Goetz MB. Atypical roentgenographic manifestations of Pneumocystis carinii pneumonia. Arch Intern Med 1992;152(7):1390–8.

29. Gruden JF, Huang L, Webb WR, et al. AIDS-related Kaposi sarcoma of the lung: radiographic findings and staging system with bronchoscopic correlation. Radiology 1995;195(2):545–52.

30. Richards PJ, Riddell L, Reznek RH, et al. High resolution computed tomography in HIV patients with suspected Pneumocystis carinii pneumonia and a normal chest radiograph. Clin Radiol 1996;51(10):689–93.

31. Kovacs JA, Ng VL, Masur H, et al. Diagnosis of *Pneumocystis carinii* pneumonia: improved detection in sputum with use of monoclonal antibodies. N Engl J Med 1988;318(10):589–93.

32. Huang L, Hecht FM, Stansell JD, et al. Suspected *Pneumocystis carinii* pneumonia with a negative induced sputum examination: is early bronchoscopy useful? Am J Respir Crit Care Med 1995;151(6): 1866–71.

33. Oren I, Finkelstein R, Hardak E, et al. Polymerase chain reaction-based detection of *Pneumocystis jirovecii* in bronchoalveolar lavage fluid for the diagnosis of *Pneumocystis* pneumonia. Am J Med Sci 2011;342(3):182–5.

34. Alvarez-Martínez MJ, Miró JM, Valls ME, et al. Sensitivity and specificity of nested and real-time PCR for the detection of *Pneumocystis jiroveci* in clinical specimens. Diagn Microbiol Infect Dis 2006;56(2): 153–60.

35. Panel on Opportunistic Infections in HIV-Infected Adults and Adolescents. Guidelines for the prevention and treatment of opportunistic infections in HIV-infected adults and adolescents: recommendations from the centers for disease control and prevention, the national institutes of health, and the HIV medicine association of the infectious diseases society of America. Available at: http://aidsinfo.nih.gov/contentfiles/lvguidelines/adult_oi.pdf. Accessed November 22, 2016.

36. Wharton JM, Coleman DL, Wofsy CB, et al. Trimethoprim-sulfamethoxazole or pentamidine for *Pneumocystis carinii* pneumonia in the acquired immunodeficiency syndrome: a prospective randomized trial. Ann Intern Med 1986;105(1):37–44.

37. Benfield T, Atzori C, Miller RF, et al. Second-line salvage treatment of AIDS-associated *Pneumocystis jirovecii* pneumonia. J Acquir Immune Defic Syndr 2008;48(1):63–7.

38. Bozzette SA, Sattler FR, Chiu J, et al. A controlled trial of early adjunctive treatment with corticosteroids for *Pneumocystis carinii* pneumonia in the acquired immunodeficiency syndrome. N Engl J Med 1990; 323(21):1451–7.

39. Gagnon S, Boota AM, Fischl MA, et al. Corticosteroids as adjunctive therapy for severe *Pneumocystis carinii* pneumonia in the acquired immunodeficiency syndrome. N Engl J Med 1990;323(21):1444–50.

40. Kielstein P, Hotzel H, Schmalreck A, et al. Occurrence of *Cryptococcus* spp. in excreta of pigeons and pet birds. Mycoses 2000;43(1–2): 7–15.

41. Mirza SA, Phelan M, Rimland D, et al. The changing epidemiology of cryptococcosis: an update from population-based active surveillance in 2 large metropolitan areas, 1992–2000. Clin Infect Dis 2003;36(6):789–94.

42. Chuck SL, Sande MA. Infections with *Cryptococcus neoformans* in the acquired immunodeficiency syndrome. N Engl J Med 1989;321(12):794–9.

43. Meyohas MC, Roux P, Bollens D, et al. Pulmonary cryptococcosis: localized and disseminated infections in 27 patients with AIDS. Clin Infect Dis 1995; 21(3):628–33.

44. Batungwanayo J, Taelman H, Bogaerts J, et al. Pulmonary cryptococcosis associated with HIV-1 infection in Rwanda: a retrospective study of 37 cases. AIDS 1994;8(9):1271–6.

45. Kralovic SM, Rhodes JC. Utility of routine testing of bronchoalveolar lavage fluid for cryptococcal antigen. J Clin Microbiol 1998;36(10):3088–9.

46. Malabonga VM, Basti J, Kamholz SL. Utility of bronchoscopic sampling techniques for cryptococcal disease in AIDS. Chest 1991;99(2):370–2.

47. Rivera V, Gaviria M, Muñoz-Cadavid C, et al. Validation and clinical application of a molecular method for the identification of *Cryptococcus neoformans/Cryptococcus gattii* complex DNA in human clinical specimens. Braz J Infect Dis 2015;19(6):563–70.

48. Skalski J, Limper A. Fungal, viral, and parasitic pneumonias associated with human immunodeficiency virus. Semin Respir Crit Care Med 2016; 37(2):257–66.

49. Garnacho-Montero J, Amaya-Villar R, Ortiz-Leyba C, et al. Isolation of *Aspergillus* spp. from the respiratory tract in critically ill patients: risk factors, clinical presentation and outcome. Crit Care 2005;9(3): R191–9.

50. Pagano L, Caira M, Candoni A, et al. Invasive aspergillosis in patients with acute myeloid leukemia: a SEIFEM-2008 registry study. Haematologica 2010; 95(4):644–50.

51. Mylonakis E, Barlara TF, Flanigan T, et al. Pulmonary aspergillosis and invasive disease in AIDS. Chest 1998;114(1):251–62.

52. Patterson TF, Thompson GR, Denning DW, et al. Practice guidelines for the diagnosis and management of aspergillosis: 2016 update by the infectious diseases society of America. Clin Infect Dis 2016; 63(4):e1–60.

53. Wheat LJ, Azar MM, Bahr NC, et al. Histoplasmosis. Infect Dis Clin North Am 2016;30(1):207–27.

54. Sarosi GA, Johnson PC. Disseminated histoplasmosis in patients infected with human immunodeficiency virus. Clin Infect Dis 1992;14(S1):S60–7.

55. Johnson P, Khardori N, Najjar A, et al. Progressive disseminated histoplasmosis in patients with the acquired immunodeficiency syndrome. Am J Med 1988;85(2):152–8.

56. Wheat LJ, Slama TG, Zeckel ML. Histoplasmosis in patients with the acquired immune deficiency syndrome. Am J Med 1986;78(2):203–10.

57. McKinsey DS, Spiegel RA, Hutwagner L, et al. Prospective study of histoplasmosis in patients infected

with human immunodeficiency virus: incidence, risk factors, and pathophysiology. Clin Infect Dis 1997; 24(6):1195–203.

58. Connolly PA, Durkin MM, Lemonte AM, et al. Detection of *Histoplasma* antigen by a quantitative enzyme immunoassay. Clin Vaccine Immunol 2007; 14(12):1587–91.

59. Hage CA, Davis TE, Fuller D, et al. Diagnosis of histoplasmosis by antigen detection in BAL fluid. Chest 2010;137(3):623–8.

60. Limper AH, Knox KS, Sarosi GA, et al. An official American Thoracic Society statement: treatment of fungal infections in adult pulmonary and critical care patients. Am J Respir Crit Care Med 2011; 183(1):96–128.

61. Ampel NM, Dols CL, Galgiani JN. Coccidioidomycosis during human immunodeficiency virus infection: results of a prospective study in a coccidioidal endemic area. Am J Med 1993;94(3): 235–40.

62. Masannat FY, Ampel NM. Coccidioidomycosis in patients with HIV-1 infection in the era of potent antiretroviral therapy. Clin Infect Dis 2010;50(1):1–7.

63. Pappas PG, Pottage JC, Powderly WG, et al. Blastomycosis in patients with the acquired immunodeficiency syndrome. Ann Intern Med 1992;116(10): 847–53.

64. Patel RG, Patel B, Petrini MF, et al. Clinical presentation, radiographic findings, and diagnostic methods of pulmonary blastomycosis: a review of 100 consecutive cases. South Med J 1999;92(3): 289–95.

65. Queiroz-Telles F, Escuissato D. Pulmonary paracoccidioidomycosis. Semin Respir Crit Care Med 2011; 32(6):764–74.

66. Sarti ECFB, de Oliveira SM, dos Santos LF, et al. Paracoccidioidal infection in HIV patients at an endemic area of paracoccidioidomycosis in Brazil. Mycopathologia 2012;173:145–9.

67. Paniago AMM, de Freitas ACC, Aguiar ESA, et al. Paracoccidioidomycosis in patients with human immunodeficiency virus: review of 12 cases observed in an endemic region in Brazil. J Infect 2005;51(3): 248–52.

68. Silva-Vegara ML, Teixeira AC, Curi VGM, et al. Paracoccidioidomycosis associated with human immunodeficiency virus infection: report of 10 cases. Med Mycol 2003;41(3):259–63.

69. Morejón KML, Machado AA, Martinez R. Paracoccidioidomycosis in patients infected with and not infected with human immunodeficiency virus: a case-control study. Am J Trop Med Hyg 2009; 80(3):359–66.

70. Marchiori E, Gasparetto EL, Escuissato DL, et al. Pulmonary paracoccidioidomycosis and AIDS: high-resolution CT findings in five patients. J Comput Assist Tomogr 2007;31(4):605–7.

71. Moreto TC, Marques MEA, de Oliveira MLSC, et al. Accuracy of routine diagnostic tests used in paracoccidioidomycosis patients at a university hospital. Trans R Soc Trop Med Hyg 2011;105(8):473–8.

72. Samson RA, Yilmaz N, Houbraken J, et al. Phylogeny and nomenclature of the genus *Talaromyces* and taxa accommodated in *Penicillium* subgenus *Biverticillium*. Stud Mycol 2011;70(1):159–83.

73. Vanittanakom N, Cooper CR, Fisher MC, et al. *Penicillium marneffei* infection and recent advances in the epidemiology and molecular biology aspects. Clin Microbiol Rev 2006;19(1):95–110.

74. Sirisanthana T, Supparatpinyo K. Epidemiology and management of penicilliosis in human immunodeficiency virus-infected patients. Int J Infect Dis 1998; 3(1):48–53.

75. Supparatpinyo K, Khamwan C, Baosoung V, et al. Disseminated *Penicillium marneffei* infection in Southeast Asia. Lancet 1994;344(8915):110–3.

76. Duong TA. Infection due to *Penicillium marneffei*, an emerging pathogen: review of 155 reported cases. Clin Infect Dis 1996;23(1):125–30.

77. Kawila R, Chaiwarith R, Supparatpinyo K. Clinical and laboratory characteristics of penicilliosis marneffei among patients with and without HIV infection in Northern Thailand: a retrospective study. BMC Infect Dis 2013;13:464.

78. Sirisanthana T, Supparatpinyo K, Perriens J, et al. Amphotericin B and itraconazole for treatment of disseminated *Penicillium marneffei* infection in human immunodeficiency virus-infected patients. Clin Infect Dis 1998;26(5):1107–10.

79. Chaiwarith R, Charoenyos N, Sirisanthana T, et al. Discontinuation of secondary prophylaxis against penicilliosis marneffei in AIDS patients after HAART. AIDS 2007;21(3):365–7.

80. Gori S, Drouhet E, Gueho E, et al. Cutaneous disseminated mycosis in a patient with AIDS due to a new dimorphic fungus. J Mycol Med 1998; 8(2):57–63.

81. Tang XH, Zhou H, Zhang XQ, et al. Cutaneous disseminated emmonsiosis due to *Emmonsia pasteuriana* in a patient with cytomegalovirus enteritis. JAMA Dermatol 2015;151(11):1263–4.

82. Feng P, Yin S, Zhu G, et al. Disseminated infection caused by *Emmonsia pasteuriana* in a renal transplant recipient. J Dermatol 2015;42(12):1179–82.

83. Pelegrín I, Ayats J, Xiol X, et al. Disseminated adiaspiromycosis: case report of a liver transplant patient with human immunodeficiency infection, and literature review. Transpl Infect Dis 2011; 13(5):507–14.

84. Pelegrín I, Alastruey-Izquierdo A, Ayats J, et al. A second look at *Emmonsia* infection can make the difference. Transpl Infect Dis 2014;16(3):519–20.

85. Malik R, Capoor MR, Vanidassane I, et al. Disseminated *Emmonsia pasteuriana* infection in

India: a case report and a review. Mycoses 2016; 59(2):127–32.

86. Kenyon C, Bonorchis K, Corcoran C, et al. A dimorphic fungus causing disseminated infection in South Africa. N Engl J Med 2013;369(15):1416–24.

87. Schwartz IS, Govender NP, Corcoran C, et al. Clinical characteristics, diagnosis, management, and outcomes of disseminated emmonsiosis: a retrospective case series. Clin Infect Dis 2015;61(6): 1004–12.

Fungal Pneumonia in Patients with Hematologic Malignancy and Hematopoietic Stem Cell Transplantation

Alisha Y. Young, MD[a], Miguel M. Leiva Juarez, MD[b],
Scott E. Evans, MD[b],*

KEYWORDS

- Fungal pneumonia • Neutropenia • Hematologic malignancy • Stem cell transplant
- Immunocompromised host pneumonia • Galactomannan

KEY POINTS

- Fungal pneumonias cause significant morbidity and mortality in patients with hematologic malignancies (HM) and recipients of hematopoietic stem cell transplantations (HSCT).
- Neutropenia, cytotoxic chemotherapy, graft-versus-host disease, genetic polymorphisms, and other immune derangements increase the risk of developing life-threatening fungal pneumonias.
- Chest imaging is often nonspecific but may aid in diagnoses. Bronchoscopy with bronchoalveolar lavage is recommended in patients at high risk of fungal pneumonia with new infiltrates on chest imaging, unexplained respiratory symptoms, or persistent fever.
- Immunoassays for fungal cell wall components, such as galactomannan and $(1,3)$-β-D-glucan, may aid the early diagnosis of invasive fungal infections in patients with HM/HSCT.
- Investigations into novel preventive strategies and host-directed therapies are ongoing.

INTRODUCTION

Immunocompetent hosts are estimated to inhale hundreds of fungal conidia daily, but most fungal pathogens are cleared without development of clinical infection.[1,2] By contrast, many patients with hematologic malignancies (HM) or those who have received hematopoietic stem cell transplantation (HSCT) have impaired antifungal defenses, and account for a disproportionate number of fungal pneumonias in North America and Europe.[3,4] Despite the use of mold-active prophylaxis since the 1990s, invasive fungal infections (IFI) remain a leading cause of morbidity in patients with HM/HSCT, with unacceptably high attributable mortality.[3,5–7] This review describes the immune deficits that enhance susceptibility to fungal pneumonia in patients with HM/HSCT, as well as the diagnosis

Disclosures: A.Y. Young and M.M. Leiva Juarez declares no relevant conflicts of interest. Dr S.E. Evans is an author on US patent 8,883,174 entitled "Stimulation of Innate Resistance of the Lungs to Infection with Synthetic Ligands." S.E. Evans owns stock in Pulmotect, which holds the commercial options on these patent disclosures.
^a Division of Pulmonary, Critical Care and Sleep Medicine, Department of Internal Medicine, The University of Texas Health Sciences Center, 6431 Fannin Street, MSB 1.434, Houston, TX 77030, USA; ^b Division of Internal Medicine, Department of Pulmonary Medicine, The University of Texas MD Anderson Cancer Center, 1515 Holcombe Boulevard, Unit 1100, Houston, TX 77030, USA
* Corresponding author.
E-mail address: seevans@mdanderson.org

Clin Chest Med 38 (2017) 479–491
http://dx.doi.org/10.1016/j.ccm.2017.04.009
0272-5231/17/© 2017 Elsevier Inc. All rights reserved.

and management of the fungal pneumonia in this patient population.

MICROBIAL EPIDEMIOLOGY

Most endemic fungal pneumonias in the North America are caused by thermally dimorphic *Histoplasma capsulatum, Coccidioides immitis,* and *Blastomyces dermatitidis,*[6] resulting in IFIs in immunocompetent and immunocompromised hosts.[9] No large epidemiologic registry of endemic fungal pneumonia in patients with HM exists, although smaller studies suggest that patients with HM develop endemic fungal pneumonias substantially more often than the general population,[4,10] and that these infections are more likely to be severe and/or lethal.[8] Interestingly, Transplant-Associated Infection Surveillance Network (TRANSNET) data suggest a very low rate of endemic fungal pneumonias in patients with HSCT, potentially due to aggressive exposure avoidance during peak vulnerability.[11]

As in **Table 1**, several registries of patients with HM/HSCT estimate annual incidence of opportunistic IFIs in the range of 1.3% to 10.0% for patients receiving treatment in tertiary centers, despite widespread use of antifungal prophylaxis.[12–14] *Aspergillus* spp account for a substantial majority of the documented events, with *Aspergillus fumigatus* identified more than *Aspergillus flavus*, whereas *Aspergillus terreus* and *Aspergillus ustus* are increasingly noted in severely immunocompromised populations.[15] Recent decades have demonstrated increasing pneumonias caused by Mucorales (80% are *Rhizopus, Mucor, Rhizomucor,* and *Lichtheimia* spp) and *Fusarium* spp (primarily *Fusarium solani, Fusarium oxysporum,* and *Fusarium moniliforme*) in profoundly neutropenic patients with HM/HSCT.[5,7,16–18]

HEMATOLOGIC MALIGNANCY/ HEMATOPOIETIC STEM CELL TRANSPLANTATION RISK FACTORS FOR FUNGAL PNEUMONIA

As in the general population, risk factors for endemic fungal pneumonia in patients with HM/ HSCT primarily relate to exposure to geographically localized biomaterials.[19–21] Thus, a thorough residential, recreational, travel, and occupational

Table 1
Proven or probable invasive fungal infections in HM/HSCT surveillance studies

Study	Patients, Centers	IFI Incidence	IFI-Attributed Mortality, %
USA (1989–2008) Lewis et al,[34] 2013	1213 HM autopsies (371 IFIs), single center	N/A	49
Austria (1995–2005) Auberger et al,[12] 2008	1095 HM/HSCT, single center	11.3%	35
SEIFEM, Italy (1999–2003) Pagano et al,[116] 2006	11,802 HM, 18 centers	4.6%	39
SEIFEM B, Italy (1999–2003) Pagano et al,[117] 2007	3228 HSCT, 11 centers	1.2% Auto, 7.8% Allo	65
TRANSNET, USA (2001–2005) Kontoyiannis et al,[17] 2010	16,200 HSCT, 23 centers	1.2% Auto, 5.8%–8.1% Allo	35
PATH Alliance, North America (2004–2007) Neofytos et al,[118] 2009	250 HSCT with IFI, 16 centers	N/A	47
Japan (2006–2008) Kurosawa et al,[55] 2012	2821 HM (597 HSCT), 22 centers	0.8% Auto, 5.4% Allo	37
SIMIFF, Italy (2009–2011) Montagna et al,[57] 2014	113 HM/HSCT, 119 non-HM with IFI, 23 centers	N/A	44
CAESAR, China (2011) Sun et al,[119] 2015	4192 HM, 35 centers	2.5%	12
Assessment of Antifungal Therapy in Hematological Disease, China (2011) Sun et al,[41] 2015	1401 HSCT, 31 centers	4.0% Auto, 8.9% Allo	13

Abbreviations: Allo, allogeneic stem cell transplantation; Auto, autologous stem cell transplantation; HM, hematologic malignancy; HSCT, hematopoietic stem cell transplantation; IFI, invasive fungal infections; N/A, not applicable.

history is essential to assessing risk levels in patients with HM/HSCT.[8] Interestingly, although neutropenia enhances susceptibility to most endemic fungi, this association is less clear for *H capsulatum*,[22,23] possibly because neutrophils are fungistatic, rather than fungicidal, for this endemic pathogen.

In immunocompetent hosts, inhaled fungi initiate immune responses from lung macrophages, dendritic cells, and epithelial cells, principally through pattern recognition receptors, such as Toll-like receptors and C-type lectins.[22,24,25] Cytokines from resident cells drive neutrophilic infiltration and stimulate T-cell–dependent type 1 and type 17 inflammatory responses that promote clearance of conidia[23] or sequestration within granulomata.[19,21] Impairment of any of these functions in HM/HSCT may allow opportunistic fungi to evade rapid elimination[19,22,25] or reactivate from granulomata years after exposure.[23] Patients with HM/HSCT face complex and concurrent immune defects derived both from disease[26,27] and treatment-specific insults. **Table 2** reports IFI incidence by type of HM and the associated immune impairments are discussed in the following sections.

Impaired Mucosal Immune Function

The sinopulmonary epithelium constitutes the first barrier to pathogen translocation and may be disrupted by many HM/HSCT-related processes, including effects of cytotoxic chemotherapy, radiation, preexisting infections, graft-versus-host disease (GVHD) and placement of nasogastric or endotracheal tubes. Beyond the physical barrier disruption of these processes, these insults may also impair epithelial expression of antimicrobial effectors, such as lactoferrin, lysozyme, or cathelicidin.[25] Alternately, HM may directly impair mucosal immunity, as when acute myeloid leukemia cells cause alterations of mucosal volatile species generation.[28]

Neutrophil Defects

Neutropenia that is profound (<500 cells/μL), prolonged (>10 days), or cyclic increased the risk for fungal pneumonia.[29–31] In animal models[32] and HM autopsies,[33] lung tissue from neutropenic hosts demonstrates hyphal growth, angioinvasion, and hemorrhagic infarctions, but minimal inflammation. This is distinct from the high inflammation/low fungal burden seen in non-neutropenic patients with HM and GVHD[33] or non-neutropenic patients with HM on prolonged corticosteroid therapy.[34]

Quantitative neutrophil deficits are compounded in patients with HM/HSCT by functional defects. Common cancer-related insults, such as radiation, corticosteroids, hypovolemia, acidosis, and hyperglycemia, can impair neutrophil chemotaxis, myeloperoxidase activity,[35] and neutrophil extracellular trap formation.[36] These functional impairments may explain in part why up to 40% of patients with HM/HSCT do not have documented neutropenia at the time of fungal pneumonia diagnosis.[37] Relatedly, corticosteroids or

Table 2
Incidence of invasive fungal infections by hematologic diagnosis

Hematologic Diagnosis	SEIFEM, Pagano et al,[116] 2006, %	Japan, Kurosawa et al,[52] 2012, %	CAESAR, Sun et al,[119] 2015, %
Acute myeloid leukemia	12	3	4.4
Acute lymphoblastic leukemia	6.5	4	2.4
Acute hyperleukocytic leukemia	NR	NR	6.3
Acute promyelocytic leukemia	NR	NR	0
Myelodysplastic syndrome	NR	2.5	5.3
Chronic myeloid leukemia	2.5	NR	2.4
Chronic lymphocytic leukemia	0.5	NR	3.5
Hodgkin lymphoma	0.7	1.1	0
Non-Hodgkin lymphoma	1.6	0.3	1.5
Multiple myeloma	0.5	0.8	0.1
Other	NR	NR	4.8
Cumulative	*4.6* *538/11802*	*1.3* *38/2821*	*2.5* *103/4192*

Abbreviation: NR, not reported.

colony-stimulating factors may increase the neutrophil count to more than 500 cells/µL without reversing the underlying immune deficits.[38,39]

Non-neutropenic Leukocyte Defects

T-cell depletion or dysfunction contributes substantially to the risk of fungal pneumonia, even in the absence of neutropenia.[36] T-cell–depleted HSCT and use of antithymocyte globulin place patients at high risk. Radiation, corticosteroids, cyclosporine, azathioprine, tacrolimus, cytotoxic purine analogs (eg, fludarabine), nucleoside analog (eg, cytarabine, gemcitabine, 5-fluorouracil), certain monoclonal antibodies (eg, alemtuzumab), and tumor necrosis factor antagonists can cause profound depletion and dysfunction of T cells that can last many months after treatment is completed.[5,13,17,29,30,40–42] Moreover, patients with Hodgkin disease, T-cell lymphoma, and some leukemias have disease-impaired cell-mediated immunity even in the absence of cytotoxic therapy,[43] possibly due to microenvironment immunosuppressive or exhaustion mechanisms.[44,45]

Although not historically thought to contribute significantly to antifungal defense, recent studies have identified protective antibodies against *Aspergillus, Histoplasma,* and *Pneumocystis* species[46] that promote complement activation and phagocytosis, and inhibit adhesion and germination. Many HMs are complicated by immunoglobulin dyscrasias, including impaired production, inappropriate class-switching, and increased antibody catabolism.[43,47] These effects appear to reduce host defenses against fungal infections, including invasive pulmonary aspergillosis.[35]

Memory Defects After Hematopoietic Stem Cell Transplantation

Near total depletion of the recipients' T and B lymphocytes is the goal of pretransplant conditioning. In addition to acute impairments, it largely abrogates immune memory from a lifetime exposure to pathogens, environmental antigens, and vaccines.[48] Even years after successful engraftment, many HSCT recipients experience immune impairment, as passive immunity from the donor provides insufficient protection. This is manifest in abnormal CD4:CD8 T-cell ratios and in immunoglobulin production that is deficient, dysregulated, and demonstrates altered kinetics.[49] The regeneration of sufficient quantities of T and B lymphocytes takes months to years, and maturation of fungal-specific immune responses takes longer still. Naïve B lymphocytes in HSCT recipients require environmental or vaccine exposure to fungal antigens and interactions with CD4+ T cells to generate fungal-specific antibodies and propagate protective memory B cells.

Graft-Versus-Host Disease

GVHD causes substantial morbidity following allogeneic HSCT, leading to prolonged use of immunosuppressive agents, increased risk of fungal infection, and increased mortality.[50–52] In addition to impairments caused by GVHD-suppressive agents, chronic GVHD is directly linked to macrophage dysfunction, impaired neutrophil chemotaxis, and immunoglobulin subclass deficiencies.[48] These defects may take years to recover after apparent resolution of GVHD.

Genetic Polymorphisms

Certain HM patient haplotypes are associated with altered immune responses and increased incidence of IFIs, prompting several novel genetic investigations into host susceptibility to fungal pneumonia.[53–56] **Table 3** lists a select number of polymorphisms in genes encoding mediators of immunity that have been associated with altered risk of fungal disease in patients with HM.

Table 3
Selected genetic polymorphisms associated with altered susceptibility to invasive aspergillosis in patients with HM/HSCT

Allele of Interest	Association with *Aspergillus* Infections
IL-10 promoter[53]	IL-10 1082(AA) genotype is associated with reduced IPA in HM
TNF receptor type 2 promoter[54]	Variable number tandem repeats associated with increased IPA in HM
TLR4[55]	Donor TLR4 S4 haplotypes increased risk for IA in HSCT recipients
Dectin-1[56]	Dectin-1 Y238X polymorphism associated with increased IA in HSCT
Plasminogen[120]	Homozygosity for D472 N polymorphism associated with increased IA in HSCT

Abbreviations: HM, hematologic malignancy; HSCT, hematologic stem cell transplantation; IA, invasive aspergillosis; IL-10, interleukin-10; IPA, invasive pulmonary aspergillosis; TLR4, Toll-like receptor 4; TNF, tumor necrosis factor.

Although these polymorphisms have not yet been incorporated into risk stratification algorithms for the patients with HM/HSCT, these genetic associations are likely to enhance understanding of antifungal immunity and may provide improved personalization of fungal prophylaxis and treatment in the future.

DIAGNOSIS OF HEMATOLOGIC MALIGNANCIES/HEMATOPOIETIC STEM CELL TRANSPLANTATION FUNGAL PNEUMONIA

Diagnosis of fungal pneumonia in any population can be challenging, due to nonspecific clinical presentations, slow growth rates in culture, and cross-reactions in fungal antigen testing.[20] These issues are amplified in patients with HM/HSCT, as the previously described immune defects frequently result in atypical presentations. Fever, fatigue, or exertional dyspnea may be the only presenting symptoms, whereas sputum and radiographic consolidations may be absent.[43,57] Many of the cardinal clinical features of pneumonia depend on robust immune responses that may be impaired in patients with HM/HSCT, thus a high clinical suspicion is key to making the correct diagnosis.

Chest Radiography

Chest radiography is routinely performed in patients with HM/HSCT with new fever or respiratory complaints. Chest radiograph is sufficient to detect some nodular or cavitary lesions, but up to 10% of patients with invasive pulmonary aspergillosis present with a normal radiograph. Consequently, computed tomography (CT) imaging is the modality recommended by the European Organization for Research and Treatment of Cancer/Invasive Fungal Infections Cooperative Group and the National Institute of Allergy and Infectious Diseases Mycoses Study Group (EORTC/MSG) Consensus Group in patients with HM/HSCT.[29] EORTC/MSG criteria list 3 chest CT findings as highly suspicious for fungal pneumonia[29]: a dense, well-circumscribed lesion or lesions (eg, a nodule with or without a halo sign), the air-crescent sign, or a cavity. The reverse halo sign or the atoll sign also should raise suspicion for fungal pneumonia.[58] However, imaging studies in this high-risk group are often nonspecific and indistinguishable from other pulmonary infections. Rather than the classically described findings, patients with HM/HSCT commonly present with centrilobular nodules, ill-defined consolidations, ground-glass infiltrates, and pleural effusions.[59]

It has been suggested that CT angiography may be more sensitive than conventional CT in detecting fungal pneumonia in patients with HM/HSCT,[60] but it is not standard practice. fludeoxyglucose-PET/CT cannot reliably differentiate malignancy from infectious pulmonary nodules. This is particularly problematic in geographic regions known to have high burdens of endemic fungi.[61] Serial CTs may be used to monitor the response to antifungal therapy, although it may take months for IFI-related radiologic abnormalities to resolve or stabilize. In neutropenic patients, radiographic findings may paradoxically worsen after initiating antifungal therapy or recovery from neutropenia due to increases in tissue inflammation.[59]

Biopsy Considerations

The definitive diagnosis of IFI requires a tissue biopsy from a sterile site demonstrating tissue invasion or culture positivity for fungal species.[29] For fungal pneumonia, a sterile specimen of lung parenchyma can be obtained via transbronchial biopsy, CT-guided transthoracic needle aspiration, or video-assisted/open surgical biopsy. Bronchoalveolar lavage (BAL) fluid is not considered sterile material in the EORTC/MSG criteria. In patients with HM/HSCT in whom previous bronchoscopic procedures were nondiagnostic, CT-guided biopsy of lung lesions larger than 1 cm offers high diagnostic yield often detecting fungal disease.[62] Unfortunately, lung biopsy is frequently impossible in patients with HM/HSCT, due to thrombocytopenia.

The EORTC/MSG classifications of IFI as possible, probable, or proven, addresses immunocompromised hosts when a lung biopsy is not possible.[29,63] Possible/probable designations allow diagnoses based on host risk factors, radiographic features, nonsterile cultures, and culture-independent assays. The definitions emphasize a multifaceted approach to diagnosing fungal pneumonia in patients with HM/HSCT, acknowledging their frequently nonspecific clinical and radiographic presentations and impaired seroreactivity.

Bronchoscopy

BAL is well tolerated, safe, and provides a reasonable diagnostic yield in patients with HM/HSCT, even in the setting of neutropenia and thrombocytopenia.[64–67] The yield for infectious pathogens appears comparable in patients with HM and patients with HSCT,[68] but the clinical utility of this study appears greatest when performed within 4 days of developing respiratory symptoms.[64] Fungal pathogens may be visualized directly on BAL samples via such techniques as Gomori methenamine silver staining or may be grown in culture, although the sensitivity of culture may be impaired by ongoing antifungal therapy at the time of BAL. As discussed further later in this article, BAL samples also can be submitted for fungal antigen detection.

Galactomannan

Galactomannan (GM) is an *Aspergillus* cell wall constituent released during hyphal growth in tissue. Galactomannan antigenemia is detectable via enzyme immunoassay up to a week before the onset of clinical manifestations of invasive aspergillosis, but is generally not observed in uninfected patients or those with *Aspergillus* colonization.[69,70] The utility of serum GM assays in asymptomatic immunocompromised populations has been an area of intensive investigation, and a recent Cochrane review[71] suggests that serial analysis may identify patients with IFI earlier than without screening. Some authorities suggest weekly or twice-weekly screening of serum for GM during the first 100 days after allogeneic HSCT and during HM-related neutropenia. However, serum GM screening of (lower-risk) patients with autologous HSCT does not appear to impact clinical outcomes.[72] Further, GM surveillance is generally limited to those not receiving antifungal prophylaxis, because the low pretest risk of invasive aspergillosis renders serum GM surveillance of asymptomatic patients unreliable.[73]

In addition to serum surveillance, GM assays on BAL fluid may enhance diagnoses of invasive pulmonary aspergillosis in patients with HM/HSCT with unexplained symptoms or abnormal radiographs. A recent meta-analysis suggests that BAL GM offers similar or better sensitivity and specificity than serum testing.[74] **Fig. 1** presents the diagnostic performance in recent studies,[75–97] revealing the strong diagnostic yield of BAL GM analysis in immunocompromised patients suspected of having pneumonia.

In the setting of established pulmonary aspergillosis, serum GM also can be used to monitor therapeutic responses.[98] Decreasing GM after 2 weeks of antifungal therapy in patients with concordant clinical responses demonstrates better survival that in those without GM declines. Failure of GM to decrease with therapy should prompt investigations to ensure adequacy of therapy.

(1,3)-β-D-glucan

(1,3)-β-D-glucan (BG) is a cell wall component of most fungal species, notably excluding Mucorales and *Cryptococcus* spp, detectable in blood during IFIs. A recent meta-analysis of studies in patients with HM[99] found serum BG to have very good sensitivity but relatively low specificity for IFI. The diagnostic performance appears better among patients with HM requiring intensive care unit admissions, and is unaffected by ongoing antifungal treatment,[100] unlike serum GM. The specificity of BG for IFI appears somewhat better in allogeneic HSCT recipients.[101] Blood transfusions, renal replacement therapy, β-lactam antibiotics, and bacterial infection[100] may cause false-positive BG results in commercially available BG assays.

MANAGEMENT OF HEMATOLOGIC MALIGNANCY/HEMATOPOIETIC STEM CELL TRANSPLANTATION FUNGAL PNEUMONIA

As infections in severely immunocompromised patients with HM/HSCT may rapidly progress to disseminated and/or fatal disease, prompt initiation of preemptive or empiric therapy is warranted when fungal pneumonia is suspected. In high-risk patients, it is not recommended to withhold therapy while awaiting results of serologic or culture studies. Unless bronchoscopy is immediately available (<2 hours), antifungal therapy should similarly not be withheld until diagnostic procedures have been completed, even acknowledging that antifungal treatments may reduce the sensitivity of BAL.

Antifungal Therapies

Concordant with the 2011 American Thoracic Society guidelines for treatment of fungal infections,[102] the initial treatment of patients with HM/HSCT with suspected invasive pulmonary aspergillosis consists of liposomal amphotericin B or intravenous voriconazole until improvement occurs, followed by transition to oral voriconazole or itraconazole. Intravenous posaconazole, caspofungin or micafungin may be required as salvage therapy in refractory disease. Once patients demonstrate clinical improvement, these salvage therapies can be followed by oral voriconazole or itraconazole until resolution of disease.

Reversal of immune suppression, such as neutropenia or chemotherapy, is generally important for successful treatment. Surgical excision should be considered in patients with HM/HSCT with focal disease or those with chronic necrotizing aspergillosis who fail antifungal treatment.[103]

Patients with HM/HSCT with probable or proven histoplasmosis or blastomycosis are typically managed with an amphotericin preparation then transitioned to extended therapy with oral itraconazole once their symptoms begin to improve. A brief course of systemic glucocorticoid may be considered in the setting of severe pulmonary histoplasmosis or blastomycosis. In cases with

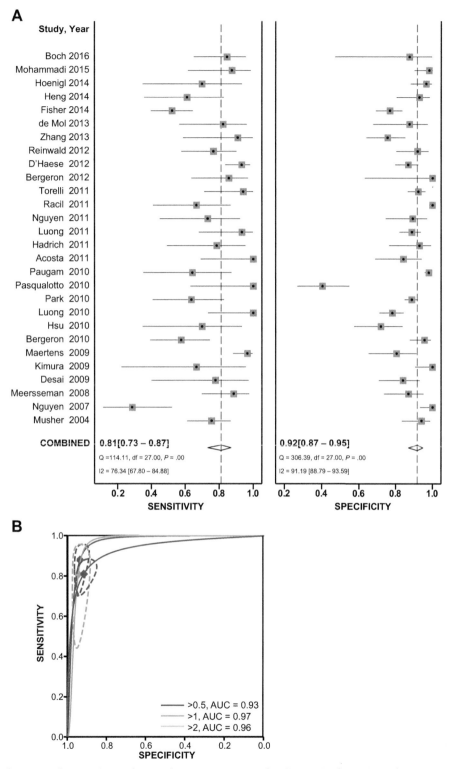

Fig. 1. Performance characteristics of BAL galactomannan assay for diagnosis of invasive pulmonary aspergillosis in patients with HM/HSCT. (*A*) Forest plots for sensitivity and specificity of BAL galactomannan EIA for probable or possible invasive pulmonary aspergillosis. Shown are estimated sensitivity and specificity (*gray squares*), 95% confidence intervals (*gray lines*), and combined sensitivity and specificity (*red dashed lines*). (*B*) Summary receiver operating characteristic curves for the studies in (*A*) at an optical index cutoff of greater than 0.5 (*red*), greater than 1 (*blue*), and greater than 2 (*green*) for probable or possible invasive aspergillosis. *Dashed lines*, 95% confidence intervals. AUC, area under the curve; EIA, enzyme immunoassay.

persistent immune suppression, urine or serum histoplasma antigen testing may be useful to detect breakthrough infections.

Mild, limited pulmonary coccidioidomycosis can often be managed with azole monotherapy, although treatment may be needed for as long as 18 months. Patients with diffuse pulmonary disease often require initial treatment with an amphotericin preparation until clinical improvement is demonstrated, followed by long-term treatment with oral fluconazole or itraconazole. Patients who remain immunocompromised may even require lifelong itraconazole therapy.

Limited evidence exists to recommend specific treatments for Mucorales or other less frequent fungal pneumonias in patients with HM/HSCT. Early initiation of amphotericin-based therapy appears to improve outcomes in zygomycosis.[104] In general, amphotericin preparations are accepted as the first line of therapy for these organisms, with posaconazole and isavuconazole used for salvage therapy.[105,106] When feasible, surgical debridement should be considered, especially to avoid fatal hemoptysis in perihilar disease.[106]

Host-Directed Therapies

Successful management of fungal pneumonia in patients with HM/HSCT often depends on reversal of immunocompromising conditions. This includes withdrawal of immunosuppressive or cytotoxic medications, or ideally, reversal of host defects/control of the underlying disease.

A major research focus has been correction of granulocytopenia. Preparations of granulocyte colony-stimulating factor (G-CSF) and granulocyte-macrophage CSF are commercially available, and can reduce the duration of neutropenia.[39,107] Although evidence suggests CSFs prevent some pneumonias in neutropenic populations,[84] they are not generally recommended as a treatment of established infections. Current data support administration of G-CSF if a patient's risk of developing febrile neutropenia is greater than 20%.[39] Infusion of donor granulocytes has also been proposed as an adjunct therapy for patients with febrile neutropenia. Although this strategy holds promise, it remains investigational.[108] Beyond increasing leukocyte counts, others have investigated manipulation of existing leukocytes through administration of recombinant cytokines. Exogenous interferon-gamma has demonstrated some success in reducing infections in patients with congenital neutropenia, and recent studies suggest efficacy against opportunistic infections following HSCT.[109,110]

Induction of antimicrobial responses directly from lung cells offers a novel alternative strategy to prevent, and possibly treat, pneumonias in patients with HM/HSCT. Lung epithelial cells are relatively chemotherapy resistant and possess the capacity to detect pathogens, to modulate local immune responses, and to generate microbicidal responses through the production of antimicrobial peptides and reactive species.[111–114] Advances in the understanding of the molecular mechanisms of these responses have allowed development of inhaled therapeutics that induce protective innate immune responses from the lung epithelium. In animal models of pneumonia, this approach provides protection against lethal pathogens, even when there is concurrent neutropenia.[112,115] One such treatment, known as PUL-042, demonstrates inducible protection against gram-positive, gram-negative, fungal, and viral pneumonias in animal models and is now in clinical trials. Augmentation of innate immune responses offers several hypothetical advantages in terms of rapid effect and broad specificity, but efficacy has not been established in humans.

SUMMARY

Fungal pneumonias cause substantial morbidity among patients with HM/HSCT. A high index of suspicion for invasive fungal infection should be maintained in immunocompromised patients with nonspecific symptoms and pursued with multiple diagnostic modalities, including CT, early bronchoscopy, and complementary tests. Early initiation and ongoing monitoring of antifungal therapy are essential to ensuring acceptable clinical outcomes.

REFERENCES

1. Margalit A, Kavanagh K. The innate immune response to Aspergillus fumigatus at the alveolar surface. FEMS Microbiol Rev 2015;39(5):670–87.
2. Latgé JP. Aspergillus fumigatus and aspergillosis. Clin Microbiol Rev 1999;12(2):310–50.
3. Bitar D, Lortholary O, Le Strat Y, et al. Population-based analysis of invasive fungal infections, France, 2001-2010. Emerg Infect Dis 2014;20(7): 1149–55.
4. Azie N, Neofytos D, Pfaller M, et al. (Prospective Antifungal Therapy) Alliance® registry and invasive fungal infections: update 2012. Diagn Microbiol Infect Dis 2012;73(4):293–300.
5. Caira M, Trecarichi EM, Mancinelli M, et al. Uncommon mold infections in hematological patients: epidemiology, diagnosis and treatment. Expert Rev Anti Infect Ther 2011;9(7):881–92.

6. Brown GD, Denning DW, Gow NA, et al. Hidden killers: human fungal infections. Sci Transl Med 2012;4(165):165rv113.

7. Hammond SP, Baden LR, Marty FM. Mortality in hematologic malignancy and hematopoietic stem cell transplant patients with mucormycosis, 2001 to 2009. Antimicrob Agents Chemother 2011;55(11): 5018–21.

8. Malcolm TR, Chin-Hong PV. Endemic mycoses in immunocompromised hosts. Curr Infect Dis Rep 2013;15(6):536–43.

9. Woods JP. Revisiting old friends: developments in understanding *Histoplasma capsulatum* pathogenesis. J Microbiol 2016;54(3):265–76.

10. Centers for Disease Control and Prevention (CDC). Increase in reported coccidioidomycosis–United States, 1998-2011. MMWR Morb Mortal Wkly Rep 2013;62(12):217–21.

11. Kauffman CA, Freifeld AG, Andes DR, et al. Endemic fungal infections in solid organ and hematopoietic cell transplant recipients enrolled in the Transplant-Associated Infection Surveillance Network (TRANSNET). Transpl Infect Dis 2014; 16(2):213–24.

12. Auberger J, Lass-Flörl C, Ulmer H, et al. Significant alterations in the epidemiology and treatment outcome of invasive fungal infections in patients with hematological malignancies. Int J Hematol 2008;88(5):508–15.

13. Cadena J, Thompson GR, Patterson TF. Invasive aspergillosis: current strategies for diagnosis and management. Infect Dis Clin North Am 2016; 30(1):125–42.

14. Wahid SF. Indications and outcomes of reduced-toxicity hematopoietic stem cell transplantation in adult patients with hematological malignancies. Int J Hematol 2013;97(5):581–98.

15. Smith JA, Kauffman CA. Pulmonary fungal infections. Respirology 2012;17(6):913–26.

16. Kwon-Chung KJ. Taxonomy of fungi causing mucormycosis and entomophthoramycosis (zygomycosis) and nomenclature of the disease: molecular mycologic perspectives. Clin Infect Dis 2012;54(Suppl 1):S8–15.

17. Kontoyiannis DP, Marr KA, Park BJ, et al. Prospective surveillance for invasive fungal infections in hematopoietic stem cell transplant recipients, 2001-2006: overview of the Transplant-Associated Infection Surveillance Network (TRANSNET) Database. Clin Infect Dis 2010;50(8):1091–100.

18. Tacke D, Koehler P, Markiefka B, et al. Our 2014 approach to mucormycosis. Mycoses 2014;57(9): 519–24.

19. Wheat LJ, Azar MM, Bahr NC, et al. Histoplasmosis. Infect Dis Clin North Am 2016;30(1):207–27.

20. Stockamp NW, Thompson GR. Coccidioidomycosis. Infect Dis Clin North Am 2016;30(1):229–46.

21. Castillo CG, Kauffman CA, Miceli MH. Blastomycosis. Infect Dis Clin North Am 2016;30(1):247–64.

22. Calderone RA, Cihlar RL. Fungal pathogenesis: principles and clinical applications. New York: Marcel Dekker; 2002.

23. Horwath MC, Fecher RA, Deepe GS. Histoplasma capsulatum, lung infection and immunity. Future Microbiol 2015;10(6):967–75.

24. Romani L. Immunity to fungal infections. Nat Rev Immunol 2011;11(4):275–88.

25. Ben-Ami R, Lewis RE, Kontoyiannis DP. Enemy of the (immunosuppressed) state: an update on the pathogenesis of *Aspergillus fumigatus* infection. Br J Haematol 2010;150(4):406–17.

26. Colmone A, Amorim M, Pontier AL, et al. Leukemic cells create bone marrow niches that disrupt the behavior of normal hematopoietic progenitor cells. Science 2008;322(5909):1861–5.

27. Pagano L, Akova M, Dimopoulos G, et al. Risk assessment and prognostic factors for mould-related diseases in immunocompromised patients. J Antimicrob Chemother 2011;66(Suppl 1):i5–14.

28. Mussai F, De Santo C, Abu-Dayyeh I, et al. Acute myeloid leukemia creates an arginase-dependent immunosuppressive microenvironment. Blood 2013;122(5):749–58.

29. De Pauw B, Walsh TJ, Donnelly JP, et al. Revised definitions of invasive fungal disease from the European Organization for Research and Treatment of Cancer/Invasive Fungal Infections Cooperative Group and the National Institute of Allergy and Infectious Diseases Mycoses Study Group (EORTC/MSG) Consensus Group. Clin Infect Dis 2008; 46(12):1813–21.

30. Kontoyiannis DP. Antifungal prophylaxis in hematopoietic stem cell transplant recipients: the unfinished tale of imperfect success. Bone Marrow Transplant 2011;46(2):165–73.

31. Gerson SL, Talbot GH, Hurwitz S, et al. Prolonged granulocytopenia: the major risk factor for invasive pulmonary aspergillosis in patients with acute leukemia. Ann Intern Med 1984;100(3):345–51.

32. Balloy V, Huerre M, Latgé JP, et al. Differences in patterns of infection and inflammation for corticosteroid treatment and chemotherapy in experimental invasive pulmonary aspergillosis. Infect Immun 2005;73(1):494–503.

33. Chamilos G, Luna M, Lewis RE, et al. Invasive fungal infections in patients with hematologic malignancies in a tertiary care cancer center: an autopsy study over a 15-year period (1989-2003). Haematologica 2006;91(7):986–9.

34. Lewis RE, Cahyame-Zuniga L, Leventakos K, et al. Epidemiology and sites of involvement of invasive fungal infections in patients with haematological malignancies: a 20-year autopsy study. Mycoses 2013;56(6):638–45.

35. Kontoyiannis DP, Georgiadou SP, Wierda WG, et al. Impaired bactericidal but not fungicidal activity of polymorphonuclear neutrophils in patients with chronic lymphocytic leukemia. Leuk Lymphoma 2013;54(8):1730–3.

36. Lass-Flörl C, Roilides E, Löffler J, et al. Minireview: host defence in invasive aspergillosis. Mycoses 2013;56(1):103–13.

37. Abers MS, Ghebremichael MS, Timmons AK, et al. A critical reappraisal of prolonged neutropenia as a risk factor for invasive pulmonary aspergillosis. Open Forum Infect Dis 2016;3(1):ofw036.

38. Cherif H, Axdorph U, Kalin M, et al. Clinical experience of granulocyte transfusion in the management of neutropenic patients with haematological malignancies and severe infection. Scand J Infect Dis 2013;45(2):112–6.

39. Skoetz N, Bohlius J, Engert A, et al. Prophylactic antibiotics or G(M)-CSF for the prevention of infections and improvement of survival in cancer patients receiving myelotoxic chemotherapy. Cochrane Database Syst Rev 2015;(12):CD007107.

40. Mulanovich VE, Kontoyiannis DP. Fungal pneumonia in patients with hematologic malignancies: current approach and management. Curr Opin Infect Dis 2011;24(4):323–32.

41. Sun Y, Meng F, Han M, et al. Epidemiology, management, and outcome of invasive fungal disease in patients undergoing hematopoietic stem cell transplantation in China: a multicenter prospective observational study. Biol Blood Marrow Transplant 2015;21(6):1117–26.

42. Harrison N, Mitterbauer M, Tobudic S, et al. Incidence and characteristics of invasive fungal diseases in allogeneic hematopoietic stem cell transplant recipients: a retrospective cohort study. BMC Infect Dis 2015;15:584.

43. Khayr W, Haddad RY, Noor SA. Infections in hematological malignancies. Dis Mon 2012;58(4):239–49.

44. Andersen MH. The targeting of immunosuppressive mechanisms in hematological malignancies. Leukemia 2014;28(9):1784–92.

45. Jiang Y, Li Y, Zhu B. T-cell exhaustion in the tumor microenvironment. Cell Death Dis 2015;6:e1792.

46. Casadevall A, Pirofski LA. Immunoglobulins in defense, pathogenesis, and therapy of fungal diseases. Cell Host Microbe 2012;11(5):447–56.

47. Segal BH, Bow EJ, Menichetti F. Fungal infections in nontransplant patients with hematologic malignancies. Infect Dis Clin North Am 2002;16(4):935–64, vii.

48. Prevention CfDCa, America IDSo, Transplantation ASoBaM. Guidelines for preventing opportunistic infections among hematopoietic stem cell transplant recipients. MMWR Recomm Rep 2000; 49(RR-10):1–125. CE121–7.

49. Center for International Blood and Marrow Transplant Research (CIBMTR), National Marrow Donor Program (NMDP), European Blood and Marrow Transplant Group (EBMT), et al. Guidelines for preventing infectious complications among hematopoietic cell transplant recipients: a global perspective. Bone Marrow Transplant 2009;44(8):453–558.

50. Arnaout K, Patel N, Jain M, et al. Complications of allogeneic hematopoietic stem cell transplantation. Cancer Invest 2014;32(7):349–62.

51. Filipovich AH, Weisdorf D, Pavletic S, et al. National Institutes of Health consensus development project on criteria for clinical trials in chronic graft-versus-host disease: I. Diagnosis and staging working group report. Biol Blood Marrow Transplant 2005; 11(12):945–56.

52. Kurosawa M, Yonezumi M, Hashino S, et al. Epidemiology and treatment outcome of invasive fungal infections in patients with hematological malignancies. Int J Hematol 2012;96(6):748–57.

53. Sainz J, Hassan L, Perez E, et al. Interleukin-10 promoter polymorphism as risk factor to develop invasive pulmonary aspergillosis. Immunol Lett 2007;109(1):76–82.

54. Sainz J, Pérez E, Hassan L, et al. Variable number of tandem repeats of TNF receptor type 2 promoter as genetic biomarker of susceptibility to develop invasive pulmonary aspergillosis. Hum Immunol 2007;68(1):41–50.

55. Kurosawa M, Yonezumi M, Hashino S, et al. Epidemiology and treatment outcome of invasive fungal infections in patients with hematological malignancies. Int J Hematol 2012;96:748–57.

56. Cunha C, Di Ianni M, Bozza S, et al. Dectin-1 Y238X polymorphism associates with susceptibility to invasive aspergillosis in hematopoietic transplantation through impairment of both recipient- and donor-dependent mechanisms of antifungal immunity. Blood 2010;116(24):5394–402.

57. Montagna MT, Lovero G, Coretti C, et al. SIMIFF study: Italian fungal registry of mold infections in hematological and non-hematological patients. Infection 2014;42(1):141–51.

58. Legouge C, Caillot D, Chrétien ML, et al. The reversed halo sign: pathognomonic pattern of pulmonary mucormycosis in leukemic patients with neutropenia? Clin Infect Dis 2014;58(5):672–8.

59. Kojima R, Tateishi U, Kami M, et al. Chest computed tomography of late invasive aspergillosis after allogeneic hematopoietic stem cell transplantation. Biol Blood Marrow Transplant 2005; 11(7):506–11.

60. Stanzani M, Sassi C, Lewis RE, et al. High resolution computed tomography angiography improves the radiographic diagnosis of invasive mold disease in patients with hematological malignancies. Clin Infect Dis 2015;60(11):1603–10.

61. Reyes N, Onadeko OO, Luraschi Monjagatta Mdel C, et al. Positron emission tomography in the evaluation of pulmonary nodules among patients living in a coccidioidal endemic region. Lung 2014;192(4):589–93.

62. Gupta S, Sultenfuss M, Romaguera JE, et al. CT-guided percutaneous lung biopsies in patients with haematologic malignancies and undiagnosed pulmonary lesions. Hematol Oncol 2010;28(2): 75–81.

63. Ascioglu S, Rex JH, de Pauw B, et al. Defining opportunistic invasive fungal infections in immunocompromised patients with cancer and hematopoietic stem cell transplants: an international consensus. Clin Infect Dis 2002;34(1):7–14.

64. Shannon VR, Andersson BS, Lei X, et al. Utility of early versus late fiberoptic bronchoscopy in the evaluation of new pulmonary infiltrates following hematopoietic stem cell transplantation. Bone Marrow Transplant 2010;45(4):647–55.

65. Hummel M, Rudert S, Hof H, et al. Diagnostic yield of bronchoscopy with bronchoalveolar lavage in febrile patients with hematologic malignancies and pulmonary infiltrates. Ann Hematol 2008; 87(4):291–7.

66. Kim SW, Rhee CK, Kang HS, et al. Diagnostic value of bronchoscopy in patients with hematologic malignancy and pulmonary infiltrates. Ann Hematol 2015;94(1):153–9.

67. Boersma WG, Erjavec Z, van der Werf TS, et al. Bronchoscopic diagnosis of pulmonary infiltrates in granulocytopenic patients with hematologic malignancies: BAL versus PSB and PBAL. Respir Med 2007;101(2):317–25.

68. Gilbert CR, Lerner A, Baram M, et al. Utility of flexible bronchoscopy in the evaluation of pulmonary infiltrates in the hematopoietic stem cell transplant population–a single center fourteen year experience. Arch Bronconeumol 2013;49(5):189–95.

69. Wingard JR. Have novel serum markers supplanted tissue diagnosis for invasive fungal infections in acute leukemia and transplantation? Best Pract Res Clin Haematol 2012;25(4):487–91.

70. Hoenigl M, Salzer HJ, Raggam RB, et al. Impact of galactomannan testing on the prevalence of invasive aspergillosis in patients with hematological malignancies. Med Mycol 2012;50(3):266–9.

71. Leeflang MM, Debets-Ossenkopp YJ, Wang J, et al. Galactomannan detection for invasive aspergillosis in immunocompromised patients. Cochrane Database Syst Rev 2015;(12):CD007394.

72. Jathavedam A, Duré DC, Taur Y, et al. Limited utility of serum galactomannan assay after auto-SCT. Bone Marrow Transplant 2009;44(1):59–61.

73. Duarte RF, Sánchez-Ortega I, Cuesta I, et al. Serum galactomannan-based early detection of invasive aspergillosis in hematology patients receiving effective antimold prophylaxis. Clin Infect Dis 2014;59(12):1696–702.

74. Wheat LJ, Walsh TJ. Diagnosis of invasive aspergillosis by galactomannan antigenemia detection using an enzyme immunoassay. Eur J Clin Microbiol Infect Dis 2008;27(4):245–51.

75. Acosta J, Catalan M, del Palacio-Peréz-Medel A, et al. A prospective comparison of galactomannan in bronchoalveolar lavage fluid for the diagnosis of pulmonary invasive aspergillosis in medical patients under intensive care: comparison with the diagnostic performance of galactomannan and of (1→ 3)-β-d-glucan chromogenic assay in serum samples. Clin Microbiol Infect 2011;17(7):1053–60.

76. Bergeron A, Porcher R, Menotti J, et al. Prospective evaluation of clinical and biological markers to predict the outcome of invasive pulmonary aspergillosis in hematological patients. J Clin Microbiol 2012;50(3):823–30.

77. Boch T, Buchheidt D, Spiess B, et al. Direct comparison of galactomannan performance in concurrent serum and bronchoalveolar lavage samples in immunocompromised patients at risk for invasive pulmonary aspergillosis. Mycoses 2016;59(2): 80–5.

78. de Mol M, de Jongste JC, van Westreenen M, et al. Diagnosis of invasive pulmonary aspergillosis in children with bronchoalveolar lavage galactomannan. Pediatr Pulmonol 2013;48(8):789–96.

79. Desai R, Ross LA, Hoffman JA. The role of bronchoalveolar lavage galactomannan in the diagnosis of pediatric invasive aspergillosis. Pediatr Infect Dis J 2009;28(4):283–6.

80. D'Haese J, Theunissen K, Vermeulen E, et al. Detection of galactomannan in bronchoalveolar lavage fluid samples of patients at risk for invasive pulmonary aspergillosis: analytical and clinical validity. J Clin Microbiol 2012;50(4):1258–63.

81. Fisher CE, Stevens AM, Leisenring W, et al. Independent contribution of bronchoalveolar lavage and serum galactomannan in the diagnosis of invasive pulmonary aspergillosis. Transpl Infect Dis 2014;16(3):505–10.

82. Hadrich I, Mary C, Makni F, et al. Comparison of PCR-ELISA and Real-Time PCR for invasive aspergillosis diagnosis in patients with hematological malignancies. Med Mycol 2011;49(5):489–94.

83. Heng SC, Chen SC, Morrissey CO, et al. Clinical utility of *Aspergillus galactomannan* and PCR in bronchoalveolar lavage fluid for the diagnosis of invasive pulmonary aspergillosis in patients with haematological malignancies. Diagn Microbiol Infect Dis 2014;79(3):322–7.

84. Hoenigl M, Prattes J, Spiess B, et al. Performance of galactomannan, beta-d-glucan, *Aspergillus* lateral-flow device, conventional culture, and PCR tests with bronchoalveolar lavage fluid for

diagnosis of invasive pulmonary aspergillosis. J Clin Microbiol 2014;52(6):2039–45.

85. Hsu LY, Ding Y, Phua J, et al. Galactomannan testing of bronchoalveolar lavage fluid is useful for diagnosis of invasive pulmonary aspergillosis in hematology patients. BMC Infect Dis 2010;10:44.

86. Kimura S, Odawara J, Aoki T, et al. Detection of sputum Aspergillus galactomannan for diagnosis of invasive pulmonary aspergillosis in haematological patients. Int J Hematol 2009;90(4):463–70.

87. Luong ML, Clancy CJ, Vadnerkar A, et al. Comparison of an Aspergillus real-time polymerase chain reaction assay with galactomannan testing of bronchoalvelolar lavage fluid for the diagnosis of invasive pulmonary aspergillosis in lung transplant recipients. Clin Infect Dis 2011;52(10):1218–26.

88. Meersseman W, Lagrou K, Maertens J, et al. Galactomannan in bronchoalveolar lavage fluid: a tool for diagnosing aspergillosis in intensive care unit patients. Am J Respir Crit Care Med 2008; 177(1):27–34.

89. Mohammadi S, Khalilzadeh S, Goudarzipour K, et al. Bronchoalveolar galactomannan in invasive pulmonary aspergillosis: a prospective study in pediatric patients. Med Mycol 2015;53(7):709–16.

90. Musher B, Fredricks D, Leisenring W, et al. Aspergillus galactomannan enzyme immunoassay and quantitative PCR for diagnosis of invasive aspergillosis with bronchoalveolar lavage fluid. J Clin Microbiol 2004;42(12):5517–22.

91. Nguyen MH, Jaber R, Leather HL, et al. Use of bronchoalveolar lavage to detect galactomannan for diagnosis of pulmonary aspergillosis among nonimmunocompromised hosts. J Clin Microbiol 2007;45(9):2787–92.

92. Nguyen MH, Leather H, Clancy CJ, et al. Galactomannan testing in bronchoalveolar lavage fluid facilitates the diagnosis of invasive pulmonary aspergillosis in patients with hematologic malignancies and stem cell transplant recipients. Biol Blood Marrow Transplant 2011;17(7):1043–50.

93. Pasqualotto AC, Xavier MO, Sánchez LB, et al. Diagnosis of invasive aspergillosis in lung transplant recipients by detection of galactomannan in the bronchoalveolar lavage fluid. Transplantation 2010;90(3):306–11.

94. Paugam A, Baixench MT, Lebuisson A, et al. Diagnosis of invasive pulmonary aspergillosis: value of bronchoalveolar lavage galactomannan for immunocompromised patients. Pathol Biol (Paris) 2010; 58(1):100–3 [in French].

95. Racil Z, Kocmanova I, Toskova M, et al. Galactomannan detection in bronchoalveolar lavage fluid for the diagnosis of invasive aspergillosis in patients with hematological diseases—the role of factors affecting assay performance. Int J Infect Dis 2011;15(12):e874–81.

96. Torelli R, Sanguinetti M, Moody A, et al. Diagnosis of invasive aspergillosis by a commercial real-time PCR assay for Aspergillus DNA in bronchoalveolar lavage fluid samples from high-risk patients compared to a galactomannan enzyme immunoassay. J Clin Microbiol 2011;49(12):4273–8.

97. Zhang XB, Chen GP, Lin QC, et al. Bronchoalveolar lavage fluid galactomannan detection for diagnosis of invasive pulmonary aspergillosis in chronic obstructive pulmonary disease. Med Mycol 2013; 51(7):688–95.

98. Neofytos D, Railkar R, Mullane KM, et al. Correlation between circulating fungal biomarkers and clinical outcome in invasive aspergillosis. PLoS One 2015;10(6):e0129022.

99. Lamoth F, Cruciani M, Mengoli C, et al. β-Glucan antigenemia assay for the diagnosis of invasive fungal infections in patients with hematological malignancies: a systematic review and meta-analysis of cohort studies from the Third European Conference on Infections in Leukemia (ECIL-3). Clin Infect Dis 2012;54(5):633–43.

100. Azoulay E, Guigue N, Darmon M, et al. (1, 3)-β-D-glucan assay for diagnosing invasive fungal infections in critically ill patients with hematological malignancies. Oncotarget 2016;7(16):21484–95.

101. Reischies FM, Prattes J, Woelfler A, et al. Diagnostic performance of 1,3-beta-d-glucan serum screening in patients receiving hematopoietic stem cell transplantation. Transpl Infect Dis 2016; 18(3):466–70.

102. Limper AH, Knox KS, Sarosi GA, et al. An official American Thoracic Society statement: treatment of fungal infections in adult pulmonary and critical care patients. Am J Respir Crit Care Med 2011; 183(1):96–128.

103. Wu GX, Khojabekyan M, Wang J, et al. Survival following lung resection in immunocompromised patients with pulmonary invasive fungal infection. Eur J Cardiothorac Surg 2016;49(1):314–20.

104. Chamilos G, Lewis RE, Kontoyiannis DP. Delaying amphotericin B-based frontline therapy significantly increases mortality among patients with hematologic malignancy who have zygomycosis. Clin Infect Dis 2008;47(4):503–9.

105. Kontoyiannis DP, Lewis RE. How I treat mucormycosis. Blood 2011;118(5):1216–24.

106. Farmakiotis D, Kontoyiannis DP. Mucormycoses. Infect Dis Clin North Am 2016;30(1):143–63.

107. Dale DC. Colony-stimulating factors for the management of neutropenia in cancer patients. Drugs 2002;62(Suppl 1):1–15.

108. Estcourt LJ, Stanworth SJ, Hopewell S, et al. Granulocyte transfusions for treating infections in people with neutropenia or neutrophil dysfunction. Cochrane Database Syst Rev 2016;(4): CD005339.

109. Safdar A. Strategies to enhance immune function in hematopoietic transplantation recipients who have fungal infections. Bone Marrow Transplant 2006; 38(5):327–37.
110. Safdar A, Rodriguez GH, Lichtiger B, et al. Recombinant interferon gamma1b immune enhancement in 20 patients with hematologic malignancies and systemic opportunistic infections treated with donor granulocyte transfusions. Cancer 2006; 106(12):2664–71.
111. Bals R, Hiemstra PS. Innate immunity in the lung: how epithelial cells fight against respiratory pathogens. Eur Respir J 2004;23(2):327–33.
112. Cleaver JO, You D, Michaud DR, et al. Lung epithelial cells are essential effectors of inducible resistance to pneumonia. Mucosal Immunol 2014;7(1): 78–88.
113. Gribar SC, Richardson WM, Sodhi CP, et al. No longer an innocent bystander: epithelial toll-like receptor signaling in the development of mucosal inflammation. Mol Med 2008;14(9–10):645–59.
114. Evans SE, Xu Y, Tuvim MJ, et al. Inducible innate resistance of lung epithelium to infection. Annu Rev Physiol 2010;72:413–35.
115. Leiva-Juarez MM, Ware HH, Kulkarni VV, et al. Inducible epithelial resistance protects mice against leukemia-associated pneumonia. Blood 2016;128(7):982–92.
116. Pagano L, Caira M, Candoni A, et al. The epidemiology of fungal infections in patients with hematologic malignancies: the SEIFEM-2004 study. Haematologica 2006;91(8):1068–75.
117. Pagano L, Caira M, Nosari A, et al. Fungal infections in recipients of hematopoietic stem cell transplants: results of the SEIFEM B-2004 study–Sorveglianza Epidemiologica Infezioni Fungine Nelle Emopatie Maligne. Clin Infect Dis 2007; 45(9):1161–70.
118. Neofytos D, Horn D, Anaissie E, et al. Epidemiology and outcome of invasive fungal infection in adult hematopoietic stem cell transplant recipients: analysis of Multicenter Prospective Antifungal Therapy (PATH) Alliance registry. Clin Infect Dis 2009; 48(3):265–73.
119. Sun Y, Huang H, Chen J, et al. Invasive fungal infection in patients receiving chemotherapy for hematological malignancy: a multicenter, prospective, observational study in China. Tumour Biol 2015;36(2):757–67.
120. Zaas AK, Liao G, Chien JW, et al. Plasminogen alleles influence susceptibility to invasive aspergillosis. PLoS Genet 2008;4(6):e1000101.

Candidemia in the Intensive Care Unit

Oleg Epelbaum, MD[a],*, Rachel Chasan, MD, MPH[b]

KEYWORDS

- Candidemia • Invasive candidiasis • *Candida* • Intensive care unit • Critical care • Fungal infection

KEY POINTS

- *Candida* is the most common invasive mycosis in critically ill patients.
- Candidemia in the intensive care unit extends the length of stay, increases health care costs, and carries a high crude mortality.
- The contribution of non-albicans *Candida* species to this infection is on the rise.
- The role of antifungal administration before culture confirmation of candidemia in critical care units remains debatable.
- Echinocandins are the drug class of choice for the treatment of established intensive care unit candidemia.

INTRODUCTION

Invasive candidiasis (IC), distinct from localized, mucocutaneous candidiasis, is a prevalent and burdensome infection of particular importance to intensive care unit (ICU) physicians. Its initial association with chemotherapy-induced neutropenia has progressively widened to encompass a broad spectrum of ICU patients in parallel with advances in organ support techniques, therapeutic immunosuppression, and antibacterial pharmacotherapy. Candidemia, the most common means by which IC is diagnosed clinically, is the principal focus of this review, although it should be borne in mind that organ involvement can take on many forms, including peritoneal, ocular, pulmonary, and central nervous system manifestations. IC presents several challenges to the ICU community. Recognition and, therefore, treatment of this infection are frequently delayed, with dramatic clinical deterioration and death often preceding the detection of *Candida* in blood cultures. Identification of individual patients at highest risk for developing candidemia remains an imperfect science, and the role of untargeted (ie, before microbiological confirmation) antifungal therapy in the ICU is yet to be fully defined. Antifungal resistance among typical *Candida* isolates and the emergence of novel, multi-drug-resistant species such as *Candida auris* complicate therapeutic decision making. The absence of well-established molecular techniques for early detection of candidemia hinders efforts to reduce the heavy clinical and economic impact of this infection. What follows is a review of nonneutropenic candidemia in the ICU with an emphasis on the aforementioned diagnostic and management challenges.

EPIDEMIOLOGY
Background

Candida is the most common invasive fungus in critically ill patients, and the candidemia rate in ICUs is about 10 to 20 times that of non-ICU

Disclosure Statement: The authors have nothing to disclose.
[a] Division of Pulmonary, Critical Care, and Sleep Medicine, Westchester Medical Center, New York Medical College, 100 Woods Road, Macy Pavilion Room 1042, Valhalla, NY 10595, USA; [b] Division of Infectious Diseases, Icahn School of Medicine at Mount Sinai, One Gustave L. Levy Place, Box 1090, New York, NY 10029, USA
* Corresponding author.
E-mail address: oleg.epelbaum@wmchealth.org

Clin Chest Med 38 (2017) 493–509
http://dx.doi.org/10.1016/j.ccm.2017.04.010
0272-5231/17/© 2017 Elsevier Inc. All rights reserved.

chestmed.theclinics.com

settings.[1,2] Among critical care areas, the highest incidence belongs to burn units.[3] Candidemia can impose a significant operational and budgetary burden on an ICU: it was shown to prolong ICU stay by nearly 13 days in one study while adding an estimated $8570 (€7800) in attributable costs in another, driven primarily by sepsis treatment itself.[4,5] Although more than 15 species of Candida have been implicated in human disease, almost all episodes of candidemia can be ascribed to 1 of 5 species: Candida albicans, Candida glabrata, Candida tropicalis, Candida parapsilosis, and Candida krusei (Table 1). C albicans is the most prevalent isolate globally, responsible for approximately 40% to 60% of cases.[6,7] In a growing number of reports, particularly more contemporary ones, C albicans constitutes the minority of Candida isolates.[6,8,9] The most prevalent non-albicans species varies geographically. In European and Australian ICUs, C glabrata, less virulent than C albicans and associated with increasing age and solid organ transplants, is generally the most common non-albicans isolate, accounting for about 20% of infections.[2,3,10] Isolation of C tropicalis, which is on par with C albicans in terms of virulence, is comparatively infrequent (~9%). A 2006 series from an Italian ICU with a large immunosuppressed contingent reported a 23% rate of the hypovirulent C parapsilosis, and a very recent Chinese ICU cohort representing diverse pathology recapitulated the same finding.[9,11,12] In South America, on the other hand, these proportions are reversed: C tropicalis is the most common non-albicans isolate (~20%), whereas C glabrata accounts for 9%.[13] These differences in species distribution may help explain the disparate ICU candidemia crude mortality figures reported from Europe and South America: 50% and 70%,

respectively.[7,10,13] Determining the attributable mortality of ICU candidemia, the net contribution of this infection to mortality beyond that expected from overall clinical status, is hampered by a paucity of data and lack of patient matching. In a retrospective, matched cohort study of Belgian ICU patients with high critical illness scores (mean Acute Physiology and Chronic Health Evaluation [APACHE] II of 25), the attributable mortality of candidemia was only 5% in comparison to 20% for a likewise matched Chinese surgical ICU population with severe sepsis and lower APACHE scores.[14,15] Studied prospectively, a global ICU cohort exhibited a nonsignificant difference of less than 5% in hospital mortality between candidemic and noncandidemic subjects after propensity score matching.[16] On the other hand, attributable mortality as high as 49% was observed in a case-control study of non-ICU candidemic adults.[17] Possible reasons for the disparity between results within and outside the ICU include earlier and more appropriate initiation of therapy in the ICU as well as the greater baseline disease severity of the critically ill, which reduces the incremental significance of any individual contributor.[18] Differences in local practices, patient types, severity of illness, and study periods may similarly account for contrasting attributable mortalities across ICU studies.

Albicans versus Non-Albicans Species

The shifting epidemiology of Candida toward non-albicans species reported by some, although not all, institutions is clinically relevant because of the high rates of fluconazole resistance among C glabrata isolates and the intrinsic fluconazole resistance of C krusei.[19,20] This development has

Table 1
Epidemiologic and clinical characteristics of the 5 most common Candida species

Species	Geographic Concentration	Age Predilection	Relative Virulence	Characteristic Clinical Associations	Fluconazole Susceptibility
C albicans	Global	None	High	Endophthalmitis	+++
C glabrata	Europe, US, Australia	Older	Intermediate	SOT	+
C tropicalis	SA, US, Asia	None	High	Immunosuppression	++
C parapsilosis	Europe, SA, Australasia	Younger	Low	Medical devices	+++
C krusei	Europe, US	None	Intermediate	Hematological malignancy	–

Abbreviations: SA, South America; SOT, solid organ transplant.
Data from Refs.[37,116–120]

spurred recent interest in identifying variables associated with non-albicans candidemia in ICU patients. Shorr and colleagues[21] were among the first investigators to explore this question, but their retrospective analysis failed to produce any factors independently associated with non-albicans candidemia either inside or outside of the ICU. Subsequent studies restricted to the critically ill yielded several compelling associations with non-albicans spp, such as central venous catheter (CVC) placement and duration, prior fluconazole exposure and its length, increasing age, and previous gastrointestinal instrumentation.[22–24] When *C glabrata*, the most prevalent non-albicans isolate in the United States and Europe, was examined separately, the risk factor profile remained remarkably similar with the notable addition of preceding exposure to broad-spectrum antibacterial agents and shorter ICU time to fungemia.[25,26]

Surgical versus Nonsurgical Patients

Comparisons between the incidence rates and densities of candidemia in medical ICUs versus surgical ICUs suggest that it occurs more frequently in the latter. In a multicenter French study, the incidence rate was higher in surgical ICUs (7.3 episodes/1000 admissions) than in medical ICUs (5.3 episodes/1000 admissions); in contrast, the incidence density was nearly identical at ~0.60 episodes per 1000 patient-days.[3] The above incidence rate of 7.3/1000 admissions to surgical critical care is within the incidence range of 7 to 9/1000 admissions derived from several other surgical ICU populations.[15,27] A higher incidence density of 0.98/1000 patient-days has been reported, however, by a large surgical ICU collaborative composed of North American centers.[28] Despite the seemingly higher burden of candidemia in surgical ICUs, crude mortality numbers favored postoperative patients compared with nonoperative cases in a cohort of well-matched critically ill subjects: 45% and 85%, respectively.[29] Not surprisingly, abdominal and thoracic operations are the most common surgical categories among patients with IC, whereas trauma and neurosurgical cases are relatively infrequent.[27] Risk factors for candidemia in surgical critical care largely mirror those identified for ICU patients generally, although higher duration of invasive mechanical ventilation and concomitant bacterial infection, especially with mixed flora, figure prominently in the surgical literature.[15,30] Unique to the care of cardiac surgery patients is the finding that cardiopulmonary bypass time greater than 120 minutes confers 8 times greater odds of developing candidemia to those patients,

much higher than those conferred by diabetes mellitus, for example, to the same patients (odds ratio = 2.4).[30]

MYCOLOGY

Candida spp are detected in the laboratory by their macroscopic growth as cream- to yellow-colored colonies (**Fig. 1**) or by microscopic visualization of budding yeast cells (**Fig. 2**, inset). *C albicans* is a dimorphic fungus capable of existence in either the yeast or the mycelial form depending on environmental conditions such as temperature. *C albicans* is also noteworthy for the ability to form true hyphae or elongated buds called pseudohyphae (see **Fig. 2**, main panel). Its hyphae originate from slender projections known as germ tubes, which are a distinguishing feature of this species and are used for identification (**Fig. 3**).

PATHOGENESIS
Clinical Factors

Like many ubiquitous fungi, *Candida* spp can inhabit normal human hosts as gut commensals and colonizers of mucocutaneous surfaces without causing disease. Superficial candidiasis occurs in the presence of defects in both the innate and the adaptive cell-mediated immune responses that are vital antifungal defenses. An example of the former is vulvovaginal candidiasis in uncontrolled diabetes mellitus promoted by impaired neutrophil chemotaxis present in diabetics.[31] The latter is exemplified by the oroesophageal candidiasis typical of patients with AIDS and its associated depletion of CD4+

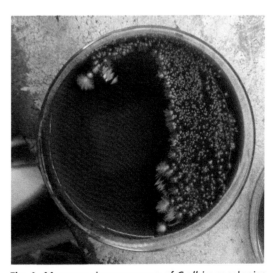

Fig. 1. Macroscopic appearance of *C albicans* colonies plated on blood agar.

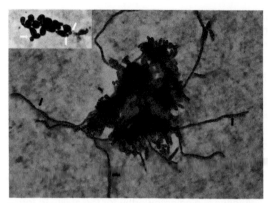

Fig. 2. Photomicrograph of Gram stain of *Candida* from blood specimen showing pseudohyphae (*black arrows*). Inset shows individual *C albicans* yeast cells, some of which exhibit budding (*white arrows*) (Gram stain, original magnification ×1000).

lymphocytes. Besides immune dysfunction, IC requires an interruption in the integumentary system or intestinal lining that allows local candidal overgrowth to gain access to the bloodstream or other normally impregnable sites. Although studies of candidemia, including ICU acquired, have suggested the potential for nosocomial transmission of Candida from patients and health care workers, they nevertheless support autoinfection as the predominant route of fungemia.[32–34] Existing data favor the intestine over the skin as the initial source of endogenous *Candida* spp ultimately recovered from blood cultures.[35] Elegant mouse

experiments have shown that neither neutropenia with preserved gut integrity nor intestinal interruption without neutropenia is sufficient for the development of disseminated candidiasis in a murine model.[36] In humans, this combination of factors is found in neutropenic enterocolitis (typhlitis), which may account for the classic predisposition of neutropenic oncology patients to candidemia. In critically ill patients, breakdown of the enteric barrier commonly occurs in the absence of neutropenia such as following abdominal surgery, which has been identified as a major risk factor for candidemia.[37] Clearly, immune defects other than neutropenia, such as those conferred by diabetes, renal failure, and greater severity of critical illness, all established risk factors for ICU candidemia, are sufficient when it comes to the ICU population.[38] The difference may lie in the additive contribution of ICU interventions, particularly the introduction of mechanical hardware, including CVCs, renal replacement therapy circuits, endotracheal tubes, and urinary catheters. CVCs, especially as access for total parenteral nutrition (TPN) and renal replacement therapy, have been identified repeatedly as risk factors.[38,39] Another dimension is the heavy burden of *Candida* colonization in the critically ill facilitated by the presence of iatrogenic devices and the widespread use of broad-spectrum antibacterial agents, the latter likewise a risk factor for candidemia.[40] Underlining the importance of colonization intensity, a study of critically ill surgical patients demonstrated 100% sensitivity for eventual IC of a *Candida* colonization index (CI) of ≥ 0.5, defined as the number of colonized non-blood body sites over the total number of sites cultured.[41] When the CI was corrected for the number of sites exhibiting heavy growth, the specificity also reached 100%.

Virulence Factors

The reason some ICU patients with known risk factors for candidemia develop this disease while others do not is likely a function of the complex interplay of fungal pathogenicity and host immune defenses. Relevant features of both sides of this equation are best described for *C albicans*, with 2 of its virulence factors deserving of special mention. *C albicans* is a dimorphic fungus capable of existence in both yeast and filamentous (hyphal or pseudohyphal) form. Mouse experiments have demonstrated that restricting *C albicans* to the nonfilamentous (ie, yeast) state renders it largely nonvirulent perhaps by reducing its ability to withstand phagocytosis.[42] Another mechanism of immune evasion by albicans and non-albicans *Candida* is the formation of a biofilm on natural

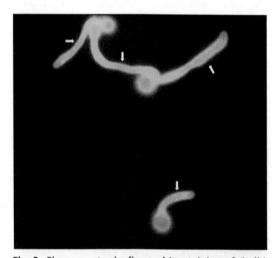

Fig. 3. Fluorescent calcofluor-white staining of *C albicans* highlights its characteristic germ tube structures (*arrows*). (*Courtesy of* Public Health Image Library, no. 295, CDC, Atlanta, GA, with permission; and Dr Brian Harrington, CDC/Mercy Hospital, Toledo, OH.)

(eg, mucosal) and artificial (eg, catheter) surfaces, which is a cohesive community of organisms embedded in an extracellular matrix.[43] Such aggregation acts as a shield from host immunity and attenuates the efficacy of antifungal agents. Biofilm producers are well suited for persistence on medical devices, the ubiquitous use of which in ICUs makes them a particularly fertile environment for IC. It is worth noting that biofilm production is less commonly associated with C albicans than with non-albicans species.[44] Among non-albicans Candida, this property is likeliest in bloodstream isolates recovered in the context of a CVC and TPN.

Host Factors

Recent research has shed considerable light on susceptibility to IC conferred by genetic immune alterations, principally in the cell-mediated arm, although the importance of humoral immunity has also gained greater appreciation.[45] Some of the discovered defects follow Mendelian inheritance. Namely, homozygotic deficiency of caspase recruitment domain-containing protein 9 (CARD9) has been linked to a predisposition to deep fungal infections, including IC.[46] CARD9 is a participant in multiple signaling pathways involved in antifungal defenses, the terminal effectors of which may be such cytokines as interleukin-6 (IL-6) and IL-17.[47] Possible connection to the latter is intriguing in light of evidence that the T helper 1 (Th1)-IL-17 component of the $CD4^+$ helper T-cell response is an important player in antifungal immunity. On a related note, deficiency of interferon-γ, a macrophage activator elaborated by Th1 cells, is associated with persistence of candidemia, whereas robust levels of tissue necrosis factor-α, a key mediator of the Th1 response, may be vital for the effective phagocytosis of Candida.[48,49] Polymorphisms of toll-like receptors 1 and 2 appear to be among the determinants of whether certain individuals harbor favorable or unfavorable antifungal cytokine profiles.[48,50]

SPECIFIC CLINICAL SCENARIOS
Catheter-Related Bloodstream Infection

The bloodstream is the third most common site of infection in ICUs worldwide, reported in 15% of an international critically ill population in a point-prevalence study.[51] Nosocomial bloodstream infections (BSIs) are intimately related to the presence of a CVC; it is not surprising, therefore, that about 50% of BSIs occur in the ICU. Central line–associated bloodstream infections (CLABSIs) are associated with increased mortality and health

care costs.[52,53] Along with Pseudomonas aeruginosa, Candida spp have been shown to independently predict death among patients with nosocomial BSIs.[54] The seminal work of Pronovost and colleagues[55] originally published in 2006 has demonstrated that the implementation of a protocol-based approach to combating CLABSIs in the ICU leads to marked and durable reduction in their incidence. Concurrent with the wide adoption of this approach has been a decline in the CLABSI rate for each of the commonest pathogens, including Candida, in adult ICUs.[56] On the other hand, the contribution of Candida to CLABSIs relative to other pathogens has actually increased and nearly doubled in the meantime. Surveillance data over the 7-year period between 1995 and 2002 attributed 9% of all nosocomial BSIs to Candida, placing them fourth on the pathogen list, whereas a point-prevalence survey conducted in 2011 found Candida responsible for 22% of nosocomial BSIs, ahead of all other pathogens.[57,58] Although the main explanation for this trend has yet to be elucidated, it is reasonable to speculate that it may be a function of differences in the mechanism of CVC seeding. Usual bacterial CLABSIs are thought to arise primarily from inoculation by cutaneous flora on the part of operator or patient, which can be reduced by adherence to placement and maintenance checklists. In the case of Candida, available evidence points to the intestine as the primary fungal reservoir, hematogenous spread from which to the CVC possibly being an alternate route of Candida CLABSI development.[35] Refinement of CVC insertion and maintenance practices would be unlikely to impact this pathogenetic sequence. Data examining the need for, and the timing of, removal of CVCs in the setting of candidemia are limited to observational studies. Many of them favor early catheter removal, but drawing firm conclusions about mortality or other clinically meaningful outcomes of this recommended practice remains problematic.[59]

Septic Shock

Septic shock in the setting of candidemia is a much less common occurrence overall than bacteremic septic shock, the latter diagnosed almost 40 times more often across US and Canadian ICUs.[60,61] Of all-comers with candidemia, about one-quarter progress to septic shock.[62] When it does occur, Candida septic shock carries a high crude mortality reported to be in the range of approximately 60% to 90%, and its development portends a worse outcome in candidemic patients.[61,63–65] ICU studies of candidemia complicated by septic shock have identified failure of source control, delay in antifungal therapy, and increasing APACHE score as risk factors associated with higher mortality in this condition.[64,65] Features predictive of progression to septic shock among candidemic ICU patients are not well established. One small study identified shorter time in the ICU before candidemia to be an independent predictor of such progression.[63]

Ocular Involvement

The focus of metastatic seeding by candidemia most relevant to routine critical care practice is ocular candidiasis. Extension into the vitreous body distinguishes endophthalmitis from the more superficial eye infection known as chorioretinitis. Incidence rates of candidal endophthalmitis published in the contemporary literature (1.6%–2.9%) indicate that this complication is less common in current ICU practice than reported in older studies (≥13%).[66–68] The causative species is almost exclusively C albicans.[37] Most patients with ocular candidiasis and the ability to communicate do not report visual symptoms, and the appearance of funduscopic findings is often delayed.[66] These disease features have led to the recommendation for dilated ophthalmologic examination of all patients with candidemia early in the course of treatment with the caveat that later examinations may be more sensitive.[69] Resolution of funduscopic abnormalities with prolonged systemic antifungal therapy is expected, although intraocular instillation of antifungals and partial vitrectomy may have an adjunctive role in refractory cases.[70,71]

DIAGNOSTIC CONSIDERATIONS
Culture

Growth in culture remains the gold standard for diagnosing candidal infections, but this method suffers from delayed results, the potential for inadequate sampling by clinicians, and possible suppression by antifungal therapy. Obtaining cultures from sterile nonblood sites is associated with procedural risks. In an attempt to address these shortcomings, the matrix-assisted laser desorption ionization time-of-flight mass spectrometry (MALDI-TOF) system has been developed for the rapid speciation of bacterial and fungal pathogens. With this system, the laboratory can identify the yeast directly from the blood culture bottle without the requirement for a plate subculture. In a recent study evaluating the role of MALDI-TOF in identifying non-albicans Candida spp, this technology correctly speciated 19/20 cases directly from blood culture and all 82 isolates grown on plates.[72]

Prediction Rules

The delayed diagnosis of IC by traditional culture methods and the association of treatment delay with adverse outcomes have prompted efforts to identify patients most likely to benefit from untargeted therapy. One of the difficulties inherent in this endeavor is that ICU patients tend to possess multiple risk factors for IC and quickly develop some degree of Candida colonization. A classic early example of a prediction tool for IC is the aforementioned Candida CI studied in a small, single-center cohort of surgical ICU patients in 1989.[41] A CI threshold of 0.5 achieved a negative predictive value (NPV) of 100% and a positive predictive value (PPV) of 66%, whereas the use of a corrected CI level of 0.4 increased the PPV to 100% without a drop in NPV. Although this seemingly ironclad link between Candida colonization and candidemia has since been challenged by a larger prospective study across multiple surgical ICUs, preemptive treatment administered for a corrected CI ≥0.4 eliminated surgical ICU-acquired IC in one French hospital.[28,73] Later investigators led by Ostrosky-Zeichner and colleagues[74] aimed to expand the study population beyond the especially high-risk critically ill surgical patients and recognized that systematic colonization surveillance, although potentially valuable, is laborious and not practical in every setting. They derived and retrospectively validated a prediction rule using mixed medical-surgical ICU subjects based not on colonization but rather on predisposing clinical factors. Positivity of the best-performing rule was defined by at least one major criterion, namely receipt of antibacterials or the presence of a CVC within 3 days, plus at least 2 of the following minor criteria: surgery, immunosuppression, pancreatitis, TPN, steroid use, and hemodialysis (HD). This model resulted in high specificity (90%) and NPV (97%), whereas the sensitivity lagged far behind at 34%. External validation of the Ostrosky-Zeichner rule at a single US institution yielded a higher sensitivity (range 66%–74%) but a lower specificity of 61%.[75] That institution achieved a superior sensitivity of 84% with its own rule that eliminated HD, added pre-ICU length of stay, and limited surgery to the abdominal cavity. Results of external validation in 4 Australian ICUs, on the other hand, were more closely aligned with the original study: sensitivity 47% and specificity 79%.[76] A corrected CI of 0.4 outperformed the Ostrosky-Zeichner rule in Australia when used alone and raised the rule's specificity from 79% to 97% when the 2 were combined. The NPV remained greater than 90%

for the Ostrosky-Zeichner rule in both US and Australian validation samples.

Candida Score

The so-called Candida score (CS) builds on the notion that both colonization status and clinical predisposition may play predictive roles in IC, assigning one point each for multifocal colonization, surgery, and TPN, and 2 points for severe sepsis.[77] Optimal sensitivity and specificity of 81% and 74%, respectively, were reached at a cutoff of 2.5 with an area under the curve (AUC) of the receiver operating characteristic (ROC) of 0.85 in the medical-surgical ICU derivation cohort. When validated prospectively in a very large sample using a threshold level of 3, the CS outperformed a CI of $\geq$0.5 in the ability to predict IC starting on day 7 of ICU stay: AUC ROC 0.77 versus 0.63, respectively.[78] Calculation of the CS in French ICU patients exhibiting severe sepsis or septic shock produced no cases of IC when the value was $\leq$3.[79]

Serum Biomarkers

The fungal cell wall product $(1\rightarrow3)$-β-D-glucan (BG) is a promising alternative or adjunct to scores and indices for predicting IC as the cause of sepsis in the critically ill. At a cutoff level of 80 pg/mL, the BG assay had a sensitivity of 93% and a specificity of 94% for IC as the cause of new ICU sepsis.[80] The corresponding AUC ROC was 0.98. In comparison, the sensitivity, specificity, and AUC ROC of CS and CI in the same study were 86%/89%/0.80 and 64%/70%/0.63, respectively. Questions persist about the impact of cross-reactivity with other invasive mycoses, false positives caused by certain antibiotics and blood products,[81] as well as the optimal cutoff level when applied to the ICU population.

Unlike BG, mannan (MN) is a genus-specific Candida cell wall component released into the bloodstream during invasive infection. The Candida antigen test detects MN in blood samples using enzyme-linked immunosorbent assay. The presence of MN in the bloodstream is transient because of rapid clearance, a property that limits its sensitivity, but this may be enhanced by concurrent testing for anti-MN antibodies. Concerns have arisen, however, about false positive antibody results in colonized but uninfected patients.[82] A review of published studies of MN and anti-MN testing in IC, many of which included ICU patients, yielded a pooled sensitivity and specificity of 83% and 86%, respectively, for both markers together.[83] These percentages amounted to a substantial increase in sensitivity (from 58%) compared with the MN assay alone without a major sacrifice in specificity (from 93%).

Other Nonculture Methods

An immunofluorescence assay has been developed to detect antibodies against C albicans germ tubes (CAGTA). In a study of ICU patients with abdominal abnormality, this test had a sensitivity of 53% and specificity of 64% for the diagnosis of IC.[84] The addition of either MN or anti-MN testing produced a modest increase in sensitivity (65%–68%) at the expense of a slight drop in specificity (55%–58%). Candida DNA polymerase chain reaction (PCR) is another potential diagnostic tool, but PCR use may be challenging in invasive mycoses because of the low organism burden and the presence of the fungal cell wall, which impedes DNA release.[85] False positivity in cases of colonization is a concern supported by a specificity of 33% for IC in an ICU population at high risk for Candida colonization.[84] In a meta-analysis of all relevant articles published through 2009, however, the specificity of PCR for IC was greater than 90%, as it was in a later study of lower-risk ICU patients.[86,87] In that ICU study, the performance characteristics of PCR were superior to those of CAGTA, among them specificity: 97% versus 57%. Such disparate false positive rates of Candida PCR testing need to be reconciled in future studies. **Table 2** summarizes the performance characteristics of the clinical and laboratory nonculture diagnostic methods discussed above.

TREATMENT
Untargeted Therapy

Untargeted antifungal therapy against Candida can be classified according to the trigger for its initiation.[88] Prophylaxis refers to treatment based on clinical patient characteristics that confer increased vulnerability to IC (eg, Ostrosky-Zeichner rule). Preemptive therapy is administered for microbiological (eg, colonization) and/or serologic (eg, BG) evidence but not proof of infection. Therapy started in the face of persistent sepsis alone is considered empirical. Optimal untargeted therapy would apply an inexpensive agent to patients at highest risk of IC and in ICUs with high rates so that the number needed to treat to prevent one infection or death could be minimized at a favorable cost. One of the concerns associated with this approach is whether the resultant expansion in antifungal use would engender resistance and select for less susceptible species such as C glabrata.

The earliest attempts at untargeted treatment in critical care involved prophylaxis of surgical ICU

Table 2
Representative performance characteristics of nonculture clinical and laboratory tools for the identification of intensive care unit patients with current or future invasive candidiasis/candidemia

Method	Type	Threshold	Sensitivity, %	Specificity, %	PPV, %	NPV, %	AUC ROC	RR
CI[41,76,80]	CPR	0.5	64–100	47–69	5–66	92–100	0.63–0.74	—
cCI[41,76]	CPR	0.4	60–100	90–100	13–100	99–100	0.75	—
O-Z[74–76]	CPR	≥1 major ≥2 minor	34–74	61–90	4–9	97–99	0.63–0.71	4.36
CS[78,79]	CPR	3	78–86	66–89	14–57	97–98	0.77	5.98
BG[80,86]	Biomarker	80 pg/mL	77–93	57–94	22–72	94–99	—	—
MN[82,83]	Biomarker	0.25/0.5 ng/mL	43–58	67–93	17	89	—	—
MN + anti-MN[82,83]	Biomarker + Serology	0.25/0.5 ng/mL + 2.5/5/10 AU	55–83	60–86	17	90	—	—
CAGTA[83,86]	Serology	≥1/160	53–74	57–64	18–38	86–90	—	—
PCR[83,85,86]	Assay	N/A	84–96	33–97	27–93	88–99	—	—

Ranges given where data from more than one study are provided.

Ostrosky-Zeichner rule, major criteria: antibiotic use prior 3 d, CVC prior 3 d; minor criteria: surgery prior 7 d, immunosuppression prior 7 d, TPN prior 3 d, dialysis prior 3 d, steroid use 7≥ days ≥3.

Abbreviations: AU, arbitrary units; cCI, CI × (number of sites with heavy growth/total number of colonized culture sites); CI, number of colonized culture sites/total number of sites cultured; CPR, clinical prediction rule; O-Z, Ostrosky-Zeichner rule; RR, relative risk.

patients with fluconazole. In a pioneering study from the late 1990s, 400 mg of fluconazole daily given to all surgical ICU admissions was associated with a 7% absolute risk reduction of IC compared with placebo.[89] Time-to-event analysis significantly favored the fluconazole group. Following initiation of universal fluconazole prophylaxis in their ICU, these investigators reported no increase in colonization by *C glabrata* or *C krusei* and an overall very low incidence of IC, although they did find a substantial rate of reduced fluconazole susceptibility in isolates from the few cases that occurred in the prophylaxis era.[90] Reductions in the rate of candidemia have subsequently been reported following initiation of fluconazole prophylaxis in a medical ICU population as well as after addition of prophylactic fluconazole to an antibacterial gut decontamination regimen in a mixed ICU.[91,92] On the other hand, caspofungin prophylaxis at 15 participating US ICUs targeting patients who fulfilled a modified version of the original Ostrosky-Zeichner rule was no better than placebo at reducing the incidence of proven or probable IC in the intention-to-treat analysis.[93] Likewise, empirical fluconazole therapy administered to ICU patients with a CVC and persistent fever despite broad antibacterials failed to produce a difference compared with placebo in a composite outcome combining efficacy and safety.[94] In contrast, successful reduction of surgical ICU IC rates by implementation of corrected CI-triggered preemptive therapy has been mentioned earlier.[73] A contemporary systematic review of studies of untargeted therapy revealed that the utility of this approach in reducing IC is supported by evidence of overall low quality, much of it subject to bias and funded by pharmaceutical companies.[95] No effect on mortality was discerned nor was there an increased risk of adverse events related to treatment. Not included in this systematic review was a recent large longitudinal study of mechanically ventilated ICU patients, predominantly medical, that showed no reduction in mortality or proven IC with untargeted antifungal therapy even after careful adjustment for confounding variables.[96]

Targeted Therapy

Three classes of antifungal agents are used for the treatment of established IC: the azoles (particularly fluconazole and voriconazole), the echinocandins (caspofungin, micafungin, and anidulafungin), and amphotericin B (AmB) either as the conventional deoxycholate compound or as the liposomal formulation designed to reduce renal toxicity. An additional agent, flucytosine, is also active against *Candida* but generally not used as monotherapy. Guidelines for the treatment of IC have been recently updated by the Infectious Diseases Society of America[69]; these recommendations are summarized in **Table 3**. Main principles guiding therapy include concern for azole resistance, rising especially among non-albicans *Candida* spp; penetration of the drug into the anatomic region of infection; and medication side effects and interactions.[40] Fluconazole, for example, is metabolized by the same cytochrome P450 isoenzymes as the commonly used ICU sedatives fentanyl and midazolam, leading to decreased sedative clearance by competitive inhibition, which may be clinically relevant.[97] AmB was the treatment of choice for many years but use was limited by nephrotoxicity and infusion reactions.[98,99] Fluconazole was found to be noninferior to amB in a randomized trial of nonneutropenic patients, leading to a shift toward triazole-based therapy.[100] However, because of increasing azole resistance as well as excellent tolerability and efficacy, the echinocandins are now recommended as initial therapy.[69] Echinocandins are only available as intravenous formulations, but their potency, favorable safety profile, and rare drug interactions have led to their widespread adoption as first-line agents. In a double-blind trial comparing caspofungin with AmB for the treatment of IC, caspofungin was as effective as AmB with a significantly lower rate of adverse events.[101] A study of micafungin versus AmB yielded similar findings,[102] and a comparison of micafungin with caspofungin demonstrated its noninferiority in the treatment of IC.[103] Even in *C albicans* infections, despite less concern about resistance, echinocandins may be superior to azoles. Anidulafungin was compared with fluconazole for the treatment of IC caused by *C albicans*, and this study found anidulafungin to be the more effective agent with significantly shorter time to clearance of blood cultures.[104] Of note, all isolates of *C albicans* in this study were susceptible to the administered drug.

Although the minimum inhibitory concentrations (MICs) of echinocandins for most *Candida* spp are low, acquired resistance has been described, particularly in *C glabrata* infection.[105–107] *C parapsilosis* has demonstrated inherently higher echinocandin MICs in vitro; nevertheless, a recent study comparing the effectiveness of fluconazole versus echinocandin therapy in *C parapsilosis* candidemia found no difference in 30-day mortality.[108] Treatment with fluconazole rather than an echinocandin in these cases is therefore no longer recommended.[69,108]

Table 3
Antifungal treatment options for invasive candidiasis

Class	Names/Formulations	Dosing	Advantages	Disadvantages	Summary/Recommendation
Polyenes	AmB deoxycholate Liposomal AmB AmB lipid complex (ABLC) AmB colloidal dispersion (ABCD, not available in the US)	AmB deoxycholate: 0.5–0.7 mg/kg daily (May consider increasing to 1 mg/kg daily for less susceptible species, such as *C glabrata* and *C krusei*) Liposomal AmB: 3–5 mg/kg daily	Efficacy Clinical experience	AmB deoxycholate: nephrotoxicity (acute kidney injury, electrolyte wasting tubular acidosis), infusion-related toxicity Liposomal AmB: cost, caution in urinary tract infections due to limited renal excretion	Alternative therapy, use when echinocandin intolerance or suspected resistance
Triazoles	Fluconazole Itraconazole Voriconazole Posaconazole Isavuconazole	Fluconazole: 800 mg load followed by 400 mg daily (50% dose reduce for creatinine clearance <50) Itraconazole: only oral, not well studied in IC Voriconazole: Little advantage over fluconazole, consider use as step-down therapy particularly cases of fluconazole resistance when voriconazole sensitive (eg, *C glabrata*) Posaconazole: No indication for therapy in invasive Candida infections, limited clinical data Isavuconazole: Recently approved, excellent in vitro data but not yet sufficient clinical data for guidance	Comparable to AmB deoxycholate for treatment of candidemia Standard therapy for esophageal, oropharyngeal, vaginal candidiasis and UTIs Excellent oral bioavailability Fluconazole greatest CSF and vitreous penetration	Inhibit cytochrome P450 system, drug-drug interactions (eg, midazolam, fentanyl) Voriconazole toxicity: hepatic injury, visual side effects, CNS side effects	Similar efficacy among individual drugs against most *Candida* spp with less activity vs non-albicans *Candida* Fluconazole recommended azole, use as step-down therapy, or initial therapy in noncritical patients without suspected azole resistance

Echinocandins	Caspofungin Micafungin Anidulafungin	Caspofungin: 70 mg loading dose followed by 50 mg/d (dose reduction recommended for moderate-severe hepatic dysfunction) Micafungin: 100 mg daily without loading dose Anidulafungin: 200 mg loading dose then 100 mg daily	Minimal toxicity, safe and well tolerated Each agent studied and efficacy demonstrated in invasive infection Daily dosing Therapeutic levels achieved except in CNS, ocular infection and urinary tract No need to dose adjust for renal failure	Only parenteral formulation	Low MICs for most *Candida* spp Higher MICs in C *parapsillosis* Currently recommended first-line therapy in the ICU setting
Flucytosine		25 mg/kg 4 times daily (if normal renal function)	High concentrations achieved in CNS and high	Oral formulation only Short half-life High rate of resistance as monotherapy Bone marrow suppression, hepatitis can occur	Broad activity vs *Candida* spp (other than C *krusei*) but limited use due to need for dual therapy with another agent Generally used in cases of refractory infection in combination with AmB

Abbreviations: CNS, central nervous system; CSF, cerebrospinal fluid; UTI, urinary tract infection.
Data from Refs.[69,97–102,104,121–123]

Once clinical stability and blood culture clearance have been achieved, sensitivity testing can be used to evaluate for possible step down to oral azole therapy. If the *Candida* isolate is susceptible to fluconazole, transition to that agent is recommended, which generally takes place about 5 to 7 days after initiation of therapy.[69] This strategy was evaluated in a multicenter prospective study of 250 patients with candidemia and IC.[109] Subjects were initially treated with anidulafungin followed by the option of switching to an oral azole in the absence of persistent candidemia if they were able to tolerate oral medications, were afebrile for greater than 24 hours, and were hemodynamically stable. The end-of-treatment response was 90% in the early switch group, supporting the feasibility of such a step-down approach. The potential for azole resistance among *C glabrata* and other non-albicans spp mandates susceptibility testing of these isolates before consideration of transitioning to oral fluconazole.[37]

The less toxic liposomal formulation of AmB is recommended as an alternative in cases of intolerance to preferred agents or their limited availability.[98] Liposomal AmB is also an appropriate option if both azole and echinocandin resistance is suspected, such as in cases of candidal infection in the setting of prolonged echinocandin use.

OUTCOMES

Candidemia remains a highly lethal condition linked to several clinical, microbiological, and host factors. Many, but not all, reports have found an association between greater time to administration of appropriate antifungal therapy and increased risk of death.[65,110–113] The same association has been observed for source control, although at least in the case of CVCs, definitive statements are hampered by the absence of robust trial data. Although a correlation between *Candida* species and mortality in ICU patients has not been demonstrated, biofilm production did confer increased risk of death in one study.[114] Patient-related variables consistently reported to be determinants of mortality in ICU candidemia include APACHE scores, age, and mechanical ventilation.[65,110,111,113] It has been shown that risk factors for early (ie, 7-day) mortality may differ from those for death at 1 month. In a large prospective surveillance study, delays in the combined intervention of adequate antifungal therapy and source control predicted early mortality, whereas patient and clinical characteristics such as age, intubation, and renal replacement therapy were independent risk factors for late mortality.[115]

SUMMARY

The last decade has ushered in major changes in several aspects of ICU candidemia. It has been marked by increasing recognition of non-albicans species as prominent pathogens in this infection. Efforts to expedite diagnosis have led to advances in culture-based identification as well as in the development of molecular diagnostics. These nonculture methods generally have high NPV but low PPV. Echinocandins have supplanted azoles as first-line antifungal agents for the treatment of confirmed candidemia. Although supported by guideline recommendations, untargeted therapy and CVC removal remain areas of controversy pending future studies with improved methodology and reduced bias.

REFERENCES

1. Petri MG, König J, Moecke HP, et al. Epidemiology of invasive mycosis in ICU patients: a prospective multicenter study in 435 non-neutropenic patients. Intensive Care Med 1997;23:317–25.
2. Playford EG, Nimmo GR, Tilse M, et al. Increasing incidence of candidaemia: long-term epidemiological trends, Queensland, Australia, 1999-2008. J Hosp Infect 2010;76:46–51.
3. Bougnoux ME, Kac G, Aegerter P, et al. Candidemia and candiduria in critically ill patients admitted to intensive care units in France: incidence, molecular diversity, management, and outcome. Intensive Care Med 2008;34:292–9.
4. Olaechea PM, Palomar M, León-Gil C, et al. Economic impact of Candida colonization and Candida infection in the critically ill patient. Eur J Clin Microbiol Infect Dis 2004;23:323–30.
5. Bloos F, Bayer O, Sachse S, et al. Attributable costs of patients with candidemia and potential implications of polymerase chain reaction-based pathogen detection on antifungal therapy in patients with sepsis. J Crit Care 2013;28:2–8.
6. Cleveland AA, Harrison LH, Farley MM, et al. Declining incidence of candidemia and the shifting epidemiology of Candida resistance in two US metropolitan areas, 2008-2013: results from population-based surveillance. PLoS One 2015; 10:e0120452.
7. Leroy O, Gangneux JP, Montravers P, et al. Epidemiology, management, and risk factors for death of invasive Candida infections in critical care: a multicenter, prospective, observational study in France (2005-2006). Crit Care Med 2009;37:1612–8.
8. Horn DL, Neofytos D, Anaissie EJ, et al. Epidemiology and outcomes of candidemia in 2019 patients: data from the prospective antifungal therapy alliance registry. Clin Infect Dis 2009;48:1695–703.

9. Gong X, Luan T, Wu X, et al. Invasive candidiasis in intensive care units in China: risk factors and prognoses of Candida albicans and no-nalbicans Candida infections. Am J Infect Control 2016;44: e59–63.

10. Lortholary O, Renaudat C, Sitbon K, et al. Worrisome trends in incidence and mortality of candidemia in intensive care units (Paris area, 2002-2010). Intensive Care Med 2014;40:1303–12.

11. Bassetti M, Righi E, Costa A, et al. Epidemiological trends in nosocomial candidemia in intensive care. BMC Infect Dis 2006;6:21.

12. Abi-Said D, Anaissie E, Uzun O, et al. The epidemiology of hematogenous candidiasis caused by different Candida species. Clin Infect Dis 1997; 24:1122–8.

13. Colombo AL, Guimarães T, Sukienik T, et al. Prognostic factors and historical trends in the epidemiology of candidemia in critically ill patients: an analysis of five multicenter studies sequentially conducted over a 9-year period. Intensive Care Med 2014;40:1489–98.

14. Blot SI, Vandewoude KH, Hoste EA, et al. Effects of nosocomial candidemia on outcomes of critically ill patients. Am J Med 2002;113:480–5.

15. Xie GH, Fang XM, Fang Q, et al. Impact of invasive fungal infection on outcomes of severe sepsis: a multicenter matched cohort study in critically ill surgical patients. Crit Care 2008;12:R5.

16. González de Molina FJ, León C, Ruiz-Santana S, et al. Assessment of candidemia-attributable mortality in critically ill patients using propensity score matching analysis. Crit Care 2012;16:R105.

17. Gudlaugsson O, Gillespie S, Lee K, et al. Attributable mortality of nosocomial candidemia, revisited. Clin Infect Dis 2003;37:1172–7.

18. Falagas ME, Apostolou KE, Pappas VD. Attributable mortality of candidemia: a systematic review of matched cohort and case-control studies. Eur J Clin Microbiol Infect Dis 2006;25:419–25.

19. Pfaller MA, Andes DR, Diekema DJ, et al. Epidemiology and outcomes of invasive candidiasis due to non-albicans species of Candida in 2,496 patients: data from the prospective antifungal therapy (PATH) registry 2004-2008. PLoS One 2014;9: e101510.

20. Holley A, Dulhunty J, Blot S, et al. Temporal trends, risk factors and outcomes in albicans and non-albicans candidaemia: an international epidemiological study in four multidisciplinary intensive care units. Int J Antimicrob Agents 2009;33:554.e1-7.

21. Shorr AF, Lazarus DR, Sherner JH, et al. Do clinical features allow for accurate prediction of fungal pathogenesis in bloodstream infections? Potential implications of the increasing prevalence of non-albicans candidemia. Crit Care Med 2007;35: 1077–83.

22. Dimopoulos G, Ntziora F, Rachiotis G, et al. Candida albicans versus non-albicans intensive care unit-acquired bloodstream infections: differences in risk factors and outcome. Anesth Analg 2008;106:523–9.

23. Chow JK, Golan Y, Ruthazer R, et al. Factors associated with candidemia caused by non-albicans Candida species versus Candida albicans in the intensive care unit. Clin Infect Dis 2008;46: 1206–13.

24. Playford EG, Marriott D, Nguyen Q, et al. Candidemia in nonneutropenic critically ill patients: risk factors for non-albicans Candida spp. Crit Care Med 2008;36:2034–9.

25. Malani A, Hmoud J, Chiu L, et al. Candida glabrata fungemia: experience in a tertiary care center. Clin Infect Dis 2005;41:975–81.

26. Cohen Y, Karoubi P, Adrie C, et al. Early prediction of Candida glabrata fungemia in nonneutropenic critically ill patients. Crit Care Med 2010;38:826–30.

27. Klingspor L, Tortorano AM, Peman J, et al. Invasive Candida infections in surgical patients in intensive care units: a prospective, multicentre survey initiated by the European Confederation of Medical Mycology (ECMM) (2006-2008). Clin Microbiol Infect 2015;21:87.e1-10.

28. Blumberg HM, Jarvis WR, Soucie M, et al. Risk factors for candidal bloodstream infections in surgical intensive care unit patients: the NEMIS prospective multicenter study. Clin Infect Dis 2001;33:177–86.

29. Charles PE, Doise JM, Quenot JP, et al. Candidemia in critically ill patients: difference of outcome between medical and surgical patients. Intensive Care Med 2003;29:2162–9.

30. Michalopoulos AS, Geroulanos S, Mentzelopoulos SD. Determinants of candidemia and candidemia-related death in cardiothoracic ICU patients. Chest 2003;124:2244–55.

31. Mowat AG, Baum J. Chemotaxis of polymorphonuclear leukocytes from patients with diabetes mellitus. N Engl J Med 1971;284:621–7.

32. Reagan DR, Pfaller MA, Hollis RJ, et al. Characterization of the sequence of colonization and nosocomial candidemia using DNA fingerprinting and a DNA probe. J Clin Microbiol 1990;28:2733–8.

33. Pfaller MA, Messer SA, Houston A, et al. National epidemiology of mycoses survey: a multicenter study of strain variation and antifungal susceptibility among isolates of Candida species. Diagn Microbiol Infect Dis 1998;31:289–96.

34. Hammarskjöld F, Mernelius S, Andersson RE, et al. Possible transmission of Candida albicans on an intensive care unit: genotype and temporal cluster analyses. J Hosp Infect 2013;85:60–5.

35. Nucci M, Anaissie E. Revisiting the source of candidemia: skin or gut? Clin Infect Dis 2001;33: 1959–67.

36. Koh AY, Köhler JR, Coggshall KT, et al. Mucosal damage and neutropenia are required for Candida albicans dissemination. PLoS Pathog 2008;4:e35.

37. McCarty TP, Pappas PG. Invasive candidiasis. Infect Dis Clin North Am 2016;30:103–24.

38. Delaloye J, Calandra T. Invasive candidiasis as a cause of sepsis in the critically ill patient. Virulence 2014;5:161–9.

39. Muskett H, Shahin J, Eyres G, et al. Risk factors for invasive fungal disease in critically ill adult patients: a systematic review. Crit Care 2011;15:R287.

40. Kullberg BJ, Arendrup MC. Invasive candidiasis. N Engl J Med 2015;373:1445–56.

41. Pittet D, Monod M, Suter PM, et al. Candida colonization and subsequent infections in critically ill surgical patients. Ann Surg 1994;220:751–8.

42. Lo HJ, Köhler JR, DiDomenico B, et al. Nonfilamentous C. albicans mutants are avirulent. Cell 1997;90:939–49.

43. Silva S, Negri M, Henriques M, et al. Adherence and biofilm formation of non-Candida albicans Candida species. Trends Microbiol 2011;19:241–7.

44. Shin JH, Kee SJ, Shin MG, et al. Biofilm production by isolates of Candida species recovered from nonneutropenic patients: comparison of bloodstream isolates with isolates from other sources. J Clin Microbiol 2002;40:1244–8.

45. Casadevall A, Pirofski LA. Immunoglobulins in defense, pathogenesis, and therapy of fungal diseases. Cell Host Microbe 2012;11:447–56.

46. Lanternier F, Mahdaviani SA, Barbati E, et al. Inherited CARD9 deficiency in otherwise healthy children and adults with Candida species-induced meningoencephalitis, colitis, or both. J Allergy Clin Immunol 2015;135:1558–68.

47. Lanternier F, Pathan S, Vincent QB, et al. Deep dermatophytosis and inherited CARD9 deficiency. N Engl J Med 2013;369:1704–14.

48. Johnson MD, Plantinga TS, van de Vosse E, et al. Cytokine gene polymorphisms and the outcome of invasive candidiasis: a prospective cohort study. Clin Infect Dis 2012;54:502–10.

49. Woeherle T, Du W, Goetz A, et al. Pathogen specific cytokine release reveals an effect of TLR2 Arg753Gln during Candida sepsis in humans. Cytokine 2008;41:322–9.

50. Plantinga TS, Johnson MD, Scott WK, et al. Toll-like receptor 1 polymorphisms increase susceptibility to candidemia. J Infect Dis 2012;205:934–43.

51. Vincent JL, Rello J, Marshall J, et al. International study of the prevalence and outcomes of infection in intensive care units. JAMA 2009;302:2323–9.

52. Siempos II, Kopterides P, Tsangaris I, et al. Impact of catheter-related bloodstream infections on the mortality of critically ill patients: a meta-analysis. Crit Care Med 2009;37:2283–9.

53. Zimlichman E, Henderson D, Tamir O, et al. Health care-associated infections: a meta-analysis of costs and financial impact on the US health care system. JAMA Intern Med 2013;173:2039–46.

54. Miller PJ, Wenzel RP. Etiologic organisms as independent predictors of death and morbidity associated with bloodstream infections. J Infect Dis 1987;156:471–7.

55. Pronovost PJ, Watson SR, Goeschel CA, et al. Sustaining reductions in central line-associated bloodstream infections in Michigan intensive care units: a 10-year analysis. Am J Med Qual 2016;31:197–202.

56. Fagan RP, Edwards JR, Park BJ, et al. Incidence trends in pathogen-specific central line-associated bloodstream infections in US intensive care units, 1990-2010. Infect Control Hosp Epidemiol 2013;34:893–9.

57. Wisplinghoff H, Bischoff T, Tallent SM, et al. Nosocomial bloodstream infections in US hospitals: analysis of 24,179 cases from a prospective nationwide surveillance study. Clin Infect Dis 2004;39:309–17.

58. Magill SS, Edwards JR, Bamberg W, et al. Multistate point-prevalence survey of health care-associated infections. N Engl J Med 2014;370:1198–208.

59. Janum S, Afshari A. Central venous catheter (CVC) removal for patients of all ages with candidaemia. Cochrane Database Syst Rev 2016;(7):CD011195.

60. Quenot JP, Binquet C, Kara F, et al. The epidemiology of septic shock in French intensive care units: the prospective multicenter cohort EPISS study. Crit Care 2013;17:R65.

61. Hadley S, Lee WW, Ruthazer R, et al. Candidemia as a cause of septic shock and multiple organ failure in nonimmunocompromised patients. Crit Care Med 2002;30:1808–14.

62. Wisplinghoff H, Seifert H, Wenzel RP, et al. Inflammatory response and clinical course of adult patients with nosocomial bloodstream infections caused by Candida spp. Clin Microbiol Infect 2006;12:170–7.

63. Guzman JA, Tchokonte R, Sobel JD. Septic shock due to candidemia: outcomes and predictors of shock development. J Clin Med Res 2011;3:65–71.

64. Kollef M, Micek S, Hampton N, et al. Septic shock attributed to Candida infection: importance of empiric therapy and source control. Clin Infect Dis 2012;54:1739–46.

65. Bassetti M, Righi E, Ansaldi F, et al. A multicenter study of septic shock due to candidemia: outcomes and predictors of mortality. Intensive Care Med 2014;40:839–45.

66. Oude Lashof AM, Rothova A, Sobel JD, et al. Ocular manifestations of candidemia. Clin Infect Dis 2011;53:262–8.

67. Gluck S, Headdon WG, Tang D, et al. The incidence of ocular candidiasis and evaluation of routine ophthalmic examination in critically ill patients with candidaemia. Anaesth Intensive Care 2015;43:693–7.

68. Nolla-Salas J, Sitges-Serra A, León C, et al. Candida endophthalmitis in non-neutropenic critically ill patients. Eur J Clin Microbiol Infect Dis 1996;15:503–6.

69. Pappas PG, Kauffman CA, Andes DR, et al. Clinical practice guideline for the management of candidiasis: 2016 update by the Infectious Diseases Society of America. Clin Infect Dis 2016;62:e1–50.

70. Rodríguez-Adrián LJ, King RT, Tamayo-Derat LG, et al. Retinal lesions as clues to disseminated bacterial and candida infections: frequency, natural history, and etiology. Medicine (Baltimore) 2003; 82:187–202.

71. Shah CP, McKey J, Spirn MJ, et al. Ocular candidiasis: a review. Br J Ophthalmol 2008;92:466–8.

72. Pulcarno G, Iula DV, Vollaro A, et al. Rapid and reliable MALDI-TOF mass spectrometry identification of Candida non-albicans isolates from bloodstream infections. J Microbiol Methods 2013;94:262–6.

73. Piarroux R, Grenouillet F, Balvay P, et al. Assessment of preemptive treatment to prevent severe candidiasis in critically ill surgical patients. Crit Care Med 2004;32:2443–9.

74. Ostrosky-Zeichner L, Sable C, Sobel J, et al. Multicenter retrospective development and validation of a clinical prediction rule for nosocomial invasive candidiasis in the intensive care setting. Eur J Clin Microbiol Infect Dis 2007;26:271–6.

75. Hermsen ED, Zapapas MK, Maiefski M, et al. Validation and comparison of clinical prediction rules for invasive candidiasis in intensive care unit patients: a matched case-control study. Crit Care 2011;15:R198.

76. Playford EG, Lipman J, Kabir M, et al. Assessment of clinical risk predictive rules for invasive candidiasis in a prospective multicentre cohort of ICU patients. Intensive Care Med 2009;35:2141–5.

77. León C, Ruiz-Santana S, Saavedra P, et al. A bedside scoring system ("Candida score") for early antifungal treatment in nonneutropenic critically ill patients with Candida colonization. Crit Care Med 2006;34:730–7.

78. León C, Ruiz-Santana S, Saavedra P, et al. Usefulness of the "Candida score" for discriminating between Candida colonization and invasive candidiasis in non-neutropenic critically ill patients: a prospective multicenter study. Crit Care Med 2009;37:1624–33.

79. Leroy G, Lambiotte F, Thévenin D, et al. Evaluation of "Candida score" in critically ill patients: a prospective, multicenter, observational, cohort study. Ann Intensive Care 2011;1:50.

80. Posteraro B, De Pascale G, Tumbarello M, et al. Early diagnosis of candidemia in intensive care unit patients with sepsis: a prospective comparison of (1→3)-β-D-glucan assay, Candida score, and colonization index. Crit Care 2011;15:R249.

81. Mikulska M, Furfaro E, Viscoli C. Non-cultural methods for the diagnosis of invasive fungal disease. Expert Rev Anti Infect Ther 2015;13:103–17.

82. Sendid B, Tabouret M, Poirot JL, et al. New enzyme immunoassays for sensitive detection of circulating Candida albicans mannan and anti-mannan antibodies: useful combined test for diagnosis of systemic candidiasis. J Clin Microbiol 1999;37:1510–7.

83. Mikulska M, Calandra T, Snguinetti M, et al. The use of mannan antigen and anti-mannan antibodies in the diagnosis of invasive candidiasis: recommendations from the Third European Conference on Infections in Leukemia. Crit Care 2010;14:R222.

84. León C, Ruiz-Santana S, Saavedra P, et al. Contribution of Candida biomarkers and DNA detection for the diagnosis of invasive candidiasis in ICU patients with severe abdominal conditions. Crit Care 2016;20:149.

85. Ahmad S, Khan Z. Invasive candidiasis: a review of nonculture-based laboratory diagnostic methods. Indian J Med Microbiol 2012;30:264–9.

86. Avni T, Leibovici L, Paul M. PCR diagnosis of invasive candidiasis: systematic review and meta-analysis. J Clin Microbiol 2011;49:665–70.

87. Fortún J, Meije Y, Buitrago MJ, et al. Clinical validation of a multiplex real-time PCR assay for detection of invasive candidiasis in intensive care unit patients. J Antimicrob Chemother 2014;69:3134–41.

88. Playford EG, Lipman J, Sorrell TC. Prophylaxis, empirical and preemptive treatment of invasive candidiasis. Curr Opin Crit Care 2010;16:470–4.

89. Pelz RK, Hendrix CW, Swoboda SM, et al. Double-blind placebo-controlled trial of fluconazole to prevent Candida infections in critically ill surgical patients. Ann Surg 2001;233:542–8.

90. Magill SS, Swoboda SM, Shields CR, et al. The epidemiology of Candida colonization and invasive candidiasis in a surgical intensive care unit where fluconazole prophylaxis is utilized. Ann Surg 2009;249:657–65.

91. Faiz S, Neale B, Rios E, et al. Risk-based fluconazole prophylaxis of Candida bloodstream infection in a medical intensive care unit. Eur J Clin Microbiol Infect Dis 2009;28:689–92.

92. Garbino J, Lew DP, Romand JA, et al. Prevention of severe Candida infections in nonneutropenic, high-risk, critically ill patients: a randomized, double-blind, placebo-controlled trial in patients treated by selective digestive decontamination. Intensive Care Med 2002;28:1708–17.

93. Ostrosky-Zeichner L, Shoham S, Vazquez J, et al. MSG-01: a randomized, double-blind,

placebo-controlled trial of caspofungin prophylaxis followed by preemptive therapy for invasive candidiasis in high-risk adults in the critical care setting. Clin Infect Dis 2014;50.1210 26.

94. Schuster MG, Edwards JE, Sobel JD, et al. Empirical fluconazole versus placebo for intensive care unit patients: a randomized trial. Ann Intern Med 2008;149:83–90.

95. Cortegiani A, Russotto V, Maggiore A, et al. Antifungal agents for preventing fungal infections in non-neutropenic critically ill patients. Cochrane Database Syst Rev 2016;(1):CD004920.

96. Bailly S, Bouadma L, Azoulay E, et al. Failure of empirical systemic antifungal therapy in mechanically ventilated critically ill patients. Am J Respir Crit Care Med 2015;191:1139–46.

97. Skrobik Y, Laverdiere M. Why Candida sepsis should matter to ICU physicians. Crit Care Clin 2013;29:853–64.

98. Safdar A, Ma J, Saliba F, et al. Drug-induced nephrotoxicity caused by amphotericin B lipid complex and liposomal amphotericin B: a review and meta-analysis. Medicine (Baltimore) 2010;89:236–44.

99. Bates DW, Su L, Yu DT, et al. Mortality and costs of acute renal failure associated with amphotericin B therapy. Clin Infect Dis 2001;32:686–93.

100. Rex JH, Bennett JE, Sugar AM, et al. A randomized trial comparing fluconazole with amphotericin B for the treatment of candidemia in patients without neutropenia. N Engl J Med 1994;331:1325–30.

101. Mora-Duarte J, Betts R, Rotstein C, et al. Comparison of caspofungin and amphotericin B for invasive candidiasis. N Engl J Med 2002;347:2020–9.

102. Kuse ER, Chetchotisakd P, da Cunha CA, et al. Micafungin versus liposomal amphotericin B for candidaemia and invasive candidosis: a phase III randomized double-blind trial. Lancet 2007;369: 1519–27.

103. Pappas PG, Rotstein CM, Betts RF, et al. Micafungin versus caspofungin for treatment of candidemia and other forms of invasive candidiasis. Clin Infect Dis 2007;45:883–93.

104. Reboli AC, Schorr AF, Rotstein, et al. Anidulafungin compared to fluconazole for treatment of candidemia and other forms of invasive candidiasis caused by Candida albicans: a multivariate analysis of factors associated with improved outcome. BMC Infect Dis 2011;11:261.

105. Dannaoui E, Desnos-Ollivier M, Garcia-Hermoso D, et al. Candida spp with acquired echinocandin resistance, France, 2004-2010. Emerg Infect Dis 2012;18:86–90.

106. Alexander BD, Johnson MD, Pfeiffer CD, et al. Increasing echinocandin resistance in Candida glabrata: clinical failure correlates with presence of FKS mutations and elevated minimum inhibitory concentrations. Clin Infect Dis 2013;56:1724–32.

107. Lewis JS 2nd, Wiederhold NP, Wickes BL, et al. Rapid emergence of echinocandin resistance in Candida glabrata resulting in clinical and microbiologic failure. Antimicrob Agents Chemother 2013; 57:4559–61.

108. Chiotos K, Vendetti N, Zaoutis TE, et al. Comparative effectiveness of echinocandins versus fluconazole therapy for the treatment of adult candidaemia due to Candida parapsilosis: a retrospective observational cohort study of the Mycoses Study Group (MSG-12). J Antimicrob Chemother 2016;71(12): 3536–9.

109. Vazquez J, Reboli AC, Pappas PG, et al. Evaluation of an early step-down strategy from intravenous anidulafungin to oral azole therapy for the treatment of candidemia and other forms of invasive candidiasis: results from an open-label trial. BMC Infect Dis 2014;14:97.

110. Morrell M, Fraser VJ, Kollef MH. Delaying the empiric treatment of Candida bloodstream infection until positive blood culture results are obtained: a potential risk factor for hospital mortality. Antimicrob Agents Chemother 2005;49:3640–5.

111. Marriott DJE, Playford EG, Chen S, et al. Determinants of mortality in non-neutropenic ICU patients with candidemia. Crit Care 2009;13:R115.

112. Patel GP, Simon D, Scheetz M, et al. The effect of time to antifungal therapy on mortality in candidemia associated septic shock. Am J Ther 2009;16: 508–11.

113. Paiva JA, Pereira JM, Tabah A, et al. Characteristics and risk factors for 28-day mortality of hospital acquired fungemias in ICUs: data from the EURO-BACT study. Crit Care 2016;20:53.

114. Tumbarello M, Posteraro B, Trecarichi EM, et al. Biofilm production by Candida species and inadequate antifungal therapy as predictors of mortality for patients with candidemia. J Clin Microbiol 2007;45:1843–50.

115. Puig-Asensio M, Pemán J, Zaragoza R, et al. Impact of therapeutic strategies on the prognosis of candidemia in the ICU. Crit Care Med 2014;42: 1423–32.

116. Eggimann P, Garbino J, Pittet D. Epidemiology of Candida species infections in critically ill non-immunosuppressed patients. Lancet Infect Dis 2003;3:685–702.

117. Pfaller MA, Diekema DJ. Epidemiology of invasive candidiasis: a persistent public health problem. Clin Microbiol Rev 2007;20:133–63.

118. Arendrup MC. Epidemiology of invasive candidiasis. Curr Opin Crit Care 2010;16:445–52.

119. Silva S, Negri M, Henriques M, et al. Candida glabrata, Candida parapsilosis and Candida tropicalis: biology, epidemiology, pathogenicity and antifungal resistance. FEMS Microbiol Rev 2012;36: 288–305.

120. Pfaller MA, Diekema DJ, Gibbs DL, et al. Candida krusei, a multidrug-resistant opportunistic fungal pathogen: geographic and temporal trends from the ARTEMIS DISK antifungal surveillance program, 2001 to 2005. J Clin Microbiol 2008;46: 515–21.

121. Bruggemann RJ, Alfenaar JW, Blijlevens NM, et al. Clinical relevance of the pharmacokinetic interactions of azole antifungal drugs with other coadministered agents. Clin Infect Dis 2009;48: 1441–58.

122. Lewis RE. Current concepts in antifungal pharmacology. Mayo Clin Proc 2011;86:805–17.

123. Pfaller MA, Boyken L, Hollis RJ, et al. In vitro susceptibility of invasive isolates of Candida spp to anidulafungin, caspofungin, and micafungin: six years of global surveillance. J Clin Microbiol 2008;46:150–6.

Fungal Infections After Lung Transplantation

Cassie C. Kennedy, MD[a],*, Raymund R. Razonable, MD[b]

KEYWORDS

- Solid organ transplantation • Lung transplantation • Fungal infection • Fungal prophylaxis

KEY POINTS

- Incidence of invasive fungal infections after lung transplantation is variable, with a mean of 8.6%.
- Prevention is a key management strategy for lung transplant recipients with most lung transplant centers providing antifungal prophylaxis for at least 3 months to 6 months postoperatively.
- Although prophylaxis drug regimens vary, common themes include the use of an azole therapy with or without inhaled amphotericin B product (to prevent invasive molds and yeast infections) and trimethoprim-sulfamethoxazole (to prevent *Pneumocystis jirovecii*).
- Manifestations of invasive fungal disease include pneumonia, pleural/mediastinal space infections, anastomotic infections, and disseminated disease.

INTRODUCTION

The first lung transplant was performed in 1963.[1] Since then, lung transplantation has emerged as a potential lifesaving treatment modality for end-stage chronic obstructive pulmonary disease, interstitial lung disease, pulmonary hypertension, and cystic fibrosis. Since 1988, more than 32,224 lung transplantations have been performed in the United States.[2] The median survival after adult lung transplantation is approximately 50% at 5 years.[2]

Survival after lung transplantation is influenced by the occurrence of 2 major complications — allograft rejection and infection (and their complications). In an effort to improve allograft survival, lung transplant recipients are maintained on an often-intense immunosuppressive drug regimen to prevent rejection and maintain allograft function. The downside of this practice, however, is a heightened risk of opportunistic infections, including invasive

fungal disease.[3] Up to 8.6% of patients develop invasive fungal infections during the first year after lung transplantation, although the incidence rates reported in clinical studies have varied widely depending on multiple factors, such as patient exposures, patient populations, immunosuppressive drug use, center-dependent practices (including the use of antifungal and other antibiotic prophylaxis), duration of study follow-up, and definitions of invasive fungal infection, among other factors.[3–5]

MICROBIOLOGY AND CLINICAL MANIFESTATIONS

The most common pathogens that cause invasive fungal infections after lung transplantation are *Aspergillus* spp (44%, most commonly *Aspergillus fumigatus*), *Candida* spp (23%, most commonly *C albicans*), and other molds, such as *Scedosporium* spp (20%). Members of the *Mucorales* group (3%,

Disclosure: Dr. C.C. Kennedy is supported by the National Heart, Lung, And Blood Institute (K23HL128859) and Dr. R.R. Razonable is supported by the National Institute of Allergy and Infectious Diseases (0024031-3) of the National Institutes of Health (NIH). The content is solely the responsibility of the authors and does not necessarily represent the official views of the NIH.

[a] Division of Pulmonary and Critical Care Medicine, William J. von Liebig Center for Transplantation and Clinical Regeneration, Mayo Clinic Robert D. and Patricia E. Kern Center for the Science of Health Care Delivery, Mayo Clinic, 200 First Street Southwest, Rochester, MN 55905, USA; [b] Division of Infectious Diseases, William J. von Liebig Center for Transplantation and Clinical Regeneration, Mayo Clinic, 200 First Street Southwest, Rochester, MN 55905, USA
* Corresponding author.
E-mail address: kennedy.cassie@mayo.edu

chestmed.theclinics.com

including *Mucor* and *Rhizopus*), *Cryptococcus neoformans* (2%), and the endemic mycoses (1%, including *Histoplasma capsulatum*, *Coccidioides immitis*, and *Blastomyces dermatitidis*) account for only a small proportion of cases.[3–6] The incidence of *P jirovecii* was up to 15% (in the absence of prophylaxis) but this has declined remarkably with the widespread use of prophylaxis.[7]

A majority of invasive fungal infections occur during the first 3 months to 12 months after lung transplantation. Depending on the specific pathogen and associated risk factors, mold infections manifest clinically as ulcerative tracheobronchitis, invasive pulmonary parenchymal disease, disseminated multiorgan disease, and/or fungemia. *Candida* spp infections, on the other hand, often cause fungemia, mediastinitis, and pleural space infection. *Cryptococcus neoformans, H capsulatum*, and *Coccidioides immitis* cause pneumonia, with tendency to disseminate to other organ systems, including the brain. *P jirovecii* also typically causes pneumonia that manifests with nonproductive cough, hypoxemia, and bilateral interstitial infiltrates. A diagnosis of invasive fungal infections after lung transplantation can be established by demonstration of the fungi in affected tissues. This can be accomplished with culture of blood, respiratory fluid, and other clinical samples; antigen detection in blood, respiratory fluid, and other clinical samples (eg, galactomannan, 1,3-β-D-glucan, and cryptococcal antigen); nucleic acid testing of clinical samples; and demonstration of the fungal pathogen in affected tissues.[6]

Collectively, invasive fungal infections directly and indirectly contribute to the poor outcome after lung transplantation.[3–6] They have been associated with a higher risk of bronchiolitis obliterans.[8] The mortality rate is also generally higher, especially in those with invasive and disseminated disease. Historically, the mortality rate is up to 25% among those with fungal tracheobronchitis compared with up to 80% among those with invasive pulmonary aspergillosis.[3,4,6,7] These rates have declined with the use of more effective antifungal drugs. Currently, the overall 3-month mortality rate is up to 22% of all lung transplant recipients with invasive fungal infection,[9] whereas 1-year mortality is up to 44%.[10]

RISK FACTORS

There are several host and environmental factors that increase the risk for invasive fungal infection after lung transplantation. The constant exposure of the transplanted lung to the environment and the abnormal anatomic and physiologic function of the transplanted lung (ie, impaired ciliary function, blunted cough reflex, and denervation injury) predispose to a higher risk of invasive fungal infections. Invasive aspergillosis and other mold infections are more common in older patients, those who have airway ischemia, those who developed cytomegalovirus disease, and those with colonization with *Aspergillus* spp.[11–13] Those who received single lung transplants are also at higher risk of invasive fungal infection compared with double lung transplant recipients, because the retained lung (in single lung transplants) can serve as reservoir for potentially pathogenic fungi. Patients with structural lung diseases, such as cystic fibrosis, are often colonized with fungi, most commonly *Aspergillus* spp, prior to lung transplantation and they have a 4-fold higher risk of invasive aspergillosis.[14] Colonization of the paranasal sinuses can also serve as reservoir for fungal colonization in patients with cystic fibrosis. The need for bronchial stents also predisposes to higher risk of invasive fungal infections, including *Candida* spp and *Aspergillus* spp. An overimmunosuppressed state increases the risk, including those with neutropenia, hypogammaglobulinemia, and T-cell depletion. Lung transplant recipients are especially vulnerable to infection with fungi due to the constant direct exposure of the lung allograft to the outside environment. Environmental exposure is a well-described risk factor for invasive mold infections, especially in areas of farming and construction.[15,16]

PREVENTION

Because of the increased risk of invasive fungal infection, and its association with adverse outcomes,[3] its prevention is a standard of care after lung transplantation. Minimizing environmental exposures, such as avoidance of areas with high concentration of fungal spores (eg, areas of construction) and the use of personal protective equipment (such as masks) during anticipated periods of exposure, are recommendations to reduce the risk. In addition, minimization of indwelling urinary catheters and indwelling central vascular lines help with prevention of *Candida* spp fungemia and funguria in the perioperative period. Preventing invasive fungal infection can further be accomplished with antifungal drugs for either prophylaxis or preemptive therapy. The drugs that are used for prevention are listed in **Table 1**.

There is no widely accepted optimal method for prevention, partly due to lack of comparative clinical trials among various strategies. In worldwide surveys conducted among lung transplant centers, only 31% to 36% of centers perform preemptive

Table 1
Antifungal drugs for the prevention and treatment of fungal infections after lung transplantation

Class	Drugs	Clinical Applications	Comments
Amphotericin B products	AmB deoxycholate	Prevention: inhaled formulation; variable dose and duration (eg, 25 mg/d) Treatment: 0.25–1.5 mg/kg IV daily (dose varies depending on pathogen)	Inhaled formulation does not protect against extrapulmonary fungal infections. Systemic formulation is associated with infusion-related and renal toxicity.
	AmB lipid complex	Prevention: inhaled formulation; variable dose and duration (eg, 50 mg every 2 d or weekly) Treatment: 5 mg/kg IV daily	Inhaled formulation does not protect against extrapulmonary fungal infections. Systemic formulation is associated with infusion-related and renal toxicity but at lower risk compared with AmB deoxycholate.
	AmB liposome	Prevention: inhaled formulation; variable dose and duration (eg, 25 mg every 2 d or weekly) Treatment: 3–5 mg/kg IV daily (up to 10-mg/kg daily has been used)	Inhaled formulation does not protect against extrapulmonary fungal infections. Systemic formulation is associated with infusion-related and renal toxicity but at lower risk compared with AmB deoxycholate.
Azoles	Fluconazole	Prevention: not recommended Treatment: 200–800 mg IV or po daily	Not recommended for prophylaxis due to lack of activity against *Aspergillus* spp and other molds. Used for treatment of candida, endemic fungi, and crytococcocus. Drug interaction with CNI
	Isavuconazole	Prevention: no data Treatment: 200 mg po/IV every 8 h for 6 doses, then once daily	Limited data for use as prophylaxis Treatment of invasive aspergillosis and mucormycosis Drug interaction with CNI
	Itraconazole	Prevention and treatment: 200 mg po tid for 3 d, then bid Treatment: 200 mg po tid for 3 d, then bid	Therapeutic drug monitoring is recommended but no consensus on effective drug levels. Drug interaction with CNI
	Posaconazole	Prevention and treatment: Oral suspension — 200 mg po tid Tablet — 300 mg po bid × 2 doses, then once daily IV — 300 mg bid × 2 doses, then once daily	Active against candida, aspergillosis Can be used for zygomycosis Drug interaction with CNI
	Voriconazole	Prevention and treatment: Oral — 200 mg po bid IV — 6 mg/kg every 12 h for 24 h, then 4 mg/kg	Most common azole used for prophylaxis; therapeutic drug monitoring to guide dose Drug interaction with CNI

(continued on next page)

Table 1
(continued)

Class	Drugs	Clinical Applications	Comments
Echinocandins	Anidulafungin	Treatment: 200 mg IV loading dose, then 100 mg daily	Not recommended for long-term prophylaxis
	Caspofungin	Treatment: 70 mg IV loading dose, then 50 mg IV once daily	Not recommended for long-term prophylaxis
	Micafungin	Treatment: 100 mg IV once daily	Not recommended for long-term prophylaxis
Others	Flucytosine	Treatment: 50–150 mg/kg/d po in divided doses	Used in combination with amphotericn B for treatment of cryptococcosis Not recommended for prophylaxis Should not be used alone
	Trimethoprim-sulfamethoxazole	Prevention: variable dose (single-strength to double-strength tablet once daily to 3 times weekly) Treatment: 75–100 mg/kg/d of sulfamethoxazole or 15–20 mg/kg/d of trimethoprim in divided doses every 6 h for 14–21 d	Prevention and treatment of *P jiroveci*

Abbreviations: AmB, amphotericin B; CNI, calcineurin inhibitor; IV, intravenous.

therapy — a strategy of providing antifungal therapy only on detection of fungal infection by surveillance cultures or fungal antigen detection in clinical specimens.[17–19] Studies have shown that detection of *Aspergillus* spp on surveillance cultures during the first 3 months after lung transplantation is a good marker for initiation of preemptive therapy.[20] This preemptive strategy is based on the principle of providing antifungal drugs only to the population at highest risk of invasive fungal disease. This reduces the exposure of most patients to the adverse effects of antifungal drugs. Its downside, however, is the lack of widely acceptable measure for surveillance that could sensitively capture all fungi (other than *Aspergillus* spp) that causes invasive fungal disease. Moreover, the isolation of nonaspergillus mold colonization has not been conclusively associated with a higher risk of posttransplant invasive fungal disease.[21]

Accordingly, a majority (59%–69%) of transplant centers provide antifungal prophylaxis to lung transplant recipients.[17–19] There is wide variation, however, in this practice — that is, whether this is given to all lung transplant recipients (universal approach) or only to selected patients (targeted approach) is subject to debate. Likewise, there is no consensus on the choice of antifungal agent, route of administration, and duration of prophylaxis. In a recent survey, the most common antifungal drug used is voriconazole, followed by

itraconazole and inhaled amphotericin B.[18] This lack of consensus is partly due to the few prospective data and randomized clinical trials, the variability in lung transplant populations and their risk factors, differences in induction and maintenance immunosuppressive strategies, local availability of various antifungal agents, and other center-dependent characteristics.

Choice of Antifungal Prophylaxis

Inhaled amphotericin B is one of the most commonly used drugs for antifungal prophylaxis after lung transplantation,[22] but its use has declined with the availability of newer triazoles.[18] A broad-spectrum antifungal drug, amphotericin B is active against the most common fungi causing invasive fungal infection after lung transplantation — *Aspergillus* spp, *Candida* spp, and *Mucorales* group. The protection provided by inhaled administration of amphotericin B, however, is limited only to the aerated lungs. In pharmacokinetic studies performed in lung transplant recipients, inhaled amphotericin B deoxycholate achieves high concentrations in the lower airways of transplanted lungs, but concentrations in native lungs (in the case of single lung transplant) are lower.[23] It also achieves good concentrations in the airways, thereby providing local delivery to the bronchial anastomosis and proximal areas at risk of infection. In the immediate postoperative period, the blood supply at the anastomosis site is compromised secondary to the surgical practice of forgoing bronchial artery anastomosis to the donor lung. Therefore, this topical approach to antifungal prophylaxis is appealing to many lung transplant centers.

The optimal dosage, formulation (deoxycholate or lipid formulations), and durations of prophylaxis with inhaled amphotericin B are unknown (see **Table 1**), and, based on surveys, it is highly variable among lung transplant centers.[18] Daily administration is the most common frequency for the amphotericin B deoxycholate formulation, especially during the early period after lung transplantation when the risk of infection in the bronchial anastomosis is high. Amphotericin B deoxycholate is the most common formulation, but the lipid products are also available for use.[24] Concentrations of inhaled amphotericin B lipid complex (measured in epithelial lining fluid) and inhaled liposomal amphotericin B (measured in bronchoalveolar lavage aliquots) remain above the minimum inhibitory concentrations of *Aspergillus* spp for at least 7 days, potentially enabling once-weekly administration.[23] Inhaled amphotericin B is not systemically absorbed; hence, it is considered safe from the nephrotoxic effects of systemic amphotericin B. Inhaled formulations, however, do not provide protection against fungal infection beyond the airways and lung parenchyma, such as pleural space, mediastinum, blood, and other extrapulmonary tissues. Infections of the pleural space and mediastinum from *C albicans*, for example, are not prevented by inhaled amphotericin B administration. Such concerns over postoperative mediastinitis, pleuritis, and extrapulmonary infections argue for the need for a systemic antifungal prophylaxis. In a survey of lung transplant centers, up to 20% of centers provide a combination of inhaled amphotericin B with a systemic azole.[18]

The triazoles are the most commonly used drugs for systemic antifungal prophylaxis after lung transplantation. Voriconazole[17,25] is the most commonly used triazole, followed by itraconazole[3,5,26] and posaconazole.[18,27,28] Oral administration provides systemic antifungal concentrations that are widely distributed in various tissues, thereby providing antifungal protection to extrapulmonary sites. These antifungal drugs provide broad-spectrum antifungal activity against yeasts (including *Candida*) and most molds (including *Aspergillus*), and for posaconazole, against mucormycosis. The use of oral itraconazole, oral suspension of posaconazole, and to a lesser extent voriconazole is complicated by their unpredictable pharmacokinetics. Itraconazole, in particular, has poor to modest absorption after oral administration, and acceptable systemic levels may not be achieved with normal recommended dosages. Conversion to liquid formulation, or its coadministration with acidic fluid, may enhance the oral absorption of itraconazole. Conversely, the oral tablet form of posaconazole provides better pharmacokinetics compared with the oral suspension. Therapeutic drug monitoring to document an acceptable systemic itraconazole, posaconazole, and voriconazole levels is generally recommended,[29] but the optimal trough level that is needed for prophylactic efficacy has not been defined. Drug doses, therefore, vary depending on center-specific practices. The use of systemic triazoles is complicated by numerous drug-drug interactions, because of their potent inhibitory effects on the cytochrome p450 enzyme system. Most commonly, administration of itraconazole and voriconazole results in increased levels of tacrolimus and calcineurin inhibitors. Careful monitoring of potential drug interactions is, therefore, highly emphasized during the use of azoles. Triazoles also have hepatotoxicity, especially when initiated during the immediate postoperative period, and they have the effect of prolonging the QT interval.[14] Long-term use of voriconazole has also been associated with a heightened predisposition to squamous cell skin cancer[30] and painful periostitis characterized by the deposition of excess fluoride in the skeletal system.[31] Fluconazole is not recommended for general antifungal prophylaxis after lung transplantation due to its lack of activity against *Aspergillus* and other molds. The newest azole drug — isavuconazole — has broad-spectrum activity against *Aspergillus* spp and *Mucor* sp, but its clinical utility as antifungal prophylaxis after lung transplantation is not yet supported by solid scientific data.

The echinocandins — caspofungin, micafungin, anidulafungin — are a class of antifungal drugs that has broad-spectrum activity against *Candida* spp, *Aspergillus* spp, and other molds. They do not have any activity, however, against *Cryptococcus* sp, *H capsulatum*, *Coccidioides immitis*, and the endemic fungi. The role of echinocandins as antifungal prophylaxis is limited due to lack of oral formulation (hence, prohibitive for long-term use). Their availability only in intravenous formulation makes them useful mainly during empiric and targeted treatment of established invasive fungal infections. They are also potentially useful as antifungal prophylaxis during the early period after lung transplantation but often are switched to oral triazole prophylaxis once patients are able to take oral medications.[18]

Lifelong *P jirovecii* prophylaxis with trimethoprim-sulfamethoxazole is standard practice after lung transplant. Patients with sulfa allergy can often be desensitized after transplant. Those who cannot take trimethoprim-sulfamethoxazole can take alternatives, such as inhaled pentamidine monthly, oral dapsone, or atovaquone therapy.

Duration of Antifungal Prophylaxis

The duration of antifungal prophylaxis against invasive mold infections is variable among transplant centers. It can be as short as 3 months after lung transplantation and as long as a lifelong strategy in some centers. Most lung transplant centers provide antifungal prevention for 6 months to 12 months. This duration targets the highest risk period for anastomotic fungal infection or ulcerative tracheobronchitis, which occurs within 3 months after lung transplantation, and invasive and disseminated fungal disease, which occur most commonly during the first 6 months to 12 months.[3–6] Epidemiologic studies, however, have highlighted the occurrence of invasive fungal infections beyond this traditional period. Hence, others have attempted to extend the duration of antifungal prophylaxis. Whether this is the optimal approach is not known. This practice increases antifungal drug exposure that also directly increases cost, potential drug resistance, and adverse drug toxicities. There is also emerging data to suggest that the onset of invasive fungal infections may be delayed by use of antifungal prophylaxis. In recent multicenter observational studies, the median time to onset of invasive fungal infections was 184 days[4] but could be as long as 504 days[32] after transplantation. Another center reported the median time to onset of 363 days for aspergillosis and 419 days for other mold infections.[10] This delay in the onset of infections, potentially due to the effect of antifungal prophylaxis during the early period after lung transplantation, has led some centers to further extend the duration of antifungal prophylaxis.

ANASTOMOTIC FUNGAL INFECTIONS

The transplanted lungs are susceptible to anastomotic fungal infections due to *Candida* spp and *Aspergillus* spp in the early post-transplant period. Such infections may manifest clinically as change in spirometry, a complaint of noisy breathing, or a feeling of difficulty coughing up secretions. Diagnosis can be suspected with an irregularity of the airway or extraluminal air on chest imaging or the presence of a pseudomembrane on bronchoscopic inspection. Confirmation of diagnosis is made with anastomotic fungal cultures, stains, and biopsies. Positive *Aspergillus* cultures of respiratory secretions have been strongly associated with the subsequent occurrence of anastomotic complications, hence the need to provide universal or targeted antifungal prophylaxis to these patients.[33] The incidence of severe fungal pseudomembrane on anastomotic inspection was approximately 15%, with an overall fungal pseudomembrane occurrence in approximately half of the early bronchoscopies after lung transplantation.[34] The reported incidence of anastomotic fungal infections ranges from 4.9% to 24.6%,[35,36] with "infection" defined as the presence of necrosis or pseudomembrane on bronchoscopic inspection of the anastomosis and biopsy evidence of invasive fungal organism. In 1 series, *Aspergillus* and *Candida* comprised a majority of anastomotic infections at 2.1% and 2.8% of all recipients, respectively, and 93% of all anastomotic infections.[35] These recipients did not differ in survival from the noninfected cohort and there were no incidences of anastomotic dehiscence. In another series, 9.8% of recipients had *Candida* spp and 16.4% had *Aspergillus* anastomotic infections (including 1 recipient with both organisms).[36] The airway complication rate after fungal infection in this series was 46.7%, including bronchial stenosis and hemorrhage; the mortality rate was 20%.[36] Rare cases of Zygomycetes-associated anastomotic infections have been reported.[37] See **Fig. 1** for an example of an anastomotic dehiscence associated with a Zygomycetes infection in a lung transplant recipient. Empiric treatment of invasive fungal infection should target the most common pathogens (*Candida* spp and *Aspergillus* spp), with the use of voriconazole, amphotericin B, or an echinocandin (see **Table 1**). If Zygomycetes is suspected, amphotericin B, posaconazole, and isavuconazole may be used. The eventual definitive treatment should be tailored based on fungal culture results and antifungal susceptibility pattern.

FUNGAL PNEUMONIAS

Fungal pneumonias in lung transplant recipients are typically suspected based on chest imaging or change in spirometry. Patients may be asymptomatic or have signs and symptoms of pulmonary infection. Imaging may demonstrate an infiltrate, micronodules, or solid nodule(s). A bronchoalveolar lavage can be performed to obtain specimens for fungal stains and cultures. Invasive disease can be demonstrated by transbronchial biopsy or transthoracic needle

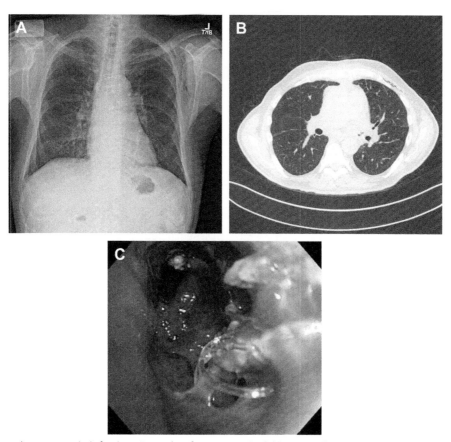

Fig. 1. Fungal anastomotic infection. Example of anastomotic dehiscence after single left lung transplant with associated positive bronchial culture for Zygomycetes. This 66-year-old male transplant recipient presented with noisy breathing and fall in spirometry 6 weeks after transplant. (*A*) Shows the chest radiograph with left bronchial irregularity and subcutaneous emphysema. (*B*) Shows the CT chest with air outside the bronchial tree and subcutaneous emphysema. (*C*) Demonstrates the findings at bronchoscopy of left bronchial anastomotic dehiscence with visible sutures. Patient responded to liposomal amphotericin B therapy and was converted to lifelong posaconazole therapy. The airway stenosed as it healed and the patient eventually required endoscopic balloon and silicone stent placement in the left airway.

aspiration. The most common pathogen causing invasive fungal pneumonia is *Aspergillus* spp. First-line treatment of invasive aspergillus pneumonia is voriconazole, and alternative treatment regimens are amphotericin B formulations (deoxycholate or lipid formulation). Echinocandins are often reserved only as salvage therapy for invasive aspergillosis. Aspergillomas are often treated with surgical resection, often with systemic antifungal therapy. See **Fig. 2** for an example of a pulmonary nodule, found on resection to be an aspergilloma in the native lung of a transplant recipient. Pneumonia due to endemic mycoses occur rarely after lung transplantation, probably due to the use of effective antifungal prophylaxis. Likewise, *P jiroveci* pneumonia has been reduced by trimethoprim-sulfamethoxazole prophylaxis.

FUNGAL MEDIASTINITIS/PLEURAL SPACE INFECTIONS

Fungal mediastinitis and fungal pleural space infections are rare after lung transplantation. Diagnosis can be suspected in cases of pleural effusion (pleural) or with sternal instability, erythema, or purulence (mediastinitis). Imaging may demonstrate fluid collection and/or pleural thickening. Diagnosis must be confirmed by fluid or tissue culture, stains, or pathology. In a large series of 776 thoracic transplant patients, mediastinitis had an incidence of 3.1% in lung and 5.2% in heart-lung recipients; *Candida* spp mediastinitis comprised 14.3% of the cases and the rest were bacterial.[38] In contrast, most pleural space infections are caused by fungal infection.[39] In a series of 455 recipients, the incidence of pleural

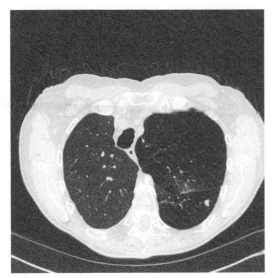

Fig. 2. Aspergilloma. Asymptomatic, 67-year-old man presents 6 months after right single lung transplant for α_1-antitrypsin deficiency with a new native lung nodule. This was found to be an aspergilloma on resection.

infections in the first 90 days was 7.5% with approximately two-thirds (61%) of these caused by fungus.[39] *Candida* spp accounted for 90.1% of these with *Aspergillus* causing 9.9%.[39] The 1-year survival of patients with a pleural space infection in this series was significantly lower than those without infection (67% vs 87%).[39] Hence, aggressive treatment should be pursued to improve outcome. Surgical débridement and evacuation of infected fluid collections is key and should be complemented by systemic antifungal therapy. Empiric antifungal treatment should target the 2 most common pathogens (*Candida* spp and *Aspergillus* spp), either with the use of extended-spectrum triazole (voriconazole) or amphotericin B or an echinocandin. Definitive treatment should be based on fungal culture results and antifungal susceptibility pattern (see **Table 1**), See **Fig. 3** for an example chest CT of a 45-year-old woman who developed a mixed fungal and bacterial pleural space infection after lung transplantation for cystic fibrosis.

DISSEMINATED FUNGAL INFECTIONS

Disseminated fungal infection in lung transplant recipients is characterized by infection of the blood stream or the involvement of multiple noncontiguous sites. The most common organisms causing invasive fungal infections in solid organ transplant recipients are *Candida* spp and less commonly *Aspergillus* spp. Much less common are infections due to *Cryptococcus neoformans*, *Scedosporium*, *Mucormycoses*, and *Fusarium*.[4,9] Invasive candidiasis is rare in lung transplant recipients (compared with other organ transplant types), and manifests clinically as blood stream infection, often in relation to indwelling vascular catheters. Azoles (including fluconazole), amphotericin B, and echinocandins are effective treatment but should be guided by fungal culture results and susceptibility testing. Angioinvasive aspergillosis is rarely detected in blood cultures but often manifests with multifocal disease, with abscess formation

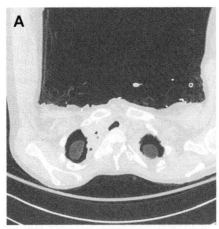
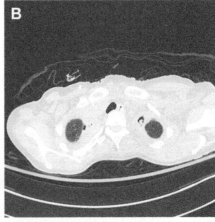

Fig. 3. Complicated postoperative bacterial and fungal pleural space infection. A 45-year-old woman with bilateral lung transplant for cystic fibrosis. At the time of transplant, the native lung apices were fused to the chest wall and diseased such that complete excision was not possible. The patient developed complicated, multiorganism pleural space infection with *Mycoplasma salivarium*, *Pseudomonas aeruginosa*, *C albicans*, and *Aspergillus fumigatus* sp. (*A*) Chest CT 9 days postoperative. (*B*) Chest CT 15 days postoperative.

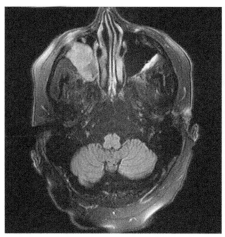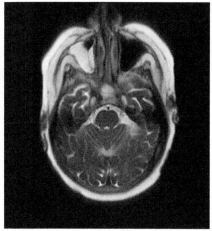

Fig. 4. Central nervous system aspergillosis. A 61-year old man 11 months post–lung transplant presented with right sided headache, double vision, and conjunctivitis. Head imaging demonstrated a right orbital mass. Biopsy demonstrated necrosis, inflammation, and numerous invading narrow-septate hyphae. Cultures grew *Aspergillus fumigatus*. Patient was treated with liposomal amphotericin B, followed by caspofungin and voriconazole, then ultimately lifelong posaconazole therapy.

in extrapulmonary sites, such as central nervous system disease. See **Fig. 4** for an example of imaging of central nervous system aspergillosis in a lung transplant recipient.

SUMMARY

Fungal infections contribute significantly to lung transplant morbidity and mortality. Prevention strategies, including antifungal prophylaxis, are commonly used but controversy remains regarding the optimal drug and duration of prophylaxis. Other common methods of preventing fungal disease (masks, avoidance, and so forth) are encouraged as are best practices to limit patient exposures to lines and hardware. Fungal infections may manifest as invasive anastomosis, lung parenchyma, pleural/mediastinal space, disseminated, or bloodstream infections. The most common pathogens are *Aspergillus* spp and *Candida* spp Empiric treatment should, therefore, target these 2 most common pathogens, but definitive treatment should always be guided by fungal cultures and antifungal susceptibility tests.

REFERENCES

1. Hardy JD, Webb WR, Dalton ML Jr, et al. Lung homotransplantation in man. JAMA 1963;186:1065–74.
2. 2016; Available at: https://www.unos.org/data/. Accessed August 15, 2016.
3. Arthurs SK, Eid AJ, Deziel PJ, et al. The impact of invasive fungal diseases on survival after lung transplantation. Clin Transplant 2010;24(3):341–8.
4. Pappas PG, Alexander BD, Andes DR, et al. Invasive fungal infections among organ transplant recipients: results of the transplant-associated infection surveillance network (TRANSNET). Clin Infect Dis 2010;50(8):1101–11.
5. Chong PP, Kennedy CC, Hathcock MA, et al. Epidemiology of invasive fungal infections in lung transplant recipients on long-term azole antifungal prophylaxis. Clin Transplant 2015;29(4):311–8.
6. Singh N, Husain S. Aspergillosis in solid organ transplantation. Am J Transplant 2013;13(Suppl 4): 228–41.
7. Martin SI, Fishman JA. Pneumocystis pneumonia in solid organ transplantation. Am J Transplant 2013; 13(Suppl 4):272–9.
8. Weigt SS, Elashoff RM, Huang C, et al. Aspergillus colonization of the lung allograft is a risk factor for bronchiolitis obliterans syndrome. Am J Transplant 2009;9(8):1903–11.
9. Doligalski CT, Benedict K, Cleveland AA, et al. Epidemiology of invasive mold infections in lung transplant recipients. Am J Transplant 2014;14(6): 1328–33.
10. Vazquez R, Vazquez-Guillamet MC, Suarez J, et al. Invasive mold infections in lung and heart-lung transplant recipients: Stanford University experience. Transpl Infect Dis 2015;17(2):259–66.
11. Cahill BC, Hibbs JR, Savik K, et al. Aspergillus airway colonization and invasive disease after lung transplantation. Chest 1997;112(5):1160–4.
12. Gavalda J, Len O, San Juan R, et al. Risk factors for invasive aspergillosis in solid-organ transplant recipients: a case-control study. Clin Infect Dis 2005; 41(1):52–9.

13. Husni RN, Gordon SM, Longworth DL, et al. Cytomegalovirus infection is a risk factor for invasive aspergillosis in lung transplant recipients. Clin Infect Dis 1998;26(3):753–5.

14. Luong ML, Chaparro C, Stephenson A, et al. Pre-transplant aspergillus colonization of cystic fibrosis patients and the incidence of post-lung transplant invasive aspergillosis. Transplantation 2014;97(3):351–7.

15. Raviv Y, Kramer MR, Amital A, et al. Outbreak of aspergillosis infections among lung transplant recipients. Transpl Int 2007;20(2):135–40.

16. Sole A, Morant P, Salavert M, et al. Aspergillus infections in lung transplant recipients: risk factors and outcome. Clin Microbiol Infect 2005;11(5):359–65.

17. Husain S, Paterson DL, Studer S, et al. Voriconazole prophylaxis in lung transplant recipients. Am J Transplant 2006;6(12):3008–16.

18. Neoh CF, Snell GI, Kotsimbos T, et al. Antifungal prophylaxis in lung transplantation–a world-wide survey. Am J Transplant 2011;11(2):361–6.

19. He SY, Makhzoumi ZH, Singer JP, et al. Practice variation in aspergillus prophylaxis and treatment among lung transplant centers: a national survey. Transpl Infect Dis 2015;17(1):14–20.

20. Hosseini-Moghaddam SM, Chaparro C, Luong ML, et al. The effectiveness of culture-directed preemptive anti-aspergillus treatment in lung transplant recipients at one year after transplant. Transplantation 2015;99(11):2387–93.

21. Silveira FP, Kwak EJ, Paterson DL, et al. Post-transplant colonization with non-aspergillus molds and risk of development of invasive fungal disease in lung transplant recipients. J Heart Lung Transplant 2008;27(8):850–5.

22. Drew RH, Dodds Ashley E, Benjamin DK Jr, et al. Comparative safety of amphotericin B lipid complex and amphotericin B deoxycholate as aerosolized antifungal prophylaxis in lung-transplant recipients. Transplantation 2004;77(2):232–7.

23. Monforte V, Roman A, Gavalda J, et al. Nebulized amphotericin B concentration and distribution in the respiratory tract of lung-transplanted patients. Transplantation 2003;75(9):1571–4.

24. Palmer SM, Drew RH, Whitehouse JD, et al. Safety of aerosolized amphotericin B lipid complex in lung transplant recipients. Transplantation 2001;72(3):545–8.

25. Mitsani D, Nguyen MH, Shields RK, et al. Prospective, observational study of voriconazole therapeutic drug monitoring among lung transplant recipients receiving prophylaxis: factors impacting levels of and associations between serum troughs, efficacy, and toxicity. Antimicrob Agents Chemother 2012;56(5):2371–7.

26. Kato K, Nagao M, Nakano S, et al. Itraconazole prophylaxis for invasive aspergillus infection in lung transplantation. Transpl Infect Dis 2014;16(2):340–3.

27. Robinson CL, Chau C, Yerkovich ST, et al. Posaconazole in lung transplant recipients: use, tolerability, and efficacy. Transpl Infect Dis 2016;18(2):302–8.

28. Patterson TF, Thompson GR 3rd, Denning DW, et al. Practice guidelines for the diagnosis and management of aspergillosis: 2016 update by the infectious diseases society of America. Clin Infect Dis 2016;63(4):e1–60.

29. Thakuria L, Packwood K, Firouzi A, et al. A pharmacokinetic analysis of posaconazole oral suspension in the serum and alveolar compartment of lung transplant recipients. Int J Antimicrob Agents 2016;47(1):69–76.

30. Goyal RK. Voriconazole-associated phototoxic dermatoses and skin cancer. Expert Rev Anti Infect Ther 2015;13(12):1537–46.

31. Wermers RA, Cooper K, Razonable RR, et al. Fluoride excess and periostitis in transplant patients receiving long-term voriconazole therapy. Clin Infect Dis 2011;52(5):604–11.

32. Neofytos D, Fishman JA, Horn D, et al. Epidemiology and outcome of invasive fungal infections in solid organ transplant recipients. Transpl Infect Dis 2010;12(3):220–9.

33. Herrera JM, McNeil KD, Higgins RS, et al. Airway complications after lung transplantation: treatment and long-term outcome. Ann Thorac Surg 2001;71(3):989–93 [discussion: 993–4].

34. Weder W, Inci I, Korom S, et al. Airway complications after lung transplantation: risk factors, prevention and outcome. Eur J Cardiothorac Surg 2009;35(2):293–8 [discussion: 298].

35. Hadjiliadis D, Howell DN, Davis RD, et al. Anastomotic infections in lung transplant recipients. Ann Transplant 2000;5(3):13–9.

36. Nunley DR, Gal AA, Vega JD, et al. Saprophytic fungal infections and complications involving the bronchial anastomosis following human lung transplantation. Chest 2002;122(4):1185–91.

37. McGuire FR, Grinnan DC, Robbins M. Mucormycosis of the bronchial anastomosis: a case of successful medical treatment and historic review. J Heart Lung Transplant 2007;26(8):857–61.

38. Abid Q, Nkere UU, Hasan A, et al. Mediastinitis in heart and lung transplantation: 15 years experience. Ann Thorac Surg 2003;75(5):1565–71.

39. Wahidi MM, Willner DA, Snyder LD, et al. Diagnosis and outcome of early pleural space infection following lung transplantation. Chest 2009;135(2):484–91.

Allergic and Noninvasive Infectious Pulmonary Aspergillosis Syndromes

Eavan G. Muldoon, MD, MPH[a,b,*], Mary E. Strek, MD[c],
Karen C. Patterson, MD[d]

KEYWORDS

- Aspergillus • ABPA • Aspergillus bronchitis • Chronic fungal infection of lung

KEY POINTS

- Allergic bronchopulmonary aspergillosis (ABPA) is a hyperimmune response to the presence of fungi in the airway in patients with asthma, which leads to permanent airway damage and often requires immunosuppression for adequate treatment.
- As a result of defects in immune clearance and mechanical clearance, patients with cystic fibrosis (CF) are particularly vulnerable to developing ABPA, which may hasten their clinical decline.
- In severe asthma with fungal sensitization (SAFS), exposures to fungi can account for asthma exacerbations; the diagnosis often requires escalation to maximal asthma therapy.
- Chronic pulmonary aspergillosis (CPA) is a spectrum of noninvasive infectious aspergillus diseases, which range from simple nodules to indolent aspergillomas to progressive cavitating and fibrotic lung disease.
- A diagnosis of aspergillus bronchitis should be considered in patients with lingering bronchitis symptoms and repeatedly positive fungal cultures.

INTRODUCTION

Despite the ubiquity of *Aspergillus* spp and that the spores are inhaled daily, only a small proportion of the population develops clinical disease. *Aspergillus* spp can cause a spectrum of disease from allergy, which does not represent true infection, to colonization, chronic infection, and finally invasive disease.[1] This article reviews the noninvasive *Aspergillus* syndromes, focusing on clinical presentation, diagnosis, management, and potential complications.

ALLERGIC ASPERGILLOSIS
Allergic Bronchopulmonary Aspergillosis

ABPA occurs almost exclusively in patients with asthma or CF, where fungal sensitization elicits a robust hypersensitivity response characterized by elevated total serum immunoglobulin (Ig) E and *Aspergillus*-specific IgE and IgG antibodies (**Table 1**). ABPA is estimated to occur in 2.5% of patients with asthma and should be suspected in patients with difficult to control or corticosteroid dependent disease or in those who expectorate

Disclosure Statement: The authors have nothing to disclose.
[a] National Aspergillosis Centre, University Hospital of South Manchester, Southmoor Road, Wythenshawe, Manchester M23 9LT, UK; [b] Division of Infection, Immunity and Respiratory Medicine, University of Manchester, Manchester, UK; [c] Section of Pulmonary and Critical Care, Department of Medicine, University of Chicago, 5481 South Maryland Avenue, Chicago, IL 60637, USA; [d] Division of Pulmonary, Allergy and Critical Care, University of Pennsylvania, 3400 Spruce Street, 828 West Gates Building, Philadelphia, PA 19104, USA
* Corresponding author. National Aspergillosis Centre, University Hospital of South Manchester, Southmoor Road, Wythenshawe, Manchester M23 9LT, United Kingdom.
E-mail address: eavan.muldoon@manchester.ac.uk

Clin Chest Med 38 (2017) 521–534
http://dx.doi.org/10.1016/j.ccm.2017.04.012
0272-5231/17/© 2017 Elsevier Inc. All rights reserved.

Table 1
Features of allergic aspergillus pulmonary diseases

Subtype	Defining Clinical Features	Diagnostic Immunologic Features	Treatment
ABPA in asthma	Persistent or escalating asthma symptoms and bronchiectasis (+/− mucus plugging and tree in bud changes) noted on chest imaging; fungal cultures may be positive for *Aspergillus spp.*	• Markedly elevated total IgE • Positive skin prick testing and/or elevated serum aspergillus-specific IgE levels • +/− Elevated aspergillus-specific IgG levels • Eosinophilia is common but not required	• Systemic corticosteroids • ICS, Bronchodilators • Trial of antifungal agents in some cases • +/− Omalizumab • Fungal avoidance if high antigen exposure
ABPA in CF	Similar to non-CF ABPA + progressive pulmonary decline, which can be permanent.	Similar to non-CF ABPA.	Similar to non-CF ABPA
SAFS	Asthma requiring high-dose ICS and often an additional controller medication + fungal sensitization; does not meet criteria for ABPA.	Positive skin prick and/or elevated serum antifungal IgE levels.	• Maximum inhaler therapy • +/− Omalizumab • Antifungal agents remain investigational

Abbreviation: ICS, inhaled corticosteroids.

mucus plugs or demonstrate bronchiectasis and/or mucus plugging on chest imaging.[2–4] It is important to establish the diagnosis of ABPA because this has an impact on therapy and potentially reduces morbidity and complications that might otherwise ensue.

Diagnosis of allergic bronchopulmonary aspergillosis

Diagnostic criteria for ABPA have been updated recently after a conference of the International Society for Human and Animal Mycology.[5] Although they have yet to be formally validated, neither were the previous proposed criteria they replaced. The updated criteria include (1) a predisposing underlying condition of either asthma or CF, (2) an elevated total IgE level greater than 1000 IU/mL AND either a positive *Aspergillus* skin test or detectable *Aspergillus fumigatus*–specific IgE, and (3) at least 2 of the following 3 criteria of serum precipitating or *Aspergillus*–specific IgG antibodies, characteristic radiographic findings, and elevated total eosinophil count (see **Table 1**). These criteria allow patients to be diagnosed with ABPA in the absence of radiographic changes. Recent administration of systemic corticosteroids may decrease total IgE levels and/or eosinophil counts, thus obscuring the diagnosis. A recent prospective study of *Aspergillus*-specific IgG levels in 102 treatment-naive patients with

ABPA compared with 48 controls found these IgG antibodies to be useful in the diagnosis of ABPA, with a sensitivity and specificity of 89% and 100%, respectively.[6] IgG levels were unreliable, however, for monitoring treatment response.

ABPA should be suspected in patients who have worsening asthma despite conventional therapy or require systemic corticosteroids. Although ABPA may be suggested by chest x-ray findings, a high-resolution CT (HRCT) may better detect the radiographic features of ABPA.[5] Transient radiographic findings include consolidation, nodules, tram-track opacities, and finger-in-glove and other fleeting opacities. Permanent changes include bronchiectasis that is often central, pleuropulmonary fibrosis, and parallel lines and ring shadows.

The Infectious Diseases Society of America practice guidelines on aspergillosis recommend screening for APBA in asthma patients on an annual basis, especially in those with frequent exacerbations.[4] Recommended screening is with *A fumigatus*–specific IgE levels.[5] If positive, a total serum IgE level should be sent. If the level is greater than 1000 IU/mL, an *Aspergillus* skin test, peripheral eosinophil count, *A fumigatus* precipitins, and/or specific IgG level should be obtained. If 2 of 4 of these tests are positive, an HRCT is performed. If the HRCT is normal, a diagnosis of seropositive ABPA is made.

Management of allergic bronchopulmonary aspergillosis

The management of ABPA includes monitoring lung function with regular spirometry and serologic assessment of total serum IgE levels, which should fall with treatment. Doubling IgE levels indicates potential relapse. Therapy for ABPA aims to both control inflammation and decrease fungal burden.[4,7] Corticosteroids are begun and tapered off or to the lowest dose possible. While some experts have favored a higher dose of systemic corticosteroids (prednisolone 0.75 mg/kg/day × 6 weeks) for a longer duration (taper over 6–12 months), data from a recently published randomized study of glucocorticoids in acute-stage ABPA complicating asthma showed that medium-dose oral corticosteroids (prednisolone 0.5 mg/kg/day × 2 weeks tapered off over 3–5 months) were as effective with decreased adverse effects compared with higher dose corticosteroids.[8] There are case reports that attest to the benefit of omalizumab in patients with ABPA but the dose may be high and thus the therapy expensive if the total serum IgE is elevated.[7,9] Experts recommend a trial of omalizumab in ABPA patients who are either dependent on or intolerant of corticosteroid therapy.[10] There is continued interest in the use of antifungal therapy to reduce fungal burden, and there is a tendency for the disease to relapse after the antifungal agent is discontinued.[4,7,11] Itraconazole is first-line therapy. Voriconazole, posaconazole, and inhaled amphotericin B are used for those who fail or are intolerant of itraconazole.[12,13] Avoidance of ongoing fungal exposure is recommended. With significant bronchiectasis, airway clearance regimens, including nebulized hypertonic saline (7%, 4 mL twice daily), may be of benefit. Because this may induce bronchospasm, the initial dose should be observed and given after a short-acting β_2-agonist.

Complications of allergic bronchopulmonary aspergillosis

Permanent bronchiectasis with restriction and a reduced diffusing capacity of lung for carbon monoxide and/or severe fixed airflow obstruction are hallmarks of advanced disease. Patients with these conditions may benefit from regular daily airway clearance regimens, including inhaled bronchodilator therapy. Colonization with gram-negative or atypical mycobacterial organisms may be noted. The treatment of atypical mycobacteria should follow established guidelines for diagnosis of infection and is best done in conjunction with infectious disease specialists. The treatment of gram-negative organisms with oral or inhaled antibiotics based on sensitivity testing should be considered in patients with ongoing respiratory symptoms, declining lung function, and/or significant radiographic bronchiectasis. Hemoptysis can occur and, if massive, be life-threatening, in which case intervention therapy with bronchial artery embolization (BAE) is indicated. A small proportion of patients develop CPA.[2]

Allergic Bronchopulmonary Aspergillosis in Cystic Fibrosis

Fungi are frequently isolated from the respiratory tract in patients with CF.[14] The significance of their presence and role in the progression of CF lung disease, however, are not always clear. Potential pulmonary responses to Aspergillus in CF include colonization, sensitization, ABPA, Aspergillus bronchitis, and aspergilloma.[15] It is estimated that 6% to 15% of patients with CF will develop ABPA.[16] In addition, 13% of ABPA patients without CF have been reported to be carriers of a CFTR gene mutation, suggesting a putative role of the CF transmembrane conductance regulator (CFTR) in the pathogenesis.[17]

Fungal colonization is the first step toward the development of ABPA, which occurs in patients who develop allergic helper T cell 2 type 2–based responses to the presence of Aspergillus.[18] Due to impaired mucociliary clearance, viscous respiratory secretions, and bronchiectasis, inhaled Aspergillus conidia are less likely to be cleared from the airways of CF patients and may germinate. Additional risk factors for colonization in CF include increasing age, corticosteroid use, antibiotic exposure, and Pseudomonas spp colonization.[14,19] CFTR-deficient cells are also less efficient at ingesting and eliminating conidia than cells with normal CFTR function.[20] The frequency of isolation of Aspergillus spp in CF seems to be increasing, having doubled in the United States between 1995 and 2005.[21]

Diagnosis of allergic bronchopulmonary aspergillosis in cystic fibrosis

The diagnostic criteria for ABPA are similar to those for non-CF populations (see **Table 1**). Serologic and skin testing should be performed after a corticosteroid holiday. New diagnostic criteria have been proposed incorporating newer molecular techniques.[22] Aspergillus sensitization is distinguished from ABPA by normal serum Aspergillus IgG levels. In addition, although not part of ABPA criteria, galactomannan antigen is usually present in respiratory secretions, whereas it is negative in sensitization alone.[22] Processing CF samples to maximize isolation and identification of fungi has not been universally standardized.[23] This makes it difficult to include sputum culture in the diagnostic criteria. Bacterial overgrowth can be problematic, and selective media is necessary to increase fungal identification.[24] Polymerase chain reaction (PCR) can increase fungal identification by 60%.[25]

Management of allergic bronchopulmonary aspergillosis in cystic fibrosis

There is a paucity of evidence on how best to treat ABPA in CF. The mainstay of therapy remains systemic corticosteroids. Triazole antifungal therapy for ABPA in CF has not been rigorously evaluated. For *Aspergillus* colonization, the only randomized controlled trial failed to show any benefit from use of itraconazole, although only 43% of patients achieved therapeutic itraconazole levels.[26] In contrast, results from a single-center, open-label study suggested benefit with itraconazole by decreasing inflammatory markers in respiratory specimens.[27] Other triazole agents have not been evaluated. Of concern, 4% of *A fumigatus* isolates from CF patients in one European study had triazole resistance.[28]

Complications of allergic bronchopulmonary aspergillosis in cystic fibrosis

In children with CF, ABPA is associated with more severe decline in lung function compared to *Aspergillus* colonization or chronic *Pseudomonas* infection.[29] In adults colonized with *Aspergillus* spp, the severity of bronchiectasis on CT may be worse compared with those without colonization, although longitudinal studies have not borne out this association.[30,31] In lung microbiota studies, the presence of fungi in CF respiratory samples is associated with worse lung function.[32]

Severe Asthma with Fungal Sensitization

Although SAFS was formally defined in 2006,[33] acute exacerbations of asthma after exposure to a large mold inoculum have long been described.[34,35] In contrast, SAFS refers to chronically severe asthma in association with ongoing exposure leading to sensitization (see **Table 1**). Fungal sensitization is common among patients with asthma, seen in more than a quarter of patients in single and pooled studies.[33] The clinical significance of fungal sensitization in those with mild to moderate asthma is, however, unclear. The definition of severe asthma typically refers to persistent symptoms despite dual therapy with high-dose inhaled corticosteroids and a long acting β_2-agonist.[33,36,37] Although obstruction may be present on pulmonary function testing, asthma severity is not defined by the presence, degree, or reversibility of forced expiratory volume in the first second of expiration reduction.

The pathogenesis of SAFS is poorly understood, and the distinction between association and causation remains unclear. Colonization is not a tenet of disease and is not a requirement for sensitization.[38] Although a genetic predisposition may underlie sensitization to environmental fungal antigens, to date no discrete genetic alterations have been identified in SAFS. *Aspergillus* spp are commonly implicated, although other respiratory and nonpulmonary fungi have also been implicated as sensitizing agents for SAFS.[36] Fungal sensitization can be demonstrated by skin prick testing for immediate fungal hyperreactivity, or by serum fungal–specific IgE titers. A multitude of skin prick antigens are available and should be tested, because the array of fungal species implicated is SAFS is large.[36] In recent years, direct immunoassays have replaced radioallergosorbent testing for detection of circulating serum antifungal IgE.[36,39] The lack of standardization of antigen preparation limits the reliability of both skin and serum tests. In addition, an individual's response, even to an identical antigen challenge, can vary over time. Therefore, performing both skin and serum tests is recommended to increase sensitivity to demonstrate fungal sensitization.[36]

A diagnosis of SAFS also requires the exclusion of ABPA. Although SAFS and ABPA lie along a continuum of disease related to fungal sensitization, there are distinguishing immunologic and clinical features. A variety of fungi may drive SAFS, whereas ABPA is most commonly due to *Aspergillus* spp.[40] Sensitization to fungal antigens, typically spores, drives SAFS, where a hyperimmune response typically due to colonization is the hallmark of ABPA. The immune response is more florid and more allergic in ABPA, marked by higher total serum IgE (>1000 IU/mL), elevated *Aspergillus*-specific IgE and IgG levels, and often eosinophilia.[38] In contrast to ABPA, there are no radiographic criteria or characteristic findings in SAFS, and sputum plugs are not a feature.[37] Clinically, patients with ABPA have persistent asthma, although unlike SAFS, asthma severity is not a defining feature of disease. Diagnostic difficulty is encountered for patients whose features fall between these 2 entities. Presumably, a subset of patients with SAFS suffers irreversible airway damage from long-standing inflammation. For those with severe asthma, fungal sensitization, and bronchiectasis, but not meeting full immunologic criteria for ABPA, a diagnosis of SAFS is most reasonable. Some patients with SAFS may eventually meet immunologic criteria for ABPA, and intermittent immunoglobulin testing is likely appropriate for those with radiographic findings suggestive of ABPA.

The treatment of SAFS centers around optimizing asthma therapies to achieve symptom control.[37] Therapies typically include use of a combined inhaled corticosteroid and long-acting β_2-agonist. Two randomized controlled trials have evaluated the efficacy of antifungal therapy in SAFS. In the first, 32 months of twice-daily itraconazole (200-mg dose) compared with placebo resulted in significantly improved quality-of-life scores on treatment; however, benefit was not sustained at 4 months.[41] The second study recruited patients with at least 2 asthma exacerbations in the preceding year despite high-dose inhaled corticosteroids; 30% were also on systemic corticosteroids.[42] Twice-daily voriconazole (200-mg dose) for 3 months did not have an impact on the incidence of asthma exacerbations. Currently, the role of antifungal agents remains investigational and is not recommended in the recently published guidelines on the management of difficult asthma.[43] Although the original description of SAFS considered fungal colonization to have a minimal role in pathogenesis, a recent study demonstrated that more than half of patients with asthma, many with moderate to severe disease, were colonized with at least one fungus.[11] In a subset of patients with colonization and poorly controlled SAFS, despite an optimized asthma regimen, a trial of antifungal therapy may be biologically reasonable. Finally, by extrapolation from data of omalizumab use in severe asthma (without document fungal sensitization), anti-IgE therapy may be beneficial in SAFS, although trials demonstrating this are lacking.

NONINVASIVE INFECTIOUS ASPERGILLOSIS
Chronic Pulmonary Aspergillosis

In contrast to the allergic aspergillosis syndromes, CPA is a progressive infection of the lung (**Table 2**). Classically considered a saprophytic infection in the case of simple aspergilloma, which typically occurs in a preexisting cavity, CPA is now recognized to both represent infection and comprise a wider spectrum of pulmonary disease.[3] Clinically, CPA ranges from solid nodules, which may mimic lung cancer, to single aspergillomas, to chronic cavitary pulmonary aspergillosis (CCPA) (ie, multiple cavities with or without aspergillomas), to chronic fibrosing pulmonary aspergillosis (CFPA).[3,44,45] Overlap between these different clinical entities is common.

Clinical presentation of chronic pulmonary aspergillosis
CPA usually occurs in middle age, with a male predominance. There is often a preexisting pulmonary condition or prior history of mycobacterial disease.[3] The frequency of specific underlying chest

conditions depends on local epidemiology; in areas where tuberculosis is highly prevalent, a history of infection is common, whereas in lower prevalence areas other chronic conditions, such as chronic obstructive pulmonary disease (COPD), predominate.[46,47] CPA, by definition, occurs in patients who are not substantially immunocompromised; however, subtle immune deficiencies may be present.[45,48–50] Subacute invasive aspergillosis (previously chronic necrotizing pulmonary aspergillosis) can occur in patients with some degree of recognized immunocompromise and resembles rapidly progressive CCPA.

CPA typically presents with a prolonged history (>3 months) of cough, shortness of breath, weight loss, and/or general malaise and fatigue.[51] Fever is not common. Hemoptysis, however, is not infrequent.[52] Some patients, in particular those with *Aspergillus* nodules or single aspergillomas, may be asymptomatic. The clinical features of CPA are nonspecific and often overlap with other chronic chest conditions and infection. Many patients with CPA have risk factors for lung cancer, which must be considered in the differential. This is particularly true when the diagnosis of CPA is not clear-cut, such as with *Aspergillus* nodules.[44] PET scanning is not helpful in the distinction, because it is likely to be avid in both diseases.[44,53] The clinical presentations of tuberculosis and CPA are also similar. In resource-limited areas, CPA may be underdiagnosed and treated as smear-negative tuberculosis.[54] This can have a significant impact on patient outcomes, health care resource utilization, and antimicrobial stewardship. On the other hand, mycobacterial infections, including tuberculosis, can occur concomitantly with CPA.[47,55] Therefore, mycobacterial testing should be part of the evaluation of CPA. Histoplasmosis, paracoccidiomycosis, and coccidiomycosis also need to be considered depending on local epidemiology.[45]

Diagnosis of chronic pulmonary aspergillosis
A diagnosis of CPA is established by clinical, laboratory, microbiological, and radiographic features. The condition must be present for more than 3 months. The most characteristic radiologic feature of CPA is an aspergilloma, defined by a thick-walled cavity containing fungal debris. Except for *Aspergillus* nodules, aspergillomas may be found in all types of CPA. The radiologic appearances of CPA subtypes are outlined in **Table 2**.

Radiologic features suggestive of CPA should prompt clinicians to perform confirmatory testing. All patients should have either *Aspergillus*-specific

Table 2
Host and imaging features of chronic pulmonary aspergillosis

Subtype of Chronic Pulmonary Aspergillosis	Host Characteristics	Radiologic Appearance and Clinical Course	Representative Radiology
Single aspergilloma	Presence of immunologically protected cystic lung spaces, typically from prior pulmonary infection or inflammatory lung disease.	Single fungal ball, which is stable or slowly progressive over many months.	
CCPA	Subtle immunocompromised state, leading to deficient fungal eradication.	Multiple cavities, with or without the presence of (a) fungal ball(s).	

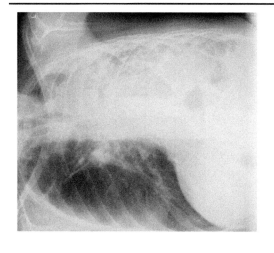

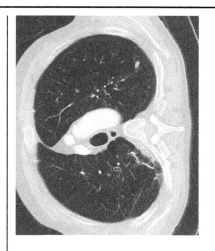

(continued on next page)

Chronic fibrosis pulmonary aspergillosis

Similar to those for CCPA; the risks for and mechanisms of fibrotic reactions are not well understood.

Extensive fibrosis with fibrotic destruction of at least 2 lobes of the lung; aspergillomas may also be present.

Aspergillus nodules

Risk factors and natural history not yet fully understood; may have subtle immune defects similar to CCPA.

Solid nodule, without cavitation. More than one may be present and can mimic other diagnoses, such as lung cancer.

Table 2
(continued)

Subtype of Chronic Pulmonary Aspergillosis	Host Characteristics	Radiologic Appearance and Clinical Course	Representative Radiology
Subacute invasive aspergillosis	Mildly immunocompromised state.	Similar appearance to CCPA, but typically progresses more quickly.	

IgG or precipitins performed.[4,45] There are numerous commercial IgG assays available; there is no clear indication which has the best diagnostic value.[54,56–58] Total and *Aspergillus*-specific IgE may have utility if the patient also has asthma but is not a mainstay of CPA diagnosis. From older literature, it seems that antibody titers have no direct relationship with disease severity.[59] Finally, although not required, a positive fungal culture can support a diagnosis of CPA. In published series, the proportion of patients with CPA who have positive respiratory cultures ranges from 56% to 81%.[51,60,61] This may be lower in those with *Aspergillus* nodules.[44] Laboratory processing of respiratory samples can affect the sensitivity of fungal culture. Collection of high-volume and undiluted specimens, sampling sputum plugs, and using fungal-specific media improve the yield of *Aspergillus* spp from respiratory specimens.[62–64] PCR is more sensitive than culture, and stronger PCR signals have higher clinical significance.[65] Because *Aspergillus* spp are ubiquitous in the environment, interpretation of *Aspergillus* spp isolation from respiratory samples, particularly from sputum, can be challenging and requires clinical correlation. Bronchoscopy samples are more reliable, being positive more frequently in infection rather than colonization.[66]

Management of chronic pulmonary aspergillosis

There is a paucity of longitudinal data on the natural history and optimal management of CPA. For asymptomatic patients with a single aspergilloma, or for CCPA with stable imaging, active surveillance alone is recommended.[4,45] Patients should be followed every 3 months to 6 months. In symptomatic patients, or in those with progressive disease by imaging or decline in pulmonary function, treatment is recommended. Although triazole antifungals are recommended as first-line therapy in CPA, there are minimal clinical trial data to support their use. Oral itraconazole therapy compared with no antifungal therapy has a significant impact on clinical and radiologic response after 6 months of therapy.[67] In another study, intravenous voriconazole (for a minimum of 2 weeks) was compared with intravenous micafungin.[68] No differences in outcomes were observed, whereas the side effect of the echinocandins were superior; the courses of therapy were very short, which call into question the relevance of the results. Oral itraconazole may prevent hemoptysis in CPA.[69] Oral voriconazole and posaconazole are accepted alternatives to itraconazole for the treatment of CPA[4,45]; there are no data yet on the use of isavuconazole. Subacute invasive aspergillosis should be treated as per invasive aspergillosis.[45]

At a minimum, patients should be treated for 6 months; in some cases, lifelong therapy is required. Patients should undergo repeat imaging 3 months to 6 months after initiation of treatment and typically less frequently thereafter, although the optimal time course for additional radiologic assessments is unknown.[4,45] Triazoles have numerous side effects, which differ among the 4 drugs. Often toxicity limits the use of azole therapy in clinical practice.[67,70,71] Additionally, interactions with other medications can be problematic; online tools are available for checking azole interactions.[71] Intravenous antifungal therapy with an echinocandin or liposomal amphotericin B may be used to initiate treatment prior to switching to an oral antifungal agent or used as salvage therapy in patients who have failed triazole therapy or have developed azole resistance.[72] In some instances, cyclic intravenous therapy has been used.[73]

In addition to antifungal agents, surgery has a management role in some cases, particularly in patients intolerant of antifungal therapy, those with resistant *Aspergillus* isolates, and/or those with focal cavitary disease.[45] The success of surgery is dependent on removal of the cavity without spillage of the contents. Resection of single aspergillomas is associated with the best surgical outcomes.[74]

Complications and outcomes of chronic pulmonary aspergillosis

The major complications of CPA include progression to CFPA, hemoptysis, and the development of resistance to antifungal therapy. Hemoptysis is common in CCPA and single aspergillomas. Although bleeding generally arises from an abnormal or novel vascular nexus of small vessels derived from the systemic circulation, bronchial artery aneurysms and pseudoaneurysms may be the source.[75] The severity ranges from mild hemoptysis to large-volume, potentially life-threatening blood loss.[52] Untreated, the reported mortality for the latter group is 50% to 100%.[76] Mild or moderate blood loss may be controlled with tranexamic acid.[77] BAE is recommended for larger volume hemoptysis.[45] The success of BAE is operator dependent, ranging between 50% and 90%.[78,79] Adverse events associated with BAE include chest wall pain and embolic phenomena and, rarely, the dissemination of infection.[45,80] Up to 50% of patients suffer recurrent hemoptysis post-BAE, and thoracic surgery should be considered in these cases.[81]

Azole resistance is an increasingly common clinical dilemma faced in the management of CPA.

Risk factors for the development of resistance include a high burden of fungal disease, subtherapeutic serum azole levels, and treatment nonadherence.[82] Even when triazole antifungal levels are therapeutic, *Aspergillus* spp can develop resistance and several genotypes can arise concomitantly.[83] Additionally, environmental strains with azole resistance (tandem repeat mutations [TR_{34}/L98H and TR_{46}/Y121F/T289A]) have been described.[84] Of great concern, panazole resistance has also been described.[85]

Fatigue and poor quality-of-life indicators are common in CPA.[86,87] The prognosis of CPA differs depending on the cohort studied.[88,89] In the largest cohort (392 patients), the 5-year survival rate was 57%.[90] Factors associated with poor prognosis included older age, a history of nontuberculous mycobacteria infection, COPD, and the presence of aspergilloma(s).

Aspergillus Bronchitis

Aspergillus bronchitis is a disease with features that mimic colonization, ABPA, and invasive tracheobronchitis. A rare aspergillosis, *Aspergillus* bronchitis is characterized as the persistence of bronchitis symptoms for at least a month, with positive fungal cultures for *Aspergillus* spp.[36,91] Respiratory symptoms include dyspnea, cough, and sputum production, which may be copious. Systemic symptoms may also be present. Typically, cultures are repeatedly positive and fungal growth is heavy.[91] Bronchoscopic inspection reveals abundant, tenacious mucus with ulceration, helping to distinguish *Aspergillus* bronchitis from simple colonization; superficial hyphal invasion may be seen on histopathology if biopsies are performed.[91] *Aspergillus*-specific IgG testing is commonly positive. Exuberant IgE and eosinophil responses are not hallmarks of this nonallergic condition.

Although *Aspergillus* bronchitis may occur in normal hosts, it is often associated with underlying pulmonary comorbidity or weakly attenuated immune states. The pathophysiology, therefore, is thought to center around a combination of anatomic alterations, leading to impaired airway clearance, and minor immune deficiency. In one series, bronchiectasis from any cause was the most common risk factor, present in 86% of patients.[91] COPD, asthma, and use of inhaled corticosteroids are also common comorbidities.[91] In addition to airways clearance deficits, alterations in mannose binding lecithin has been identified as a possible disease risk modifier for *Aspergillus* bronchitis.[91]

Antifungal treatment is the mainstay of treatment of *Aspergillus* bronchitis. Optimal treatment duration is unclear, but several months of treatment with voriconazole or itraconazole are typically used. Unfortunately, relapse is common, highlighting the role of impaired clearance in the disease. Because allergic responses are not a tenet of disease, corticosteroids do not have a role in treatment.

It is important to distinguish *Aspergillus* bronchitis from tracheobronchitis, a related but more aggressive condition marked by infection, rather than merely colonization with reactive bronchitis, of the large airways in immunocompromised patients, especially lung transplant recipients.[92] *Aspergillus* bronchitis also may be misdiagnosed as ABPA, particularly in patients with underlying bronchiectasis. Repeatedly positive sputum cultures for *Aspergillus* spp or repeated detection of *Aspergillus* DNA by PCR, in the absence of floridly elevated total and *Aspergillus*-specific IgE levels or lack of concomitant asthma, support the diagnosis of *Aspergillus* bronchitis.

SUMMARY

All of the *Aspergillus*-related diseases reviewed in this article share the potential to be misdiagnosed on account of symptoms or clinical findings that overlap with each other or with nonfungal conditions. When an aspergillosis syndrome is not considered, the delay in diagnosis may lead to permanent lung damage. ABPA can be easily overlooked, at least initially, as persistent asthma and progressive pulmonary decline in CF may be misattributed to the associated underlying diseases. ABPA must be suspected in patients with asthma that is difficult to control and with characteristic clinical and radiologic findings. In SAFS, patients demonstrate sensitization to fungi, without the hyperimmune state observed in ABPA. The condition may be driven by fungi other than *Aspergillus* spp and recognizing the role of fungal sensitization in SAFS is important, where exposures can account for exacerbations, and the diagnosis prompts escalation to a maximal asthma therapy. The clinical presentation of CPA often also mimics other pulmonary diagnoses. In some cases, malignancy needs to be excluded. Finally, a diagnosis of *Aspergillus* bronchitis is often delayed because the clinical presentation is similar to nonfungal bronchitis. The persistence of bronchitis symptoms (>1 month), failure to improve with antibiotics, and repeatedly positive fungal cultures strongly suggest the diagnosis of *Aspergillus* bronchitis.

Increased physician recognition of pulmonary aspergillosis syndromes is needed to identify patients who could benefit from an appropriate or altered therapeutic approach. Management may require multidisciplinary care with infectious disease and pulmonary physicians. Further study on more recently described clinical entities, such as SAFS and *Aspergillus* bronchitis, is required to guide best practice. The role of antifungal therapy is most established for symptomatic or progressive CPA and for *Aspergillus* bronchitis. It is important to be aware of the potential for azole resistance, which adds to the complexity of management and in some cases limits therapeutic choices.

REFERENCES

1. Hope WW, Walsh TJ, Denning DW. The invasive and saprophytic syndromes due to Aspergillus spp. Med Mycol 2005;43(Suppl 1):S207–38.
2. Denning DW, Pleuvry A, Cole DC. Global burden of allergic bronchopulmonary aspergillosis with asthma and its complication chronic pulmonary aspergillosis in adults. Med Mycol 2013;51(4):361–70.
3. Kosmidis C, Denning DW. The clinical spectrum of pulmonary aspergillosis. Thorax 2015; 70(3):270–7.
4. Patterson TF, Thompson GR 3rd, Denning DW, et al. Practice guidelines for the diagnosis and management of aspergillosis: 2016 update by the infectious diseases society of America. Clin Infect Dis 2016; 63(4):e1–60.
5. Agarwal R, Chakrabarti A, Shah A, et al. Allergic bronchopulmonary aspergillosis: review of literature and proposal of new diagnostic and classification criteria. Clin Exp Allergy 2013;43(8):850–73.
6. Agarwal R, Dua D, Choudhary H, et al. Role of Aspergillus fumigatus-specific IgG in diagnosis and monitoring treatment response in allergic bronchopulmonary aspergillosis. Mycoses 2017;60(1): 33–9.
7. Shah A, Panjabi C. Allergic bronchopulmonary aspergillosis: a perplexing clinical entity. Allergy Asthma Immunol Res 2016;8(4):282–97.
8. Agarwal R, Aggarwal AN, Dhooria S, et al. A randomized trial of glucocorticoids in acute-stage allergic bronchopulmonary aspergillosis complicating asthma. Eur Respir J 2016;47:385–7.
9. Tanou K, Zintzaras E, Kaditis AG. Omalizumab therapy for allergic bronchopulmonary aspergillosis in children with cystic fibrosis: a synthesis of published evidence. Pediatr Pulmonol 2014; 49(5):503–7.
10. Perez-de-Llano LA, Vennera MC, Parra A, et al. Effects of omalizumab in Aspergillus-associated airway disease. Thorax 2011;66(6):539–40.
11. Agbetile J, Fairs A, Desai D, et al. Isolation of filamentous fungi from sputum in asthma is associated with reduced post-bronchodilator FEV1. Clin Exp Allergy 2012;42(5):782–91.
12. Moss RB. Treatment options in severe fungal asthma and allergic bronchopulmonary aspergillosis. Eur Respir J 2014;43(5):1487–500.
13. Moreira AS, Silva D, Ferreira AR, et al. Antifungal treatment in allergic bronchopulmonary aspergillosis with and without cystic fibrosis: a systematic review. Clin Exp Allergy 2014;44(10):1210–27.
14. Pihet M, Carrere J, Cimon B, et al. Occurrence and relevance of filamentous fungi in respiratory secretions of patients with cystic fibrosis–a review. Med Mycol 2009;47(4):387–97.
15. Felton IC, Simmonds NJ. Aspergillus and cystic fibrosis: old disease - new classifications. Curr Opin Pulm Med 2014;20(6):632–8.
16. Armstead J, Morris J, Denning DW. Multi-country estimate of different manifestations of aspergillosis in cystic fibrosis. PLoS One 2014;9(6):e98502.
17. Eaton TE, Weiner Miller P, Garrett JE, et al. Cystic fibrosis transmembrane conductance regulator gene mutations: do they play a role in the aetiology of allergic bronchdopulmonary aspergillosis? Clin Exp Allergy 2002;32(5):756–61.
18. Romani L. The T cell response against fungal infections. Curr Opin Immunol 1997;9(4):484–90.
19. Amin R, Dupuis A, Aaron SD, et al. The effect of chronic infection with Aspergillus fumigatus on lung function and hospitalization in patients with cystic fibrosis. Chest 2010;137(1):171–6.
20. Chaudhary N, Datta K, Askin FB, et al. Cystic fibrosis transmembrane conductance regulator regulates epithelial cell response to Aspergillus and resultant pulmonary inflammation. Am J Respir Crit Care Med 2012;185(3):301–10.
21. Nielsen SM, Kristensen L, Søndergaard A, et al. Increased prevalence and altered species composition of filamentous fungi in respiratory specimens from cystic fibrosis patients. APMIS 2014;122(10): 1007–12.
22. Baxter CG, Dunn G, Jones AM, et al. Novel immunologic classification of aspergillosis in adult cystic fibrosis. J Allergy Clin Immunol 2013;132(3):560–6.e10.
23. Liu JC, Modha DE, Gaillard EA. What is the clinical significance of filamentous fungi positive sputum cultures in patients with cystic fibrosis? J Cyst Fibros 2013;12(3):187–93.
24. Blyth CC, Harun A, Middleton PG, et al. Detection of occult Scedosporium species in respiratory tract specimens from patients with cystic fibrosis by use of selective media. J Clin Microbiol 2010;48(1):314–6.
25. Nagano Y, Elborn JS, Millar BC, et al. Comparison of techniques to examine the diversity of fungi in adult patients with cystic fibrosis. Med Mycol 2010;48(1): 166–76.e1.
26. Aaron SD, Vandemheen KL, Freitag A, et al. Treatment of Aspergillus fumigatus in patients with cystic fibrosis: a randomized, placebo-controlled pilot study. PLoS One 2012;7(4):e36077.

27. Coughlan CA, Chotirmall SH, Renwick J, et al. The effect of Aspergillus fumigatus infection on vitamin D receptor expression in cystic fibrosis. Am J Respir Crit Care Med 2012;186(10):999–1007.

28. Burgel PR, Baixench MT, Amsellem M, et al. High prevalence of azole-resistant Aspergillus fumigatus in adults with cystic fibrosis exposed to itraconazole. Antimicrob Agents Chemother 2012;56(2):869–74.

29. Kraemer R, Deloséa N, Ballinari P, et al. Effect of allergic bronchopulmonary aspergillosis on lung function in children with cystic fibrosis. Am J Respir Crit Care Med 2006;174(11):1211–20.

30. McMahon MA, Chotirmall SH, McCullagh B, et al. Radiological abnormalities associated with Aspergillus colonization in a cystic fibrosis population. Eur J Radiol 2012;81(3):e197–202.

31. de Vrankrijker AM, van der Ent CK, van Berkhout FT, et al. Aspergillus fumigatus colonization in cystic fibrosis: implications for lung function? Clin Microbiol Infect 2011;17(9):1381–6.

32. Paganin P, Fiscarelli EV, Tuccio V, et al. Changes in cystic fibrosis airway microbial community associated with a severe decline in lung function. PLoS One 2015;10(4):e0124348.

33. Denning DW, O'Driscoll BR, Hogaboam CM, et al. The link between fungi and severe asthma: a summary of the evidence. Eur Respir J 2006;27(3):615–26.

34. Salvaggio J, Seabury J, Schoenhardt FA. New Orleans asthma. V. Relationship between Charity Hospital asthma admission rates, semiquantitative pollen and fungal spore counts, and total particulate aerometric sampling data. J Allergy Clin Immunol 1971;48(2):96–114.

35. Dales RE, Cakmak S, Judek S, et al. The role of fungal spores in thunderstorm asthma. Chest 2003;123(3):745–50.

36. Denning DW, Pashley C, Hartl D, et al. Fungal allergy in asthma-state of the art and research needs. Clin Transl Allergy 2014;4:14.

37. Agarwal R. Severe asthma with fungal sensitization. Curr Allergy Asthma Rep 2011;11(5):403–13.

38. Patterson K, Strek ME. Allergic bronchopulmonary aspergillosis. Proc Am Thorac Soc 2010;7(3):237–44.

39. Kespohl S, Maryska S, Bünger J, et al. How to diagnose mould allergy? Comparison of skin prick tests with specific IgE results. Clin Exp Allergy 2016;46(7):981–91.

40. Bhabhra R, Askew DS. Thermotolerance and virulence of Aspergillus fumigatus: role of the fungal nucleolus. Med Mycol 2005;43(Suppl 1):S87–93.

41. Denning DW, O'Driscoll BR, Powell G, et al. Randomized controlled trial of oral antifungal treatment for severe asthma with fungal sensitization: the Fungal Asthma Sensitization Trial (FAST) study. Am J Respir Crit Care Med 2009;179(1):11–8.

42. Agbetile J, Bourne M, Fairs A, et al. Effectiveness of voriconazole in the treatment of Aspergillus fumigatus-associated asthma (EVITA3 study). J Allergy Clin Immunol 2014;134(1):33–9.

43. Chung KF, Wenzel SE, Brozek JL, et al. International ERS/ATS guidelines on definition, evaluation and treatment of severe asthma. Eur Respir J 2014;43(2):343–73.

44. Muldoon LG, Churman A, Page I, et al. Aspergillus nodules; another presentation of chronic pulmonary aspergillosis. BMC Pulm Med 2016;16(1):123.

45. Denning DW, Cadranel J, Beigelman-Aubry C, et al. Chronic pulmonary aspergillosis: rationale and clinical guidelines for diagnosis and management. Eur Respir J 2016;47(1):45–68.

46. Denning DW, Pleuvry A, Cole DC. Global burden of chronic pulmonary aspergillosis as a sequel to pulmonary tuberculosis. Bull World Health Organ 2011;89(12):864–72.

47. Smith NL, Denning DW. Underlying conditions in chronic pulmonary aspergillosis including simple aspergilloma. Eur Respir J 2011;37(4):865–72.

48. Smith NL, Denning DW. Clinical implications of interferon-gamma genetic and epigenetic variants. Immunology 2014;143(4):499–511.

49. Harrison E, Singh A, Morris J, et al. Mannose-binding lectin genotype and serum levels in patients with chronic and allergic pulmonary aspergillosis. Int J Immunogenet 2012;39(3):224–32.

50. Kosmidis C, Powell G, Borrow R, et al. Response to pneumococcal polysaccharide vaccination in patients with chronic and allergic aspergillosis. Vaccine 2015;33(51):7271–5.

51. Denning DW, Riniotis K, Dobrashian R, et al. Chronic cavitary and fibrosing pulmonary and pleural aspergillosis: case series, proposed nomenclature change, and review. Clin Infect Dis 2003;37(Suppl 3):S265–80.

52. Patterson KC, Strek ME. Diagnosis and treatment of pulmonary aspergillosis syndromes. Chest 2014;146(5):1358–68.

53. Baxter CG, Bishop P, Low SE, et al. Pulmonary aspergillosis: an alternative diagnosis to lung cancer after positive [18F]FDG positron emission tomography. Thorax 2011;66(7):638–40.

54. Page ID, Richardson MD, Denning DW. Comparison of six Aspergillus-specific IgG assays for the diagnosis of chronic pulmonary aspergillosis (CPA). J Infect 2016;72(2):240–9.

55. Kunst H, Wickremasinghe M, Wells A, et al. Nontuberculous mycobacterial disease and Aspergillus-related lung disease in bronchiectasis. Eur Respir J 2006;28(2):352–7.

56. van Toorenenbergen AW. Between-laboratory quality control of automated analysis of IgG antibodies against Aspergillus fumigatus. Diagn Microbiol Infect Dis 2012;74(3):278–81.

57. Baxter CG, Denning DW, Jones AM, et al. Performance of two Aspergillus IgG EIA assays compared with the precipitin test in chronic and allergic aspergillosis. Clin Microbiol Infect 2013;19(4):E197–204.

58. Guitard J, Sendid B, Thorez S, et al. Evaluation of a recombinant antigen-based enzyme immunoassay for the diagnosis of noninvasive aspergillosis. J Clin Microbiol 2012;50(3):762–5.

59. Longbottom JL, Pepys J, Clive FT. Diagnostic precipitin test in Aspergillus pulmonary mycetoma. Lancet 1964;1(7333):588–9.

60. Camuset J, Nunes H, Dombret MC, et al. Treatment of chronic pulmonary aspergillosis by voriconazole in nonimmunocompromised patients. Chest 2007; 131(5):1435–41.

61. Nam HS, Jeon K, Um SW, et al. Clinical characteristics and treatment outcomes of chronic necrotizing pulmonary aspergillosis: a review of 43 cases. Int J Infect Dis 2010;14(6):e479–82.

62. Pashley CH, Fairs A, Morley JP, et al. Routine processing procedures for isolating filamentous fungi from respiratory sputum samples may underestimate fungal prevalence. Med Mycol 2012;50(4): 433–8.

63. Fraczek MG, Kirwan MB, Moore CB, et al. Volume dependency for culture of fungi from respiratory secretions and increased sensitivity of Aspergillus quantitative PCR. Mycoses 2014;57(2):69–78.

64. Horvath JA, Dummer S. The use of respiratory-tract cultures in the diagnosis of invasive pulmonary aspergillosis. Am J Med 1996;100(2):171–8.

65. Denning DW, Park S, Lass-Florl C, et al. High-frequency triazole resistance found in nonculturable Aspergillus fumigatus from lungs of patients with chronic fungal disease. Clin Infect Dis 2011;52(9): 1123–9.

66. Uffredi ML, Mangiapan G, Cadranel J, et al. Significance of Aspergillus fumigatus isolation from respiratory specimens of nongranulocytopenic patients. Eur J Clin Microbiol Infect Dis 2003; 22(8):457–62.

67. Agarwal R, Vishwanath G, Aggarwal AN, et al. Itraconazole in chronic cavitary pulmonary aspergillosis: a randomised controlled trial and systematic review of literature. Mycoses 2013;56(5):559–70.

68. Kohno S, Izumikawa K, Ogawa K, et al. Intravenous micafungin versus voriconazole for chronic pulmonary aspergillosis: a multicenter trial in Japan. J Infect 2010;61(5):410–8.

69. De Beule K, De Doncker P, Cauwenbergh G, et al. The treatment of aspergillosis and aspergilloma with itraconazole, clinical results of an open international study (1982-1987). Mycoses 1988;31(9): 476–85.

70. Felton TW, Baxter C, Moore CB, et al. Efficacy and safety of posaconazole for chronic pulmonary aspergillosis. Clin Infect Dis 2010;51(12):1383–91.

71. Available at: http://aspergillus.org.uk/content/antifungal-drug-interactions. Accessed 22nd August, 2016.

72. Newton PJ, Harris C, Morris J, et al. Impact of liposomal amphotericin B therapy on chronic pulmonary aspergillosis. J Infect 2016;73(5):485–95.

73. Keir GJ, Garfield B, Hansell DM, et al. Cyclical caspofungin for chronic pulmonary aspergillosis in sarcoidosis. Thorax 2014;69(3):287–8.

74. Farid S, Mohamed S, Devbhandari M, et al. Results of surgery for chronic pulmonary aspergillosis, optimal antifungal therapy and proposed high risk factors for recurrence–a National Centre's experience. J Cardiothorac Surg 2013;8:180.

75. Sbano H, Mitchell AW, Ind PW, et al. Peripheral pulmonary artery pseudoaneurysms and massive hemoptysis. AJR Am J Roentgenol 2005;184(4): 1253–9.

76. Chun JY, Morgan R, Belli AM. Radiological management of hemoptysis: a comprehensive review of diagnostic imaging and bronchial arterial embolization. Cardiovasc Intervent Radiol 2010;33(2):240–50.

77. Prutsky G, Domecq JP, Salazar CA, et al. Antifibrinolytic therapy to reduce haemoptysis from any cause. Cochrane Database Syst Rev 2012;(4):CD008711.

78. Corr P. Management of severe hemoptysis from pulmonary aspergilloma using endovascular embolization. Cardiovasc Intervent Radiol 2006;29(5):807–10.

79. Swanson KL, Johnson CM, Prakash UB, et al. Bronchial artery embolization: experience with 54 patients. Chest 2002;121(3):789–95.

80. Seki M, Maesaki S, Hashiguchi K, et al. Aspergillus fumigatus isolated from blood samples of a patient with pulmonary aspergilloma after embolization. Intern Med 2000;39(2):188–90.

81. Serasli E, Kalpakidis V, Iatrou K, et al. Percutaneous bronchial artery embolization in the management of massive hemoptysis in chronic lung diseases. Immediate and long-term outcomes. Int Angiol 2008; 27(4):319–28.

82. Howard SJ, Pasqualotto AC, Anderson MJ, et al. Major variations in aspergillus fumigatus arising within aspergillomas in chronic pulmonary aspergillosis. Mycoses 2013;56(4):434–41.

83. Camps SM, van der Linden JW, Li Y, et al. Rapid induction of multiple resistance mechanisms in Aspergillus fumigatus during azole therapy: a case study and review of the literature. Antimicrob Agents Chemother 2012;56(1):10–6.

84. Verweij PE, Chowdhary A, Melchers WJ, et al. Azole resistance in Aspergillus fumigatus: can we retain the clinical use of mold-active antifungal azoles? Clin Infect Dis 2016;62(3):362–8.

85. van Ingen J, van der Lee HA, Rijs AJ, et al. High-level pan-azole-resistant aspergillosis. J Clin Microbiol 2015;53(7):2343–5.

86. Al-Shair K, Muldoon EG, Morris J, et al. Characterisation of fatigue and its substantial impact on health

status in a large cohort of patients with chronic pulmonary aspergillosis (CPA). Respir Med 2016;114: 117–22.

87. Al-shair K, Atherton GT, Kennedy D, et al. Validity and reliability of the St. George's Respiratory Questionnaire in assessing health status in patients with chronic pulmonary aspergillosis. Chest 2013; 144(2):623–31.

88. Camara B, Reymond E, Saint-Raymond C, et al. Characteristics and outcomes of chronic pulmonary aspergillosis: a retrospective analysis of a tertiary hospital registry. Clin Respir J 2015;9(1): 65–73.

89. Jhun BW, Imamura Y, Takazono T, et al. Clinical characteristics and treatment outcomes of chronic pulmonary aspergillosis. Med Mycol 2013;51(8):811–7.

90. Lowes D, Al-Shair K, Newton PJ, et al. Predictors of mortality in chronic pulmonary aspergillosis. Eur Respir J 2017;49(2).

91. Chrdle A, Mustakim S, Bright-Thomas RJ, et al. Aspergillus bronchitis without significant immunocompromise. Ann N Y Acad Sci 2012;1272:73–85.

92. Fernandez-Ruiz M, Silva JT, San-Juan R, et al. Aspergillus tracheobronchitis: report of 8 cases and review of the literature. Medicine (Baltimore) 2012;91(5):261–73.

Laboratory Diagnostics for Fungal Infections
A Review of Current and Future Diagnostic Assays

Poornima Ramanan, MD, Nancy L. Wengenack, PhD,
Elitza S. Theel, PhD*

KEYWORDS

- Invasive fungal diagnostics • Molecular methods • Serology • Antibody • Antigen

KEY POINTS

- Classic serologic techniques, including immunodiffusion and complement fixation, in addition to fungal antigen detection methods, continue to be used routinely for diagnosis of fungal infections.
- Novel diagnostic tools, including rapid lateral-flow assays for *Cryptococcus* antigen detection, have been developed and have good performance characteristics.
- Identification of fungi from culture isolates can be rapidly and reliably achieved using a variety of molecular methods, including nucleic acid hybridization probes, matrix-assisted laser desorption ionization time of flight mass spectrometry, polymerase chain reaction (PCR), and DNA sequencing.
- The direct identification of fungi from specimens without the need to culture first is still largely limited to selected *Candida* species or to single-target PCR assays but multiplex PCR panels and direct sequencing methods are beginning to appear in the literature.

INTRODUCTION

The diagnosis of fungal infections has evolved dramatically over the past few decades. Although classic fungal culture and traditional serologic techniques continue to be relevant and necessary, the detection and identification of fungi after growth in culture and directly from specimens by molecular techniques is a rapidly evolving diagnostic field. This review focuses on the routinely used methods for detection of antibodies to and antigens from common invasive fungal agents, and presents an update on recently described molecular methods for fungal detection. This includes discussion of broad-range PCR and sequencing, matrix-assisted laser desorption ionization time of flight (MALDI-TOF) mass spectrometry and real-time PCR applications. **Table 1** summarizes the general advantages and limitations associated with each of these applications. Importantly, we do not present information on phenotypic fungal identification through culture and staining techniques. Finally, although we recognize that *Microsporidia* species are fungi, diagnostic testing for this group of organisms are not be covered because testing is often still relegated to parasitology laboratories.

REVIEW OF SEROLOGIC METHODS FOR ANTIBODY AND ANTIGEN DETECTION

Classically, detection of antifungal antibodies relied on traditional techniques, including complement fixation (CF) and immunodiffusion (ID) assays, both originally optimized in the 1940s.

Disclosure Statement: The authors have nothing to disclose.
Division of Clinical Microbiology, Department of Laboratory Medicine and Pathology, Mayo Clinic, 200 First Street, Rochester, MN 55905, USA
* Corresponding author.
E-mail address: theel.elitza@mayo.edu

Clin Chest Med 38 (2017) 535–554
http://dx.doi.org/10.1016/j.ccm.2017.04.013

Table 1
General advantages and limitations of fungal diagnostic tests

Tests	Advantages	Limitations
Antigen detection	• Rapid TAT (vs culture) • Minimally invasive specimens • Reduces the need to handle potentially infectious fungi in the laboratory • Serial monitoring may be used for early diagnosis and to gauge treatment response	• Potential for cross-reactivity between closely related fungi • Potential cross-reactivity due to therapeutic interventions • Lack of culture isolate for susceptibility testing (ie, Aspergillus sp, Fusarium sp) • Antigen performance varies depending on specimen and disease state • Pan-fungal nature of β-D-Glucan (BDG) • Mannan antigen: Low sensitivity and specificity when performed alone
Antibody detection	• Rapid TAT (vs culture) • Minimally invasive specimens • Reduces the need to handle potentially infectious fungi in the laboratory	• Lower sensitivity associated with acute infection and in severely immunosuppressed patients • Low specificity associated with antibodies to other closely related fungi • Persistent seropositivity post disease resolution and in patients residing in endemic regions
Nucleic acid probes	• High specificity and sensitivity • Rapid turnaround time (vs culture)	• Need to grow in culture first (delayed TAT) • Potential for cross-reaction with closely related fungi • Limited species-specific probe availability
MALDI-TOF MS	• Rapid TAT (vs morphologic identification) • High specificity • High throughput • Cost-effective	• Need to grow in culture first (delayed TAT) • Lack of accuracy associated with mixed colonies • Inability to perform direct-from-specimen testing • Inability to perform antimicrobial susceptibility testing • Suboptimal breadth of spectral libraries • Inability to differentiate some closely related species
Identification of isolates by DNA Sequencing	• High specificity • Ability to identify novel species • High throughput	• Need to grow in culture first (delayed TAT) • Suboptimal breadth and accuracy of sequence databases. • Longer TAT than probes or MALDI-TOF MS • High cost • Technically challenging
Identification directly from specimens by DNA sequencing	• High specificity • Rapid TAT (no need to wait for culture growth) • Ability to identify organisms that fail to grow in culture	• Low sensitivity • Highly susceptible to environmental contamination of specimens and reagents (false positives) • High cost • Technically challenging
Identification directly from specimens by Real-time PCR	• High sensitivity and specificity • Rapid TAT • Closed system that reduces potential for contamination by environmental fungi or amplicon	• Lack of assay standardization • Lack of commercially available FDA-approved assays • Available for a limited number of fungi; often single targets per assay • The significance of a positive result from a nonsterile source (eg, BAL fluid) may be clinically confounding • Lack of an isolate limits ability to perform antimicrobial susceptibility testing

Abbreviations: BAL, bronchoalveolar lavage; FDA, Food and Drug Administration; MALDI-TOF MS, matrix-assisted laser desorption ionization time of flight mass spectrometry; PCR, polymerase chain reaction; TAT, turnaround time.

Although enzyme-linked immunoassays (ELISAs) and lateral-flow immunoassays (LFAs) have been developed in an effort to enhance diagnostic accuracy and improve laboratory testing throughput, CF and ID continue to be widely used.[1] These 4 methodologies are briefly reviewed and their specific performance characteristics for select fungi are summarized separately.

Complement Fixation

CF assays are based on activity of the classic complement pathway. Briefly, patient sera is heated to inactivate innate human complement factors and subsequently mixed and incubated with antigen from the infectious agent of interest. Guinea pig complement components are added next and incubated. In the presence of antigen-specific serum antibodies, an antigen-antibody complex will be formed, which will fix the guinea pig complement and inactivate it. Conversely, in the absence of host target antibodies, complement will remain active. Hemolysin-sensitized sheep red blood cells (RBCs) are added to the reaction, incubated, and following a centrifugation step, the reaction is read for the level of RBC hemolysis. The absence of a significant level of hemolysis indicates the presence of target-specific antifungal antibodies (ie, antifungal antibodies were present in the patient sample and the antibody-antigen complex bound and inactivated the guinea pig complement) and the dilution at which this occurs is reported (**Fig. 1**A).

Immunodiffusion

ID, also referred to as Ouchterlony double diffusion or precipitin test, is a precipitation reaction that occurs in an agar gel matrix.[2] Briefly, a rosette of wells is made in the agar (**Fig. 1**B) and antigen from the infectious agent of interest is added to the center well. Patient specimens and controls are added to the surrounding wells. During the incubation step, patient antibody (if present) and the antigen diffuse out of the wells. The point at which antigen and antibody are at equilibrium, an antigen-antibody complex will develop forming a precipitate, visible as a "band" in the agar by the naked eye, without staining.

Enzyme-Linked Immunoassays

The most common type of ELISA used for detection of antibodies to infectious agents, including fungi, are noncompetitive ELISAs. Briefly, select fungal antigen(s) are adhered to the bottom of microtiter wells, to which human serum (or other appropriate specimen source) is added and incubated. If antibodies specific to the target antigen are present, they will bind and become immobilized in the microtiter well. Following a wash step to remove excess patient specimen, an enzyme-labeled, antihuman antibody specific to the Fc portion of human immunoglobulin is added, which will bind to the immobilized patient antibodies (if present). Enzyme substrate is subsequently added, the reaction (eg, colorimetric, chemiluminescent, etc.) is detected and, depending on the assay design, either a qualitative or quantitative result is reported.

Lateral-Flow Immunoassay or Device

These are immunochromatographic assays based on capillary flow of a specimen over a porous membrane separated into 3 general areas: a sample application pad, a conjugate pad, and a reaction area. Briefly, patient specimen is applied to the sample pad and flows to the conjugate region. Depending on the target analyte, the conjugate pad contains lyophilized antibody or antigen conjugated to a reporter label (eg, colloidal gold or latex nanoparticles). If the target analyte is present, it will bind the conjugated reporter and this immunocomplex will flow to the reaction pad. Immobilized on the reaction pad is a band of secondary antibody or antigen (to capture the immunocomplex) and a band of control antibody specific to the conjugated reporter molecule. This latter antibody ensures that capillary flow occurred and that the test is valid. Visible bands appear as the detector particles concentrate; the presence of a control band alone indicates that the specimen did not contain the target analyte.

DETECTION OF HOST-SPECIFIC ANTIBODIES TO AND ANTIGENS FROM SELECT FUNGI

One of the challenges associated with determining diagnostic accuracy of serologic assays for detection of invasive fungal infections (IFIs) is the absence of a gold standard comparator. Although fungal culture and histopathology remain the preferred diagnostic methods, the invasive specimen collection procedures (ie, bronchoalveolar lavage [BAL], lung biopsy) are often contraindicated in critically ill patients. Additionally, culture from such sources is considered insensitive, with positivity rates approaching only 45% to 60% in cases of invasive aspergillosis (IA).[3] Similar sensitivity limitations are observed with blood cultures from patients with IA or candidiasis, ranging from less than 10% to 50%, respectively.[3,4] Therefore, the comparison of new diagnostic assays to the current reference method for IFI can lead to inaccurate conclusions regarding the performance characteristics of contemporary methods.

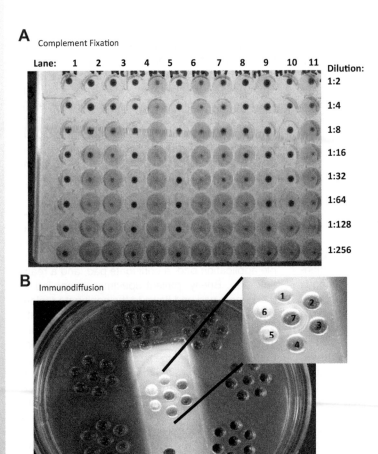

A Complement Fixation

B Immunodiffusion

Fig. 1. CF and immunodiffusion for detection of antifungal antibodies. (*A*) *Histoplasma capsulatum* yeast antigen complement fixation assay. Lanes 1 to 10 are patient samples, Lanes 11 and 12 are positive and negative controls, respectively. The dilution at which 30% or less hemolysis is observed is considered the end-point titer. (*B*) *H capsulatum* immunodiffusion assay. Wells 1 and 6 contain positive and negative control antisera, Well 7 contains *H capsulatum* H and M antigens, Wells 2 to 5 contain patient sample. The band closest to the antigen well (Well 7) is the M-band and the band closest to the serum well is the H-band.

To overcome this limitation, the European Organization for the Research and Treatment of Cancer/Mycoses Study Group developed definitions, based on clinical findings, imaging studies, and laboratory data, to categorize patients with either proven, probable, possible, or no IFI.[5] Importantly, although discussions remain regarding appropriate use of these categories, these guidelines provide a comparative standard against which any new IFI diagnostic assay can more accurately be evaluated.

Aspergillus Species

Aspergillus spp are ubiquitous in the environment and humans are regularly exposed to these hyaline molds, inhaling approximately 200 conidia daily.[6] Despite rapid clearance of conidia, either by ciliary movement or neutrophil activity, anti-*Aspergillus* antibodies are formed in healthy individuals and are detectable in most adults.[7] As discussed elsewhere in this series, the disease spectrum associated with *Aspergillus* infections is broad, ranging from allergic bronchopulmonary aspergillosis (ABPA) to chronic pulmonary aspergillosis (CPA) and invasive pulmonary aspergillosis (IPA), depending on the individual's underlying immune status. Diagnosis of IPA requires a high degree of clinical suspicion due to the nonspecific symptoms associated with this infection, and a combination of imaging studies and pathology and microbiology testing, is needed.[5] Because of the limitations associated with some of the reference methods noted previously, noninvasive methods to detect circulating *Aspergillus* spp antibodies and antigens are increasingly relied on to make the diagnosis.

Although numerous *Aspergillus* antibody detection assays have been developed (eg, immunodiffusion, indirect hemagglutination, CF), most commercially available assays are ELISA-based. Due to the high seroprevalence rate, an abnormal ELISA result for anti-*Aspergillus* antibodies is defined as antibody levels above those typically observed in healthy individuals. Although detection of this analyte may be used as a supplemental test for diagnosis of CPA or ABPA, detection of anti-*Aspergillus* antibodies in cases of acute IPA is often limited because of the profound immunocompromised state and weekend humoral response in these high-risk patients. The sensitivity of anti-*Aspergillus* immunoglobulin (Ig)G ELISAs in severely neutropenic individuals with proven or probable IPA ranges from 6% to 84% depending on the target antigen (eg, cell lysate, purified or recombinant antigens) used and the patient population tested.[8,9] The inconsistency of these data suggests that detection of antibodies to *Aspergillus* alone cannot be relied on as an accurate diagnostic marker for acute IPA in this patient population. In contrast, in patients with confirmed CPA and/or ABPA, the sensitivity and specificity of anti-*Aspergillus* antibody ELISAs are significantly higher, ranging from 85.9% to 97.0% and 75.7% to 91.3%, respectively.[10,11] Collectively, detection of elevated anti-*Aspergillus* antibodies can be used as a diagnostic marker for noninvasive disease in immunocompetent or nonneutropenic individuals. However, these assays have a limited clinical utility in immunosuppressed patients, for whom additional laboratory evidence (eg, fungal culture, radiographic signs) is necessary. Notably, detection of this analyte is absent from recently developed algorithms for differentiating *Aspergillus* colonization from invasive disease in intensive care patients.[12]

During active growth, germinating *Aspergillus* conidia and growing hyphae release galactomannan (GM), a polysaccharide of galactofuranosyl side chains on a mannan backbone. Several assays exist for detection of this biomarker in serum and BAL, including the commonly used Platelia *Aspergillus* Ag enzyme immunoassay (EIA) (Bio-Rad, Hercules, CA). This assay relies on the rat monoclonal antibody (mAb), EBA-2, to bind the $\beta(1-5)$-linked galactofuranosyl residues on circulating GM.[13] Performance of the Platelia GM EIA is variable and dependent on the patient population tested, the specimen type, the number of tests performed, the cutoff used, and the use of antifungal therapy before testing. Two recent meta-analyses found an overall sensitivity and specificity of 71% to 78% and 81% to 89%, respectively, for detection of proven IA when performed in serum.[14,15] Through subgroup analysis, Pfeiffer and colleagues[14] showed significantly higher sensitivity values for detection of IA by the Platelia GM EIA in patients with hematologic malignancies (70%) and in hematopoietic stem cell transplant recipients (HSCT; 82%), compared with patients with IA who received a solid organ

transplant (SOT; 22%). Based on these and other studies, the most recent practice guidelines for diagnosis and management of IA recommend against screening GM of low-risk patients, including SOT recipients and those with chronic granulomatous disease.[16] The lower observed sensitivity for GM detection in such patients may be related to the more robust immune response in these hosts, leading to lower fungal burden and a lack of angioinvasion.

Diagnostic accuracy of GM assays is further influenced by how often the test is performed in serum, with a significant improvement in the positive predictive value (PPV) for IA documented during biweekly (87.5%) screening of high-risk patients compared with single time-point testing (66.1%). Serial positive GM results often precede radiologic and fungal culture results for cases of proven IA by 6 to 10 days for more than 80% of HSCT recipients.[17,18] In addition to serial screening, the specimen source (BAL vs serum) significantly impacts assay performance characteristics; BAL fluid, likely due to the higher fungal biomass, is associated with GM EIA sensitivity and specificity values of 85% and 86%, respectively, compared with 65% and 95% values observed for serum.[19] Although BAL is considered the superior specimen source, other investigators have reported only modest accuracy of the GM EIA in BAL fluid for detecting IA in hematologic patients (sensitivity 50%, specificity 73%).[20] Additionally, the diagnostic accuracy of the GM EIA in high-risk patients on empiric antifungal prophylaxis is significantly diminished. A study of 217 high-risk patients on posaconazole prophylaxis who were serially screened biweekly by the GM EIA, found a PPV of only 11.8%.[21] These data suggest that asymptomatic patients on effective prophylaxis should be evaluated only by the GM EIA in cases of suspected, breakthrough IA.

Finally, the analytical specificity of the GM EIA is influenced by several factors. This assay cross-reacts with several fungi (eg, *Penicillium* spp, *Geotrichum* spp, *Histoplasma capsulatum*) and bacteria (eg, *Bifidobacterium* spp), which produce GM similar to *Aspergillus* spp or have lipoteichoic acid recognizable by the EBA-2 antibody, respectively. This is particularly confounding in the setting of mucositis and neonatal colonization with *Bifidobacterium*.[16,22,23] Infusion or ingestion of solutions containing high levels of gluconate can likewise lead to elevated GM levels in patients without IA.[22] Finally, although certain beta-lactam antibiotics (eg, amoxicillin-clavulanate) are associated with false-positive GM results, recent studies suggest that newer formulations of piperacillin-tazobactam no longer contain elevated GM levels and are now a rare case of elevated GM levels in patients receiving this drug.[23] Collectively, when used with an appreciation for the associated caveats and alongside radiography and clinical judgment, the GM EIA is helpful for the early detection of IA in serially tested, high-risk patients who are not on antifungal prophylaxis.[16] Furthermore, preemptive screening of patients using this biomarker to gauge possible early antifungal intervention may be an alternative to empiric antifungal therapy.[16]

A second, recently described antigen biomarker for *Aspergillus* spp has been identified and a rapid (~15-minute), point-of-care (POC) lateral-flow device (LFD) has been developed by Isca Diagnostics Ltd (Cornwall, UK). This novel antigen is an extracellular glucoprotein, secreted during the active growth from *Aspergillus* hyphae only; it is not secreted from conidia. The LFD uses the JF5 mAb to detect a unique protein epitope found on the surface this glycoprotein.[24] A 7-study meta-analysis report an overall sensitivity and specificity of the *Aspergillus* LFD for the detection of proven or probable IA using serum specimens as 68% and 87%, respectively.[25] This is similar to performance of the Platelia GM EIA in this specimen source. This same evaluation showed that the utilization of the *Aspergillus* LFD in BAL fluid was associated with both higher sensitivity (86%) and specificity (93%) compared with serum. Although not yet commercially available in the United States, these data are encouraging and present a possible rapid alternative to the GM EIA.

Candida Species

Several serologic assays for detection of anti-*Candida* spp antibodies are commercially available. These include the Vircell *Candida albicans* germ tube antibody (CAGTA; Vircell, Granada, Spain) assay, an indirect immunofluorescence test for detection of anti-mycelium antibodies to multiple *Candida* spp, and the Platelia *Candida* Antibody (Ab) Plus assay (Bio-Rad), an ELISA targeting anti-mannan antibodies to *Candida*. When used alone, Leon and colleagues[26] show that both the CAGTA and anti-mannan assays are associated with low sensitivity (53.5% and 25.8%, respectively) and only moderate specificity (64.3% and 89.0%, respectively) for detection of invasive candidiasis (IC). These assays were also positive in a significant percentage of individuals who were considered colonized with *Candida* (range 16.7%–70.8%) and in patients neither colonized nor infected with *Candida* (range 12.5%–21.3%).[26]

A second often sited biomarker for detection of *Candida* infection is the mannan antigen, a major cell wall component of *Candida* spp making up approximately 7% of the organism's dry cell weight.[27] The assay most commonly used to detect mannan antigen is the Platelia *Candida* Ag Plus ELISA, which uses *Candida* oligomannoside-specific rat mAbs as the capture antibody. In patients with proven IC, use of the mannan antigen assay alone is associated with low sensitivity (43.3%–58.0%) and variable specificity (67.3%–93.0%).[26,27] Additionally, this assay was found to be reactive in 20.8% of patients without *Candida* infection or colonization.

Despite the limited clinical utility of anti-*Candida* antibody and mannan antigen detection individually, multiple groups have shown that combination testing for these analytes is associated with improved diagnostic accuracy. One study highlighted that among all the possible antibody/antigen pairings, combination of CAGTA and the (1–3)-β-D-glucan antigen (BDG; described later in this article) provided the highest sensitivity (90.3%–96.8%) and negative predictive value (NPV; 96.6%–97.7%) for diagnosis of IC.[26] A recent 14-study meta-analysis described high sensitivity (83%), specificity (86%), and diagnostic odds ratio (58%) for diagnosis of IC using paired testing for anti-mannan antibodies and *Candida* mannan antigen.[27] A separate group also documented that for 73% of patients with IC, a positive result by at least one test occurred before the first positive blood culture.[28] Importantly, although these combinations provided nearly perfect sensitivity for infections with *C albicans*, *Candida glabrata*, *Candida tropicalis* and *Candida parapsilosis*, only antibody combinations with BDG detected *Candida krusei* infections.[27,29]

Cryptococcus Species

Fungal culture remains the gold standard test for detection of *Cryptococcus neoformans* or *Cryptococcus gattii* infection; however, its utility is limited by the incubation period required for fungal growth. Detection of *Cryptococcus* antigen (CrAg) has therefore become a vital diagnostic test for evaluation of cryptococcal infection. Multiple different CrAg tests are commercially available, and although they vary in the methodology (eg, latex agglutination [LA], EIA, or LFA), they all detect the glucuronoxylomannan (GXM), a capsular polysaccharide present in all 4 major *Cryptococcus* serotypes (A–D), which have recently been divided into 7 unique *Cryptococcus* species.[30] Importantly, although GXM is conserved among *Cryptococcus* agents, the relative amount of xylose and O-acetylation of this polysaccharide varies between serotypes, leading to insensitivity of CrAg assays, which are based on single mAbs (eg, Pastorex Crypto Plus [Bio-Rad], Remel CrAg latex agglutination test [Remel, Lenexa, KS]) to detect *C gattii* (serotype C) infections.[31,32] Recently, a POC CrAg LFA was developed by IMMY (Norman, OK) using 2 mAbs (ie, F12D2 and 339), which have broad reactivity against all *Cryptococcus* serotypes, leading to significantly improved overall sensitivity for detection of cryptococcal infections in both serum and cerebrospinal fluid (CSF).[33,34] In one comparative study using the CrAg Latex Agglutination System (Meridian Bioscience Inc, Cincinnati, OH) as the comparator method, the sensitivity and specificity of the IMMY CrAg LFA was 100% and 99.8%, respectively, from serum samples.[35] Importantly, antigen titers do not correlate between different methods, with the LFA often leading to much higher titers compared with other assays. Furthermore, the CrAg LFA has been shown to be an excellent tool for detection of cryptococcal meningitis, with sensitivity and specificity values of 99.3% and 99.1%, respectively, compared with traditional techniques (ie, culture and India ink stains).[36] Due to the slow clearance of GXM, however, CrAg detection assays are not recommended for the purposes of therapeutic monitoring, as titers may remain elevated despite effective treatment.[37]

CrAg detection assays may yield false results in the setting of *Trichosporon* spp and *Capnocytophaga* spp infections, and rarely in association with other confounding factors, including anaerobic transport vials and excess starch.[38–40] Although uncommon, false-negative results may occur in specimens with extremely high CrAg concentrations (prozone effect) or in cases of infection with an atypical morphology or poorly encapsulated strain of *Cryptococcus*.[41]

(1–3)-β-D-Glucan: A Pan-Fungal Biomarker

BDG is a major cell wall component of most fungi with the exception of *Cryptococcus* spp, *Blastomyces dermatitidis,* and the *Mucorales* group (eg, *Rhizopus* spp, *Mucor* spp). Four different assays for BDG detection have been developed, among which the Fungitell assay (Associates of Cape Code, Inc, East Falmouth, MA) is the only one approved for in vitro diagnostic by the Food and Drug Administration (FDA). Fungitell is a chromogenic, kinetic, quantitative ELISA, which relies on the clotting cascade of horseshoe crab (*Limulus polyphemus)* amebocytes to initiate coagulation in the presence of BDG.[42] The performance characteristics for detection of this pan-fungal biomarker by the Fungitell assay vary, with sensitivity and specificity ranging from 38% to 100%

and 45% to 99%, respectively.[42–46] Similar to the *Aspergillus* GM assay, these inconsistent results are largely a result of the heterogeneous nature of the published studies, which differ in the patient populations tested, the study-specific cutoff criteria, the number of BDG tests performed per patient, and the control populations used. Importantly, however, the BDG assay performs well in 2 high-risk populations: neutropenic patients and HSCT recipients.[44,47,48] A comparative study of 105 patients with hematological malignancy with proven (n = 14) or probable (n = 91) IA and 207 controls showed that although the BDG assay was less specific than the GM ELISA (82% vs 97%), it was significantly more sensitive (81% vs 49%).[49] A 6-study meta-analysis evaluating serial BDG testing in high-risk neutropenic patients with hematologic malignancy reported a significantly elevated diagnostic odds ratio for the presence of IFI following 2 consecutively positive BDG results (111.8) compared with a single positive value (16.3).[50] Such serial testing also was associated with an overall sensitivity, PPV, and NPV of 49.6%, 83.5%, and 94.6%, respectively. Although trending of BDG values following initiation of antifungal therapy is not well described, studies in patients with candidemia suggest that a negative slope in serially plotted BDG levels is associated with favorable outcome (90% PPV).[51] Additional studies in patients with other fungal infections are needed before application of routine BDG monitoring as an indicator of response to therapy.

BDG makes up a significant proportion of the *Pneumocystis jirovecii* cell wall and its detection often serves as a biomarker for infection with this fungal agent, in patients at risk for this infection.[52] Elevated serum BDG levels in serum of patients with human immunodeficiency virus with laboratory-proven *Pneumocystis* pneumonia (PCP) were associated with a sensitivity and specificity of 94.8% and 86.3%, respectively.[53] Although the pan-fungal nature of this biomarker does not allow providers to distinguish PCP from other causes of fungal pneumonia, the high sensitivity and NPV (>95%) associated with a positive BDG result in patients with proven PCP allows clinicians to discount *P jirovecii* infection in patients negative for BDG.[54] Some researchers suggest that BDG evaluation may be helpful in distinguishing whether *P jirovecii,* detected by PCR or by smear, is associated with disease or is present due to colonization.[55]

The limitations of BDG evaluation include the pan-fungal nature of the antigen itself, which necessitates additional evaluation and/or culture to identify the causative fungal agent and susceptibility testing. Additionally, cross-reactivity of these

BDG assays has been documented in patients with certain bacteremias (eg, *Pseudomonas aeruginosa, Enterococcus faecalis*), infusion of select antimicrobial agents (eg, beta-lactam antibiotics, pegylated asparaginase), or fractionated blood products (eg, intravenous immunoglobulin, albumin), excessive use of gauze during surgery, and hemodialysis.[16,58–59]

DIMORPHIC FUNGAL AGENTS
Histoplasma capsulatum

Among the best studied *H capsulatum* antigen detection ELISA is the assay currently performed at MiraVista Diagnostics (Indianapolis, IN). This quantitative ELISA uses polyclonal antibodies to detect an *H capsulatum* polysaccharide antigen from various sources (eg, urine, serum, CSF). The MiraVista ELISA demonstrates high clinical sensitivity in patients with acute pulmonary (APH) and disseminated histoplasmosis, 75% to 81% and 91% to 92%, respectively.[60–62] Furthermore, in a seminal multicenter collaboration, Hage and colleagues[62] reported that antigenuria and antigenemia were detected in 97% and 100% of disseminated histoplasmosis cases, respectively, whereas antigenuria was detectable in only 6% to 34% of subacute and chronic pulmonary histoplasmosis cases. Therefore, a negative *H capsulatum* urine or serum antigen result should not be relied on to rule out nondisseminated disease. Additionally, a study by Swartzentruber and colleagues[63] showed that 82.8% of patients with APH were positive for *H capsulatum* antigen in serum and/or urine, of whom 45.8% of individuals presented with antigenuria only. Collectively, this study suggests that during acute presentation, both serum and urine should be submitted for evaluation to optimize the diagnostic yield. Finally, a study evaluating the clinical significance of low positive (<0.6 ng/mL) urine antigen results by the MiraVista assay in patients without prior histoplasmosis, found that 48% of such results were falsely positive, suggesting cautious result interpretation in such scenarios.[64] *H capsulatum* antigen levels are also monitored following treatment initiation to gauge response to therapy, with declining levels indicative of disease resolution, although for some patients, low-level antigenuria may persist despite cure.[65]

An alternative *H capsulatum* antigen ELISA was recently developed and released for commercial use by IMMY Diagnostics. This assay can be performed only in urine and is based on an mAb to detect *H capsulatum* GM, and although also quantitative, due to the detection of different analytes, reported values are not interchangeable between the IMMY and MiraVista assays. One study comparing performance of the IMMY assay with the MiraVista test showed an overall qualitative agreement of 90% (135/150) in urine samples.[66] Importantly, an additional "indeterminate" qualitative interpretation was included for this IMMY assay, which is not shared by the MiraVista ELISA, and most of the specimens with discordant results (80%) fell within the IMMY indeterminate range. Zhang and colleagues[67] similarly reported high-performance characteristics of this assay, including sensitivity and specificity values of 90.5% and 96.3%, respectively, using urine specimens from patients with clinically characterized histoplasmosis. Overall, these studies suggest that IMMY assay is a suitable alternative for detection of *H capsulatum* antigen. An important limitation for all *H capsulatum* antigen tests is their high level of cross-reactivity with other dimorphic fungi, most notably *B dermatitidis*.[68]

Multiple different methods are used for detection of antibodies to *H capsulatum*; however, we focus on the CF and ID assays, as these remain the reference standards for serologic diagnosis. Briefly, CF for *H capsulatum* is performed using both whole-cell yeast antigen and mycelial antigen (ie, histoplasmin). Histoplasmin contains 3 immunodominant antigens, including the M antigen (a catalase), H antigen (a β-glucosidase), and C antigen (GM).[69] Among these, the C antigen is responsible for most of the cross-reactivity observed by CF in the presence of infection with other dimorphic agents (eg, *B dermatitidis, Coccidioides immitis/posadasii*). In contrast, the H and M antigens are largely specific for *H capsulatum* and antibodies to these antigens are detected by ID.

Serologic evaluation for histoplasmosis is associated with several caveats, including low sensitivity during acute disease and persistent seropositivity following disease resolution and in residents of endemic regions. Overall sensitivity for antibody detection by CF and ID varies from 70% to 100% and is largely dependent on the timing of specimen collection after exposure and the disease state.[70] One study revealed that 3 weeks after exposure, ID and CF were positive in 0% and 5% of individuals, respectively; this positivity increased to 50% and 77%, respectively by 6 weeks.[71] Sensitivity is highest in cases of subacute pulmonary disease (78%–89%) and chronic pulmonary disease (93%); notably antibody detection during acute disease is highly variable (40%–80%).[72] During natural infection, antibodies to the M antigen appear first and by ID, can persist for up to 3 years after disease resolution. Anti-H antigen antibodies appear in only 7% of acutely infected individuals, and can remain detectable for 1 to 2 years following recovery.[70] ID specificity is nearly 100%, and although the presence of both precipitins is diagnostic, definition of the disease state requires clinical correlation. CF results are reported semiquantitatively, although disease severity has not been associated with a defined titer and asymptomatic individuals can present with CF titers ranging from less than 1:8 to greater than 1:64.[72] Despite this, CF titers ranging from 1:8 to 1:16 are considered weakly positive, whereas a fourfold rise in titers between acute and convalescent sera or a CF titer ≥1:32 is considered indicative of acute histoplasmosis. False-negative CF results have been reported and may be due to excess rheumatoid factor and/or cold agglutinins.[73] A final caveat to consider for these assays is their performance in immunosuppressed individuals who are often at greatest risk for disseminated histoplasmosis. In patients with AIDS with disseminated histoplasmosis, CF and ID sensitivity ranges from 45% to 63% and 32% to 61%, respectively, compared with 71% to 82% and 82% to 86%, respectively, for patients without underlying immunosuppression.[74,75]

Blastomyces dermatitidis

Currently, detection of B dermatitidis antigen is available only through MiraVista Diagnostics (Indianapolis, IN). This quantitative ELISA may be used for both initial diagnosis and to monitor response to therapy. For pulmonary and disseminated blastomycosis, Durkin and colleagues[76] reported sensitivity values of 100% and 89%, respectively, for the MiraVista B dermatitidis ELISA, with an overall sensitivity of 93%. Importantly, although false-positive results were not observed in healthy volunteers, this study showed significant cross-reactivity with other dimorphic agents, including H capsulatum, Paracoccidioides brasiliensis, and Talaromyces (Penicillium) marneffei, yielding an overall specificity of 79%. Further studies suggest that detection of B dermatitidis antigenuria (90%) is significantly higher than detection of antigenemia (57%) in patients with confirmed blastomycosis.[77] The level of antigenuria is often higher in patients with pulmonary blastomycosis compared with extrapulmonary blastomycosis, possibly due to lower fungal burden and lack of fungemia in the latter condition.[77] Limited data suggest that antigen levels decline with successful therapy and may be used to monitor both treatment response and predict relapse.[78,79]

Serologic evaluation for antibodies to B dermatitidis can be achieved through ID and CF. The B dermatitidis ID assay relies on a precipitation reaction between host antibodies and B dermatitidis A antigen. A positive reaction is considered diagnostic for blastomycosis with specificity approaching 100%.[80] The sensitivity of this assay however is low, ranging from 26% to 79%. CF for B dermatitidis is no longer routinely performed, largely due to unavailability of reagents and generally poor performance characteristics, including sensitivity and specificity values both below 50%.[80,81] Although an FDA-cleared ELISA is available for detection of total antibodies to the A antigen with high sensitivity (>83%), this assay is cross-reactive with antibodies to H capsulatum, necessitating confirmatory testing of ELISA reactive results[82] More recently, an ELISA using the B dermatitidis surface protein BAD-1 as the capture antigen showed a sensitivity of 87.8% for patients with blastomycosis with a specificity of 94.0% in patients with histoplasmosis.[83] Although not commercially available, these preliminary findings are encouraging and support the need for continued evaluation of this assay.

Coccidioides immitis/posadasii

A quantitative Coccidioides antigen ELISA is available solely through MiraVista Diagnostics and can be used as an adjunct test for diagnosis of coccidioidomycosis. However, due to the limited sensitivity (71%) of this marker in urine among patients with severe coccidioidomycosis, the utility of this biomarker is limited.[84] Despite poor sensitivity in urine, this assay was found to have high sensitivity (93%) and specificity (100%) for the diagnosis of Coccidioides meningitis.[85] Similar to the previously mentioned dimorphic antigen assays, cross reactions may occur with this assay in patients with other dimorphic mycoses.[84]

Similar to H capsulatum and B dermatitidis, serologic evaluation for antibodies to Coccidioides species can be achieved through ID-based, CF-based, and ELISA-based methods. Early studies identified 2 antigens, the tube precipitation (TP, a cell wall polysaccharide) and CF (a fungal chitinase) antigen, which reacted with IgM-class and IgG-class antibodies to Coccidioides, respectively.[86] Preparations of these antigens continue to be used for most currently available Coccidioides serologic assays. Detection of IgM-class antibodies to TP antigen by ID are observed early in the course of infection, with approximately 53% of individuals positive for this analyte during the first week of illness and 97% of patients positive 3 weeks after illness onset. Notably, IgM antibodies to this antigen remained detectable in 4% of individuals with nondisseminated infection at 7 months after disease resolution, compared with residual IgM reactivity in nearly 50% of patients with disseminated disease months to years following recovery.[87] IgG-class antibodies to CF antigen are detectable 1 to 3 weeks after illness onset, and can remain detectable for years following treatment, effectively limiting the clinical utility of this marker for subsequent evaluation of relapse or reinfection.[87] Higher CF antibody titers are associated with more severe disease and declining levels can be used as a prognostic indicator.

Multiple ELISAs are commercially available for detection of anti-Coccidioides antibodies and although considered significantly more sensitive than CF/ID, conflicting data remain regarding the specificity of these tests, particularly for IgM-positive results. Using the Premier Coccidioides ELISA (Meridian Bioscience, Inc), Blair and Currier[88] showed that among 28 IgM-positive (IgG-negative) patients, 4 were culture positive for Coccidioides and 24 had a concordant ID-positive or CF-positive result or seroconverted to IgG positive on repeat testing. The group concluded that false-positive IgM results are rare and that a positive anti-Coccidioides IgM result may be used as supportive evidence for coccidioidomycosis in a patient with appropriate exposure and clinical presentation. In contrast, using the same assay, Kuberski and colleagues[89] reported that among 17 IgM-positive/IgG-negative patients, the IgM ELISA was falsely positive in 14 (82%) patients. Because of these discordant findings, some laboratories use Coccidioides ELISAs as an initial screening test, with confirmatory testing of reactive specimens by Coccidioides CF/ID.

NOVEL BIOMARKERS FOR DETECTION OF FUNGAL AGENTS

Multiple novel biomarkers and techniques have recently been described as possible alternative methods for diagnosis of IA. Among these novel assays is use of high-performance liquid chromatography tandem mass spectrometry (HPLC-MS/MS) to detect gliotoxin, a secondary metabolite released by nearly all strains of Aspergillus fumigatus.[90] A small, proof-of-concept study found promising results for detection of IA, although more detailed evaluation of this assay in a clinical setting is necessary. A second novel assay for detection of IA was recently presented by Koo and colleagues,[91] who used thermal desorption/gas chromatography-MS to detect volatile monoterpenes released from Aspergillus spp in 34 breath samples collected from patients with IA. They report a sensitivity of 94% for IA and a specificity of 93% in breath samples collected from patients with non-Aspergillus pulmonary infections.

Although further studies are needed to verify these preliminary findings, the possibility to diagnose IA using a breath specimen is exciting, particularly for patients in whom invasive specimen collection procedures are contraindicated. Finally, although new assays continue to be developed, current assays (eg, BDG, GM) continue to be optimized, including identification of preferred cutoff values for determination of "positive" versus "negative" results. Additionally, the development of automated and objective interpretive instruments for manual assays, including a laser thermal contrast scanner for use with the IMMY CrAg LFA, are forthcoming.[18,36]

Notably, an area open for research and development is biomarker detection from patients infected with Mucorales agents. To date, not a single diagnostic assay (molecular or serologic) is available for this important class of fungal agents.

Molecular Methods

Molecular methods of fungal identification are particularly attractive for fungi that fail to produce characteristic morphologic characters in a timely fashion and due to the general decline in the expertise of fungal identification by morphology among laboratory technicians. As a general rule, molecular databases for fungi lag behind bacterial databases in terms of maturity because of the diversity of fungal genera and challenges presented in manipulating this group of microorganisms.

Identification of Culture Isolates

Nucleic acid hybridization probes

Fungal nucleic acid hybridization probes are available for the identification of selected dimorphic fungi from culture. The test principle is based on the ability of complementary nucleic acid strands to align and form double-stranded complexes. The initial step involves lysis of the organism, which releases ribosomal RNA (rRNA) from the cells. A chemiluminescent-labeled DNA probe (specific for the target fungal rRNA) is then added to the lysate solution containing the fungal rRNA. If the DNA probe is complementary to the RNA target, it will bind specifically. Any remaining unbound DNA probe is hydrolyzed and removed in a wash step. The DNA-RNA hybrid is then detected by a chemiluminescence reaction and its presence is measured in relative light units using a luminometer.[92] The advantages of the nucleic acid probes include their high specificity and sensitivity, technical simplicity, and the rapid turnaround time (~2 hours from colony growth to identification).[93] Limitations of the probes include the inability of the Coccidioides probe to differentiate between *C immitis* and *C posadasii*, but species identification has little role in patient care for coccidiodomycosis.[92] There is a potential for the *Histoplasma* probe to cross-react with *Aspergillus niger* and *Chrysosporium* spp.[94,95] The probe for *B dermatitidis* may cross-react with *Paracoccidioides* brasiliensis, *Gymnascella* spp, *Emmonsia* spp, and *Chrysosporium* spp, but these are infrequently encountered and morphologic correlation with probe results can help to distinguish these organisms.[92,96,97] Probe test results should therefore be interpreted in conjunction with other laboratory and clinical data, including travel history.

Matrix-assisted laser desorption ionization time of flight mass spectrometry

MALDI-TOF mass spectrometry (MALDI-TOF MS) is a revolutionary semiautomated MS system that provides accurate, rapid, and cost-effective identification of microbial isolates. The technology, which originated in Europe, is being increasingly embraced by microbiology laboratories worldwide mainly through 2 commercial systems, the VITEK MS (bioMérieux Inc, Marcy-l'Étoile, France) and the MALDI Biotyper CA System (Bruker Daltonics Inc, Billerica, MA).[98] Although the use of this technology was first exploited for bacteria, numerous studies have demonstrated utility for the identification of fungi.[99–101] For yeasts, a colony of the organism to be identified is placed on a metal plate and overlain with matrix. The colony spot is targeted by laser, which causes desorption and ionization of proteins in a high-vacuum environment. A mass spectrum of proteins is generated when the proteins are accelerated using electric charge in a tube toward a detector (**Fig. 2**). The time of flight is recorded, with the lighter proteins traveling faster and heavier proteins traveling slower. The generated spectrum is compared with a database of spectra derived from previously characterized fungi by computer software. Identification to the genus and species level of the most closely related organisms is generated with a numerical ranking or score.[98] MALDI-TOF MS of filamentous fungi used the same procedure as for yeast, but a robust lysis and nucleic acid extraction process is generally required before spotting the organism on the MALDI-TOF MS plate. MALDI-TOF MS has many advantages, including its rapid turnaround time, accuracy, ability to test multiple organisms simultaneously, requirement for small sample size (eg, single colony of organism) and cost-effectiveness, which enables effective utilization of laboratory resources, resulting in improved clinical outcomes and significant cost savings to the patient.[102] Current limitations of MALDI-TOF MS are the need for isolated colonies (mixed infections are not identified accurately), the inability to perform direct-from-specimen testing or to provide significant information on the antifungal drug susceptibility markers. As discussed, filamentous

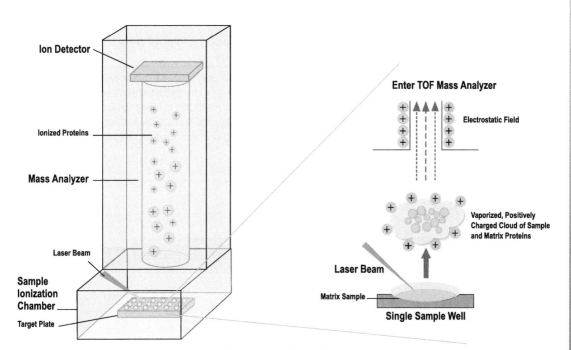

Fig. 2. Diagram of MALDI-TOF. (*Courtesy of* Mayo Foundation for Medical Education and Research, Rochester, MN; with permission.)

fungi require additional processing steps to inactivate the organism, disrupt the cell wall, and extract proteins.[101] In addition, the spectra library for filamentous fungi is not as robust as that for bacteria or yeast, which makes it difficult to identify certain filamentous fungi by this method.[103] Despite these caveats, MALDI-TOF MS has revolutionized the identification of fungi.[99] Development and expansion of custom MALDI MS spectral libraries have the potential to increase the utility of this method for fungi.

Sequence-based identification

DNA sequencing and comparative sequence analysis is an important method for the identification of fungi. Morphologic identification of fungi is sometimes sufficient for patient care but there are instances in which waiting for development of the characteristic structures is undesirable or in which several fungi are indistinguishable using morphologic characterization. For example, A fumigatus and Aspergillus lentulus are phenotypically similar but A lentulus tends to be more resistant to antifungal agents, so identification using sequencing may be important for timely direction of patient care. The utility of sequencing for the identification of yeasts and medically important filamentous fungi have been evaluated in the past.[104–106] Traditional sequencing techniques (eg, Sanger, pyrosequencing) are based on the incorporation of dideoxynucleotides into a growing strand of DNA, which prevents further extension. The resultant DNA fragments are analyzed and the sequence of the unknown isolate is interrogated against a fungal sequence library. The availability of the next-generation sequencing may expand the ability of the clinical laboratory to identify a wider variety of fungi due to its ability to interrogate a large number of targets, but cost and turnaround time may be unfavorable compared with single-target methods. The fungal rRNA gene region

consists of 4 genes: the 18S small subunit, the 5.8S subunit, the 25 to 28S large subunit, and the 5S subunit genes separated by the internal transcribed spacer (ITS) region (**Fig. 3**).[92] The most common targets used for fungal identification by DNA sequencing are the D1/D2 region of the large subunit of the 28S rRNA gene and the ITS region. Although the nuclear ribosomal large subunit is frequently used, the ITS region often has better discriminatory power at the species level for a wide variety of fungal genera.[107] However, no single target is sufficient for all fungi. For example, the ITS region does not resolve many Mucorales fungi to the species level.[108] Additional targets can also be useful for certain genera (eg, β-tubulin for Aspergillus spp or EF-1α for Fusarium spp). An ideal sequence database that contains accurate sequences of all fungal species currently does not exist. The International Sequence Database Collaboration, the largest public DNA sequence archive, has only 10% to 15% of fungal species, 14% erroneous sequences, and a revision rate of 1%.[109,110] Commercial DNA sequencing systems, such as MicroSeq (Applied Biosystems, Foster City, CA), have their own libraries that are not available to the public and are not exhaustive. Many reference laboratories develop custom-built libraries that are more accurate but may be limited by their size. Given the current limitations, the Consortium of the Barcode of Life is working on putting together a quality global reference library of DNA barcode sequences.[108]

Identification of Fungi Directly from Specimens

Real-time polymerase chain reaction testing

PCR is one of the oldest and most frequently used molecular methods in clinical microbiology laboratories. After the fungal DNA is isolated, it is amplified using primers. For organism-specific assays,

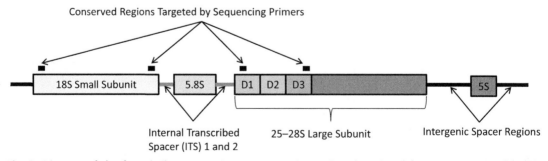

Fig. 3. Diagram of the fungal ribosome major RNA transcript region. (*Reprinted from* Petti CA, Bosshard PP, Brandt ME, et al. Interpretive criteria for identification of bacteria and fungi by DNA target sequencing; approved guideline. *CLSI* document MM18-A 28 (1); with permission of the Clinical and Laboratory Standards Institute (CLSI).)

the primers bind to DNA sequences that are unique to the organism, whereas for broad-range assays, the primer needs to bind to conserved areas that are preserved phylogenetically. The rRNA gene cluster is a frequently used target and contains both the conserved and variable areas. A detailed review of the methodology and diagnostic utility of PCR assays for fungal infections have been published elsewhere.[111,112] Traditional PCR assays are unable to quantify the amount of amplified fungal DNA.[113] The development of the real-time PCR assay has, in some instances, allowed for quantitation of the amplified DNA, which helps differentiate between colonization and invasive disease by providing a measure of fungal burden.[113] Advantages of real-time PCR over conventional testing methods include its high sensitivity and specificity, ease of performance, rapid turnaround time, and lower risk of contamination, because amplification and detection occur in an enclosed space.[111] One disadvantage of PCR testing for filamentous fungi, such as *Aspergillus* spp, is the lack of standardization, owing, in part, to the different techniques used for the isolation of fungal DNA, as fungal cell walls are difficult to lyse. This has resulted in significant discrepancies between assays, hindering its use in clinical practice. Another concern is the potential for falsely positive PCR tests resulting from contamination of surfaces, clinical samples, and reagents, as fungi are ubiquitous in the environment.[113]

Candida species
The current gold standard diagnostic test for IC is blood culture. Despite the high sensitivity of blood cultures, the prolonged turnaround time (24–120 hours) may cause delay in starting appropriate treatment. Molecular tests, such as DNA detection by PCR directly from blood, have the potential for rapid diagnosis of IC. In a meta-analysis by Avni and colleagues,[114] the sensitivity and specificity of PCR for suspected IC was 95% and 92%, respectively. The use of whole-blood samples and detection limit of fewer than 10 colony-forming units per milliliter were associated with favorable test performance. Nguyen and colleagues[115] evaluated the performance of *Candida* PCR, BDG, and blood cultures in the diagnosis of IC. In their study, the tests were similar in diagnosing candidemia, but PCR was more sensitive than blood cultures among patients with deep-seated candidiasis (88% vs 17%). *Candida* PCR assays have the advantage of offering rapid diagnosis, often identifying to species level, higher sensitivity in diagnosing deep-seated IC without candidemia, and the detection of molecular markers of drug resistance. The lack of standardization and multicenter validation of the PCR assays limit their routine use in clinical practice.[116] Introduction of the FilmArray BCID panel (BioFire Diagnostics, Salt Lake City, UT) has enabled the rapid and specific identification of 5 *Candida* species (*C albicans, C glabrata, C parapsilosis, C tropicalis,* and *C krusei*) directly from positive blood culture bottles.[117]

Aspergillus species
The role of *Aspergillus* PCR in the diagnosis of IA remains unclear. Current guidelines do not provide any recommendation regarding its use in clinical practice in the United States.[16] In a recent meta-analysis of 18 clinical trials involving immunocompromised patients, the mean sensitivity and specificity of *Aspergillus* PCR from blood for diagnosing IA was 80.5% and 78.5% for a single positive test and 58.0% and 96.2% for 2 consecutive positive test results.[118] In another meta-analysis of 25 studies, the whole blood and serum PCR assays had a sensitivity and specificity of 84% and 76%, respectively, for a single positive result and 64% and 95% for 2 positive results.[119] These results suggest that a single positive or a negative result does not confirm or exclude IA. However, 2 positive *Aspergillus* PCR results carry a higher PPV and are more likely to be indicative of active *Aspergillus* sp infection. *Aspergillus* PCR in BAL has a higher sensitivity than in blood but its clinical utility is compromised due to the inability to differentiate IPA from airway colonization. This assay may be used to rule out IPA due to its high NPV.[16] Newer strategies using a combination of biomarkers, such as the *Aspergillus* PCR and GM were associated with an earlier diagnosis (up to 7 days earlier) and lower incidence of IA in high-risk patients when compared with patients who were monitored by GM alone.[120] Although *Aspergillus* PCR appears to be a promising tool for the early diagnosis of IA and has higher sensitivity than culture, its current use is impeded by the lack of test standardization.

Pneumocystis jirovecii
As *P jirovecii* cannot be grown in cultures, the traditional methods for the laboratory diagnosis of *P jirovecii* have involved the direct examination of clinical specimens using fluorescent microscopy, direct fluorescent antibody testing, and histopathologic examination. These tests are subjective and can be limited by lower sensitivity in some settings.[92] *Pneumocystis* PCR plays an important role in the early diagnosis of PCP and has greatly improved sensitivity when compared with the traditional methods. Despite its high

sensitivity, the test does not differentiate between airway colonization and pneumonia. Oftentimes, the clinical significance of a positive PCR test may be unclear due to the frequent occurrence of *Pneumocystis* airway colonization, even in high-risk patients.[121] Studies have shown that patients with PCP have a higher concentration of *Pneumocystis* DNA in BAL fluid when compared with those who were colonized.[122] In a study by Fauchier and colleagues,[123] quantitative PCR of BAL was found to be an important tool in differentiating colonization versus pneumonia by using fungal burden estimates from cycle threshold (Ct) values. In addition, serum BDG is a useful marker to differentiate infection from colonization and was noted to have high sensitivity in detecting PCP.[53,55,124] An elevated BDG in the setting of a positive *Pneumocystis* PCR from BAL may prompt initiation of treatment.

Mucorales

The agents of mucormycosis, a potentially life-threatening infection, are not detected by the widely used fungal biomarkers GM or BDG. The key to a favorable clinical outcome lies in the development of laboratory tests that enable early diagnosis and timely treatment of mucormycosis. Several studies have looked at antigen-based and PCR-based tests for Mucorales. One study evaluated the performance of a laboratory-developed real-time PCR assay that detected 6 species of Mucorales agents in culture and tissue samples. The clinical sensitivity and specificity of the assay were 100% and 92% with culture isolates and 56% and 100% with formalin-fixed, paraffin-embedded tissues. The sensitivity and specificity for 2 fresh tissue specimens were 100%.[125] In a retrospective study that evaluated a combination of 3 quantitative PCR assays targeting *Mucor/Rhizopus*, *Lichtheimia*, and *Rhizomucor,* Mucorales DNA was detected from serum samples in 9 of 10 patients up to 68 days before a diagnosis of mucormycosis was confirmed by histopathology or culture.[126] Currently, there are no standardized blood PCR tests for the diagnosis of mucormycosis.

Dimorphic fungi

Laboratory diagnosis of coccidiomycosis is frequently done by serology, direct smear, histopathology, and culture. Serology may remain negative in early disease and in immunocompromised hosts. Direct smear and histopathology are limited by sensitivity. Culture has high sensitivity but is limited by the long turnaround time and the potential safety hazard to laboratory personnel. *Coccidioides* PCR, although not widely

available, has the advantage of rapid turnaround time with high sensitivity and specificity. It may be used for the identification of the organism from culture isolates or for the direct detection of *Coccidioides* from patient specimens. In a study that assessed the performance of a laboratory-developed *Coccidioides* PCR test on clinical specimens, the test had a sensitivity and specificity of 100% and 98.4% when compared with cultures when testing respiratory samples. The assay was also validated on fresh tissue and paraffin-embedded tissue specimens and yielded a sensitivity of 93.0% and 73.4%, respectively.[127]

Several PCR methods have been developed and evaluated for the detection of *H capsulatum* and *Blastomyces* spp from culture, direct specimen, and paraffin-embedded tissue samples.[128,129] Babady and colleagues,[130] reported the performance of a PCR assay that detected *Blastomyces dermatitides* and *H capsulatum* from culture isolates and clinical specimens. The assay demonstrated 100% specificity and 100% sensitivity for *B dermatitidis* and 100% specificity and 94% sensitivity for *H capsulatum* from culture isolates. When compared with culture, the assay had specificities and sensitivities of 99% and 86% for *B dermatitidis,* and 100% and 73% for *H capsulatum* directly from clinical specimens. Gago and colleagues[131] report a multiplex real-time PCR assay for the identification of *H capsulatum* in addition to *P jirovecii* and *C neoformans/gattii* directly from clinical specimens and from culture isolates. The assay had 100% specificity and 100% sensitivity for culture isolates and 90.7% sensitivity for clinical samples and may have clinical applications in the early diagnosis of opportunistic fungal infections in patients with compromised immunity.

Broad-range gene polymerase chain reaction and sequencing

The direct detection of fungal DNA in clinical samples by broad-range PCR and sequencing is an important, culture-independent method for the rapid identification of bacterial and fungal pathogens.[132] Unlike specific PCR assays that detect one organism, broad-range PCR assays use primers that are designed to detect a large number of organisms in a particular group. Postamplification analysis by DNA sequencing is used for identification of the fungal organism. This test is particularly useful when cultures remain negative despite clinical and histopathological evidence of infection. In general, broad-range PCR plus sequencing tests are most useful when microorganisms are visualized using pathology or microbiology stains (smear positive) but fail to grow in culture. This situation may arise when the infection is caused by fastidious or noncultivable organisms or in the setting of prior antimicrobial use.[132] Vollmer and colleagues[133] evaluated a novel broad-range PCR assay that targeted the 28S rDNA and was able to detect a broad range of clinically relevant fungi with one set of primers and probes. The test sensitivity may be hindered by the small volume of sample used for PCR when compared with culturing and the potential for PCR inhibitors due to the presence of background material from human DNA. Nonviable fungal pathogens may be picked up by the assay. Another limitation of broad-range assays is the potential for falsely positive results due to environmental or reagent contamination. If multiple organisms are amplified, DNA sequencing may not be able to give meaningful results. Despite these caveats, broad-range molecular genetic methods are highly specific, rapid, and cost-effective, and may be used as an adjunct to cultures for the detection and identification of fungal pathogens.

Magnetic resonance
The direct detection of selected *Candida* species directly from whole blood without performing a culture can be done using magnetic resonance spectroscopy. The T2Candida Panel (T2 Biosystems Inc, Lexington, MA) requires approximately 4 hours to complete and can identify *C albicans*/*C tropicalis*, *C parapsilosis*, and *C glabrata*/*C krusei*.[134]

Molecular detection of drug resistance
Molecular tests that detect gene mutations associated with antifungal drug resistance may provide rapid susceptibility information when compared with the traditional phenotypic methods. The development of echinocandin resistance in *C albicans* has been linked to amino acid substitutions in the *fks*1 subunit of the glucan synthase complex.[135] Azole resistance in *A fumigatus* is predominantly driven by fungicide exposure and is often caused by mutations in *cyp*51.[136] The genotypic tests that detect these mutations are predominantly laboratory-developed tests and are not widely available for clinical diagnostics that are presently used mainly for epidemiologic purposes.

REFERENCES

1. Crowe A. Immunodiffusion. 2nd edition. New York: Academic Press, Inc.; 1973.
2. Stevens CD. Clinical immunology and serology: a laboratory perspective. Philadelphia: F. A. Davis Company; 1996.
3. Singh N, Paterson DL. Aspergillus infections in transplant recipients. Clin Microbiol Rev 2005; 18(1):44–69.
4. Ellepola AN, Morrison CJ. Laboratory diagnosis of invasive candidiasis. J Microbiol 2005;43 Spec No:65–84.
5. De Pauw B, Walsh TJ, Donnelly JP, et al. Revised definitions of invasive fungal disease from the European Organization for Research and Treatment of Cancer/Invasive Fungal Infections Cooperative Group and the National Institute of Allergy and Infectious Diseases Mycoses Study Group (EORTC/MSG) Consensus Group. Clin Infect Dis 2008; 46(12):1813–21.
6. Dagenais TR, Keller NP. Pathogenesis of *Aspergillus fumigatus* in invasive aspergillosis. Clin Microbiol Rev 2009;22(3):447–65.
7. Bardana EJ Jr. Measurement of humoral antibodies to aspergilli. Ann N Y Acad Sci 1974;221:64–75.
8. Cornillet A, Camus C, Nimubona S, et al. Comparison of epidemiological, clinical, and biological features of invasive aspergillosis in neutropenic and nonneutropenic patients: a 6-year survey. Clin Infect Dis 2006;43(5):577–84.
9. Page ID, Richardson M, Denning DW. Antibody testing in aspergillosis–quo vadis? Med Mycol 2015;53(5):417–39.
10. Guitard J, Sendid B, Thorez S, et al. Evaluation of a recombinant antigen-based enzyme immunoassay for the diagnosis of noninvasive aspergillosis. J Clin Microbiol 2012;50(3):762–5.
11. Dumollard C, Bailly S, Perriot S, et al. Prospective evaluation of a new aspergillus IgG enzyme immunoassay kit for diagnosis of chronic and allergic pulmonary aspergillosis. J Clin Microbiol 2016; 54(5):1236–42.
12. Blot SI, Taccone FS, Van den Abeele AM, et al. A clinical algorithm to diagnose invasive pulmonary aspergillosis in critically ill patients. Am J Respir Crit Care Med 2012;186(1):56–64.
13. Klont RR, Mennink-Kersten MA, Verweij PE. Utility of aspergillus antigen detection in specimens other than serum specimens. Clin Infect Dis 2004;39(10): 1467–74.
14. Pfeiffer CD, Fine JP, Safdar N. Diagnosis of invasive aspergillosis using a galactomannan assay: a meta-analysis. Clin Infect Dis 2006;42(10): 1417–27.
15. Leeflang MM, Debets-Ossenkopp YJ, Visser CE, et al. Galactomannan detection for invasive aspergillosis in immunocompromised patients. Cochrane Database Syst Rev 2008;(4):CD007394.
16. Patterson TF, Thompson GR 3rd, Denning DW, et al. Practice guidelines for the diagnosis and management of aspergillosis: 2016 update by the Infectious Diseases Society of America. Clin Infect Dis 2016;63(4):e1–60.
17. Maertens J, Van Eldere J, Verhaegen J, et al. Use of circulating galactomannan screening for early diagnosis of invasive aspergillosis in allogeneic

stem cell transplant recipients. J Infect Dis 2002; 186(9):1297–306.

18. Maertens JA, Klont R, Masson C, et al. Optimization of the cutoff value for the aspergillus double-sandwich enzyme immunoassay. Clin Infect Dis 2007;44(10):1329–36.

19. Miceli MH, Maertens J. Role of non-culture-based tests, with an emphasis on galactomannan testing for the diagnosis of invasive aspergillosis. Semin Respir Crit Care Med 2015;36(5):650–61.

20. Affolter K, Tamm M, Jahn K, et al. Galactomannan in bronchoalveolar lavage for diagnosing invasive fungal disease. Am J Respir Crit Care Med 2014; 190(3):309–17.

21. Duarte RF, Sanchez-Ortega I, Cuesta I, et al. Serum galactomannan-based early detection of invasive aspergillosis in hematology patients receiving effective antimold prophylaxis. Clin Infect Dis 2014;59(12):1696–702.

22. Guigue N, Menotti J, Ribaud P. False positive galactomannan test after ice-pop ingestion. N Engl J Med 2013;369(1):97–8.

23. Vergidis P, Razonable RR, Wheat LJ, et al. Reduction in false-positive aspergillus serum galactomannan enzyme immunoassay results associated with use of piperacillin-tazobactam in the United States. J Clin Microbiol 2014;52(6):2199–201.

24. Thornton CR. Development of an immunochromatographic lateral-flow device for rapid serodiagnosis of invasive aspergillosis. Clin Vaccine Immunol 2008;15(7):1095–105.

25. Pan Z, Fu M, Zhang J, et al. Diagnostic accuracy of a novel lateral-flow device in invasive aspergillosis: a meta-analysis. J Med Microbiol 2015; 64(7):702–7.

26. Leon C, Ruiz-Santana S, Saavedra P, et al. Contribution of Candida biomarkers and DNA detection for the diagnosis of invasive candidiasis in ICU patients with severe abdominal conditions. Crit Care 2016;20(1):149.

27. Mikulska M, Calandra T, Sanguinetti M, et al. The use of mannan antigen and anti-mannan antibodies in the diagnosis of invasive candidiasis: recommendations from the Third European Conference on Infections in Leukemia. Crit Care 2010; 14(6):R222.

28. Yera H, Sendid B, Francois N, et al. Contribution of serological tests and blood culture to the early diagnosis of systemic candidiasis. Eur J Clin Microbiol Infect Dis 2001;20(12):864–70.

29. Martinez-Jimenez MC, Munoz P, Valerio M, et al. Candida biomarkers in patients with candidaemia and bacteraemia. J Antimicrob Chemother 2015; 70(8):2354–61.

30. Warnock DW. Name changes for fungi of medical importance, 2012 to 2015. J Clin Microbiol 2016; 55(1):53–9.

31. Percival A, Thorkildson P, Kozel TR. Monoclonal antibodies specific for immunorecessive epitopes of glucuronoxylomannan, the major capsular polysaccharide of Cryptococcus neoformans, reduce serotype bias in an immunoassay for cryptococcal antigen. Clin Vaccine Immunol 2011;18(8):1292–6.

32. Tintelnot K, Hagen F, Han CO, et al. Pitfalls in serological diagnosis of Cryptococcus gattii infections. Med Mycol 2015;53(8):874–9.

33. Prattes J, Heldt S, Eigl S, et al. Point of care testing for the diagnosis of fungal infections: are we there yet? Curr Fungal Infect Rep 2016;10:43–50.

34. Jarvis JN, Percival A, Bauman S, et al. Evaluation of a novel point-of-care cryptococcal antigen test on serum, plasma, and urine from patients with HIV-associated cryptococcal meningitis. Clin Infect Dis 2011;53(10):1019–23.

35. Binnicker MJ, Jespersen DJ, Bestrom JE, et al. Comparison of four assays for the detection of cryptococcal antigen. Clin Vaccine Immunol 2012;19(12):1988–90.

36. Boulware DR, Rolfes MA, Rajasingham R, et al. Multisite validation of cryptococcal antigen lateral flow assay and quantification by laser thermal contrast. Emerg Infect Dis 2014;20(1):45–53.

37. Perfect JR, Dismukes WE, Dromer F, et al. Clinical practice guidelines for the management of cryptococcal disease: 2010 update by the Infectious Diseases Society of America. Clin Infect Dis 2010; 50(3):291–322.

38. Chanock SJ, Toltzis P, Wilson C. Cross-reactivity between Stomatococcus mucilaginosus and latex agglutination for cryptococcal antigen. Lancet 1993;342(8879):1119–20.

39. McManus EJ, Jones JM. Detection of a Trichosporon beigelii antigen cross-reactive with Cryptococcus neoformans capsular polysaccharide in serum from a patient with disseminated trichosporon infection. J Clin Microbiol 1985;21(5): 681–5.

40. Wilson DA, Sholtis M, Parshall S, et al. False-positive cryptococcal antigen test associated with use of BBL Port-a-Cul transport vials. J Clin Microbiol 2011;49(2):702–3.

41. Opota O, Desgraz B, Kenfak A, et al. Cryptococcus neoformans meningitis with negative cryptococcal antigen: evaluation of a new immunochromatographic detection assay. New Microbes New Infect 2015;4:1–4.

42. Theel ES, Doern CD. Beta-D-glucan testing is important for diagnosis of invasive fungal infections. J Clin Microbiol 2013;51(11):3478–83.

43. Marchetti O, Lamoth F, Mikulska M, et al. ECIL recommendations for the use of biological markers for the diagnosis of invasive fungal diseases in leukemic patients and hematopoietic SCT recipients. Bone Marrow Transplant 2012;47(6):846–54.

44. Odabası Z, Mattiuzzi G, Estey E, et al. Beta-D-glucan as a diagnostic adjunct for invasive fungal infections: validation, cutoff development, and performance in patients with acute myelogenous leukemia and myelodysplastic syndrome. Clin Infect Dis 2004;39(2):199–205.

45. Pickering JW, Sant HW, Bowles CA, et al. Evaluation of a (1->3)-beta-D-glucan assay for diagnosis of invasive fungal infections. J Clin Microbiol 2005;43(12):5957–62.

46. Karageorgopoulos DE, Vouloumanou EK, Ntziora F, et al. Beta-D-glucan assay for the diagnosis of invasive fungal infections: a meta-analysis. Clin Infect Dis 2011;52(6):750–70.

47. Senn L, Robinson JO, Schmidt S, et al. 1,3-Beta-D-glucan antigenemia for early diagnosis of invasive fungal infections in neutropenic patients with acute leukemia. Clin Infect Dis 2008;46(6):878–85.

48. Ellis M, Al-Ramadi B, Finkelman M, et al. Assessment of the clinical utility of serial beta-D-glucan concentrations in patients with persistent neutropenic fever. J Med Microbiol 2008;57(Pt 3):287–95.

49. Sulahian A, Porcher R, Bergeron A, et al. Use and limits of (1-3)-beta-d-glucan assay (Fungitell), compared to galactomannan determination (Platelia Aspergillus), for diagnosis of invasive aspergillosis. J Clin Microbiol 2014;52(7):2328–33.

50. Lamoth F, Cruciani M, Mengoli C, et al. Beta-Glucan antigenemia assay for the diagnosis of invasive fungal infections in patients with hematological malignancies: a systematic review and meta-analysis of cohort studies from the Third European Conference on Infections in Leukemia (ECIL-3). Clin Infect Dis 2012;54(5):633–43.

51. Jaijakul S, Vazquez JA, Swanson RN, et al. (1,3)-beta-D-glucan as a prognostic marker of treatment response in invasive candidiasis. Clin Infect Dis 2012;55(4):521–6.

52. Thomas CF Jr, Limper AH. Current insights into the biology and pathogenesis of Pneumocystis pneumonia. Nat Rev Microbiol 2007;5(4):298–308.

53. Karageorgopoulos DE, Qu JM, Korbila IP, et al. Accuracy of beta-D-glucan for the diagnosis of Pneumocystis jirovecii pneumonia: a meta-analysis. Clin Microbiol Infect 2013;19(1):39–49.

54. Held J, Koch MS, Reischl U, et al. Serum (1-> 3)-beta-D-glucan measurement as an early indicator of Pneumocystis jirovecii pneumonia and evaluation of its prognostic value. Clin Microbiol Infect 2011;17(4):595–602.

55. Damiani C, Le Gal S, Lejeune D, et al. Serum (1->3)-beta-D-glucan levels in primary infection and pulmonary colonization with Pneumocystis jirovecii. J Clin Microbiol 2011;49(5):2000–2.

56. Marty FM, Lowry CM, Lempitski SJ, et al. Reactivity of (1->3)-beta-d-glucan assay with commonly used intravenous antimicrobials. Antimicrob Agents Chemother 2006;50(10):3450–3.

57. Metan G, Koc AN, Agkus C, et al. Can bacteraemia lead to false positive results in 1,3-beta-D-glucan test? Analysis of 83 bacteraemia episodes in high-risk patients for invasive fungal infections. Rev Iberoam Micol 2012;29(3):169–71.

58. Kanda H, Kubo K, Hamasaki K, et al. Influence of various hemodialysis membranes on the plasma (1->3)-beta-D-glucan level. Kidney Int 2001;60(1):319–23.

59. Ogawa M, Hori H, Niiguchi S, et al. False-positive plasma (1->3)-beta-D-glucan test following immunoglobulin product replacement in an adult bone marrow recipient. Int J Hematol 2004;80(1):97–8.

60. Wheat LJ, Conces D, Allen SD, et al. Pulmonary histoplasmosis syndromes: recognition, diagnosis, and management. Semin Respir Crit Care Med 2004;25(2):129–44.

61. Wheat LJ, Garringer T, Brizendine E, et al. Diagnosis of histoplasmosis by antigen detection based upon experience at the histoplasmosis reference laboratory. Diagn Microbiol Infect Dis 2002;43(1):29–37.

62. Hage CA, Ribes JA, Wengenack NL, et al. A multicenter evaluation of tests for diagnosis of histoplasmosis. Clin Infect Dis 2011;53(5):448–54.

63. Swartzentruber S, Rhodes L, Kurkjian K, et al. Diagnosis of acute pulmonary histoplasmosis by antigen detection. Clin Infect Dis 2009;49(12):1878–82.

64. Theel ES, Ramanan P. Clinical significance of low-positive histoplasma urine antigen results. J Clin Microbiol 2014;52(9):3444–6.

65. Wheat LJ, Freifeld AG, Kleiman MB, et al. Clinical practice guidelines for the management of patients with histoplasmosis: 2007 update by the Infectious Diseases Society of America. Clin Infect Dis 2007;45(7):807–25.

66. Theel ES, Harring JA, Dababneh AS, et al. Reevaluation of commercial reagents for detection of Histoplasma capsulatum antigen in urine. J Clin Microbiol 2015;53(4):1198–203.

67. Zhang X, Gibson B Jr, Daly TM. Evaluation of commercially available reagents for diagnosis of histoplasmosis infection in immunocompromised patients. J Clin Microbiol 2013;51(12):4095–101.

68. Wheat LJ, Azar MM, Bahr NC, et al. Histoplasmosis. Infect Dis Clin North Am 2016;30(1):207–27.

69. Deepe GS Jr, Durose GG. Immunobiological activity of recombinant H antigen from Histoplasma capsulatum. Infect Immun 1995;63(8):3151–7.

70. Guimaraes AJ, Nosanchuk JD, Zancope-Oliveira RM. Diagnosis of histoplasmosis. Braz J Microbiol 2006;37(1):1–13.

71. Davies SF. Serodiagnosis of histoplasmosis. Semin Respir Infect 1986;1(1):9–15.

72. Wheat LJ. Improvements in diagnosis of histoplasmosis. Expert Opin Biol Ther 2006;6(11):1207–21.

73. Johnson JE, Roberts GD. Blocking effect of rheumatoid factor and cold agglutinins on complement fixation tests for histoplasmosis. J Clin Microbiol 1976;3(2):157–60.

74. Williams B, Fojtasek M, Connolly-Stringfield P, et al. Diagnosis of histoplasmosis by antigen detection during an outbreak in Indianapolis, Ind. Arch Pathol Lab Med 1994;118(12):1205–8.

75. Tobon AM, Agudelo CA, Rosero DS, et al. Disseminated histoplasmosis: a comparative study between patients with acquired immunodeficiency syndrome and non-human immunodeficiency virus-infected individuals. Am J Trop Med Hyg 2005;73(3):576–82.

76. Durkin M, Witt J, Lemonte A, et al. Antigen assay with the potential to aid in diagnosis of blastomycosis. J Clin Microbiol 2004;42(10):4873–5.

77. Connolly P, Hage CA, Bariola JR, et al. *Blastomyces dermatitidis* antigen detection by quantitative enzyme immunoassay. Clin Vaccine Immunol 2012;19(1):53–6.

78. Chapman SW, Dismukes WE, Proia LA, et al. Clinical practice guidelines for the management of blastomycosis: 2008 update by the Infectious Diseases Society of America. Clin Infect Dis 2008; 46(12):1801–12.

79. Mongkolrattanothai K, Peev M, Wheat LJ, et al. Urine antigen detection of blastomycosis in pediatric patients. Pediatr Infect Dis J 2006;25(11): 1076–8.

80. Areno JP 4th, Campbell GD Jr, George RB. Diagnosis of blastomycosis. Semin Respir Infect 1997; 12(3):252–62.

81. Wheat LJ. Antigen detection, serology, and molecular diagnosis of invasive mycoses in the immunocompromised host. Transpl Infect Dis 2006;8(3): 128–39.

82. Bradsher RW, Pappas PG. Detection of specific antibodies in human blastomycosis by enzyme immunoassay. South Med J 1995;88(12):1256–9.

83. Richer SM, Smedema ML, Durkin MM, et al. Development of a highly sensitive and specific blastomycosis antibody enzyme immunoassay using *Blastomyces dermatitidis* surface protein BAD-1. Clin Vaccine Immunol 2014;21(2):143–6.

84. Durkin M, Connolly P, Kuberski T, et al. Diagnosis of coccidioidomycosis with use of the Coccidioides antigen enzyme immunoassay. Clin Infect Dis 2008;47(8):e69–73.

85. Kassis C, Zaidi S, Kuberski T, et al. Role of coccidioides antigen testing in the cerebrospinal fluid for the diagnosis of coccidioidal meningitis. Clin Infect Dis 2015;61(10):1521–6.

86. Nguyen C, Barker BM, Hoover S, et al. Recent advances in our understanding of the environmental, epidemiological, immunological, and clinical dimensions of coccidioidomycosis. Clin Microbiol Rev 2013;26(3):505–25.

87. Pappagianis D, Zimmer BL. Serology of coccidioidomycosis. Clin Microbiol Rev 1990;3(3):247–68.

88. Blair JE, Currier JT. Significance of isolated positive IgM serologic results by enzyme immunoassay for coccidioidomycosis. Mycopathologia 2008;166(2): 77–82.

89. Kuberski T, Herrig J, Pappagianis D. False-positive IgM serology in coccidioidomycosis. J Clin Microbiol 2010;48(6):2047–9.

90. Cerqueira LB, de Francisco TM, Gasparetto JC, et al. Development and validation of an HPLC-MS/MS method for the early diagnosis of aspergillosis. PLoS One 2014;9(4):e92851.

91. Koo S, Thomas HR, Daniels SD, et al. A breath fungal secondary metabolite signature to diagnose invasive aspergillosis. Clin Infect Dis 2014;59(12): 1733–40.

92. Wengenack NL, Binnicker MJ. Fungal molecular diagnostics. Clin Chest Med 2009;30(2):391–408, viii.

93. Alexander BD, Pfaller MA. Contemporary tools for the diagnosis and management of invasive mycoses. Clin Infect Dis 2006;43:S15–27.

94. Hall GS, Pratt-Rippin K, Washington JA. Evaluation of a chemiluminescent probe assay for identification of *Histoplasma capsulatum* isolates. J Clin Microbiol 1992;30(11):3003–4.

95. Brandt ME, Gaunt D, Iqbal N, et al. False-positive *Histoplasma capsulatum* Gen-Probe chemiluminescent test result caused by a *Chrysosporium* species. J Clin Microbiol 2005;43(3):1456–8.

96. Iwen PC, Sigler L, Tarantolo S, et al. Pulmonary infection caused by *Gymnascella hyalinospora* in a patient with acute myelogenous leukemia. J Clin Microbiol 2000;38(1):375–81.

97. Padhye AA, Smith G, Standard PG, et al. Comparative evaluation of chemiluminescent DNA probe assays and exoantigen tests for rapid identification of *Blastomyces dermatitidis* and *Coccidioides immitis*. J Clin Microbiol 1994;32(4):867–70.

98. Patel R. MALDI-TOF MS for the diagnosis of infectious diseases. Clin Chem 2015;61(1):100–11.

99. Theel ES, Hall L, Mandrekar J, et al. Dermatophyte identification using matrix-assisted laser desorption ionization-time of flight mass spectrometry. J Clin Microbiol 2011;49(12):4067–71.

100. Westblade LF, Jennemann R, Branda JA, et al. Multicenter study evaluating the Vitek MS system for identification of medically important yeasts. J Clin Microbiol 2013;51(7):2267–72.

101. Schulthess B, Ledermann R, Mouttet F, et al. Use of the Bruker MALDI Biotyper for identification of molds in the clinical mycology laboratory. J Clin Microbiol 2014;52(8):2797–803.

102. Dhiman N, Hall L, Wohlfiel SL, et al. Performance and cost analysis of matrix-assisted laser desorption ionization-time of flight mass spectrometry for routine identification of yeast. J Clin Microbiol 2011;49(4):1614–6.

103. McMullen AR, Wallace MA, Pincus DH, et al. Evaluation of the Vitek MS matrix-assisted laser desorption ionization-time of flight mass spectrometry system for identification of clinically relevant filamentous fungi. J Clin Microbiol 2016; 54(8):2068–73.

104. Hall L, Wohlfiel S, Roberts GD. Experience with the MicroSeq D2 large-subunit ribosomal DNA sequencing kit for identification of filamentous fungi encountered in the clinical laboratory. J Clin Microbiol 2004;42(2):622–6.

105. Hall L, Wohlfiel S, Roberts GD. Experience with the MicroSeq D2 large-subunit ribosomal DNA sequencing kit for identification of commonly encountered, clinically important yeast species. J Clin Microbiol 2003;41(11):5099–102.

106. Ciardo DE, Schar G, Bottger EC, et al. Internal transcribed spacer sequencing versus biochemical profiling for identification of medically important yeasts. J Clin Microbiol 2006;44(1):77–84.

107. Schoch CL, Seifert KA, Huhndorf S, et al. Nuclear ribosomal internal transcribed spacer (ITS) region as a universal DNA barcode marker for fungi. Proc Natl Acad Sci U S A 2012; 109(16):6241–6.

108. Halliday CL, Kidd SE, Sorrell TC, et al. Molecular diagnostic methods for invasive fungal disease: the horizon draws nearer? Pathology 2015;47(3): 257–69.

109. Nilsson RH, Ryberg M, Kristiansson E, et al. Taxonomic reliability of DNA sequences in public sequence databases: a fungal perspective. PLoS One 2006;1:e59.

110. Bridge PD, Roberts PJ, Spooner BM, et al. On the unreliability of published DNA sequences. New Phytol 2003;160(1):43–8.

111. Espy MJ, Uhl JR, Sloan LM, et al. Real-time PCR in clinical microbiology: applications for routine laboratory testing. Clin Microbiol Rev 2006;19(1):165–256.

112. Kourkoumpetis TK, Fuchs BB, Coleman JJ, et al. Polymerase chain reaction-based assays for the diagnosis of invasive fungal infections. Clin Infect Dis 2012;54(9):1322–31.

113. Arvanitis M, Anagnostou T, Fuchs BB, et al. Molecular and nonmolecular diagnostic methods for invasive fungal infections. Clin Microbiol Rev 2014;27(3):490–526.

114. Avni T, Leibovici L, Paul M. PCR diagnosis of invasive candidiasis: systematic review and meta-analysis. J Clin Microbiol 2011;49(2):665–70.

115. Nguyen MH, Wissel MC, Shields RK, et al. Performance of *Candida* real-time polymerase chain reaction, beta-D-glucan assay, and blood cultures in the diagnosis of invasive candidiasis. Clin Infect Dis 2012;54(9):1240–8.

116. Pappas PG, Kauffman CA, Andes DR, et al. Clinical practice guideline for the management of candidiasis: 2016 update by the Infectious Diseases Society of America. Clin Infect Dis 2016; 62(4):e1–50.

117. Altun O, Almuhayawi M, Ullberg M, et al. Clinical evaluation of the FilmArray blood culture identification panel in identification of bacteria and yeasts from positive blood culture bottles. J Clin Microbiol 2013;51(12):4130–6.

118. Cruciani M, Mengoli C, Loeffler J, et al. Polymerase chain reaction blood tests for the diagnosis of invasive aspergillosis in immunocompromised people. Cochrane Database Syst Rev 2015;(10):CD009551.

119. Arvanitis M, Ziakas PD, Zacharioudakis IM, et al. PCR in diagnosis of invasive aspergillosis: a meta-analysis of diagnostic performance. J Clin Microbiol 2014;52(10):3731–42.

120. Aguado JM, Vazquez L, Fernandez-Ruiz M, et al. Serum galactomannan versus a combination of galactomannan and polymerase chain reaction-based aspergillus DNA detection for early therapy of invasive aspergillosis in high-risk hematological patients: a randomized controlled trial. Clin Infect Dis 2015;60(3):405–14.

121. Khodadadi H, Mirhendi H, Mohebali M, et al. *Pneumocystis jirovecii* colonization in non-HIV-infected patients based on nested-PCR detection in bronchoalveolar lavage samples. Iran J Public Health 2013;42(3):298–305.

122. Etoh K. Evaluation of a real-time PCR assay for the diagnosis of *Pneumocystis pneumonia*. Kurume Med J 2008;55(3–4):55–62.

123. Fauchier T, Hasseine L, Gari-Toussaint M, et al. Detection of *Pneumocystis jirovecii* by quantitative PCR to differentiate colonization and pneumonia in immunocompromised HIV-positive and HIV-negative patients. J Clin Microbiol 2016;54(6): 1487–95.

124. Tasaka S, Kobayashi S, Yagi K, et al. Serum (1–> 3) beta-D-glucan assay for discrimination between *Pneumocystis jirovecii* pneumonia and colonization. J Infect Chemother 2014;20(11):678–81.

125. Hata DJ, Buckwalter SP, Pritt BS, et al. Real-time PCR method for detection of zygomycetes. J Clin Microbiol 2008;46(7):2353–8.

126. Millon L, Larosa F, Lepiller Q, et al. Quantitative polymerase chain reaction detection of circulating DNA in serum for early diagnosis of mucormycosis in immunocompromised patients. Clin Infect Dis 2013;56(10):e95–101.

127. Binnicker MJ, Buckwalter SP, Eisberner JJ, et al. Detection of *Coccidioides* species in clinical

specimens by real-time PCR. J Clin Microbiol 2007; 45(1):173–8.

128. Sidamonidze K, Peck MK, Perez M, et al. Real-time PCR assay for identification of *Blastomyces dermatitidis* in culture and in tissue. J Clin Microbiol 2012; 50(5):1783–6.

129. Koepsell SA, Hinrichs SH, Iwen PC. Applying a real-time PCR assay for *Histoplasma capsulatum* to clinically relevant formalin-fixed paraffin-embedded human tissue. J Clin Microbiol 2012;50(10):3395–7.

130. Babady NE, Buckwalter SP, Hall L, et al. Detection of *Blastomyces dermatitidis* and *Histoplasma capsulatum* from culture isolates and clinical specimens by use of real-time PCR. J Clin Microbiol 2011;49(9):3204–8.

131. Gago S, Esteban C, Valero C, et al. A multiplex real-time PCR assay for identification of *Pneumocystis jirovecii*, *Histoplasma capsulatum*, and *Cryptococcus neoformans/Cryptococcus gattii* in samples from AIDS patients with opportunistic pneumonia. J Clin Microbiol 2014;52(4):1168–76.

132. Petti CA. Detection and identification of microorganisms by gene amplification and sequencing. Clin Infect Dis 2007;44(8):1108–14.

133. Vollmer T, Stormer M, Kleesiek K, et al. Evaluation of novel broad-range real-time PCR assay for rapid detection of human pathogenic fungi in various clinical specimens. J Clin Microbiol 2008;46(6): 1919–26.

134. Mylonakis E, Clancy CJ, Ostrosky-Zeichner L, et al. T2 magnetic resonance assay for the rapid diagnosis of candidemia in whole blood: a clinical trial. Clin Infect Dis 2015;60(6):892–9.

135. Dudiuk C, Gamarra S, Jimenez-Ortigosa C, et al. Quick detection of FKS1 mutations responsible for clinical echinocandin resistance in *Candida albicans*. J Clin Microbiol 2015;53(7):2037–41.

136. van der Linden JW, Arendrup MC, Warris A, et al. Prospective multicenter international surveillance of azole resistance in *Aspergillus fumigatus*. Emerg Infect Dis 2015;21(6):1041–4.

Emergence of the Molds Other than *Aspergillus* in Immunocompromised Patients

CrossMark

Sana Arif, MB,BS*, John R. Perfect, MD

KEYWORDS

- Mucormycosis • *Fusarium* • *Scedosporium* • Immunocompromised • Transplant
- Dematiaceous mold • *Lomentospora prolificans*

KEY POINTS

- Clinical and radiographic presentations of sinopulmonary mold infections tend to be similar; culture and histopathology are needed to make a diagnosis.
- Mucorales infections tend to most commonly involve the lungs and sinuses. Skin involvement is usually due to trauma and is rarely seen in disseminated infection.
- Blood cultures in *Aspergillus* and Mucorales infections are usually negative. *Fusarium* and *Scedosporium* frequently yield positive blood cultures in disseminated infections.
- Although susceptibility testing can be done on emerging fungal pathogens, such as Mucorales, dematiaceous molds and *Fusarium*, no standardized break points are available as of yet.
- The management of most mold infections tends to be complex and requires a combination of surgical debridement, antifungal therapy, and possibly adjunctive therapy.

As medical science advances, more patients are becoming eligible for solid organ transplants (SOTs) and stem cell transplants (SCTs), hence, increasing the population of severely immunocompromised patients. The lack of an adequate immune system has made these patients more prone to infections from organisms that were previously considered environmental contaminants and not true pathogens. A major fraction of these pathogens are fungi such as Mucorales, dematiaceous molds, and plant pathogens such as *Fusarium*. These emerging fungi are associated with high mortality, and our understanding in regard to their pathogenesis and treatment is limited.

MUCORALES

Over the years there have been significant changes to the nomenclature used for this group of fungi.

After the establishment of the fungal kingdom (1968), they were initially classified in the phylum Zygomycota. The phylum contained 10 different orders, including Mucorales and Entomophthorales. Infections due to organisms belonging to these two orders were referred to as zygomycosis.[1]

In the 1990s, when taxonomists started to apply molecular techniques, to obtain a better understanding of fungal lineages, it was noted that the Zygomycota were actually polyphyletic. In 2007 Hibbett and colleagues[2] suggested eliminating Zygomycota as a phylum and raising 4 of its orders, including Mucorales and Entomophthorales, to the rank of subphyla. This action led to the reuse of the term *mucormycosis*.[3] Although the term sounds like it would mean infections due to the *Mucor* species, it reflects infection due to all fungi in the Mucorales order. In recent years, the terms *zygomycosis* and *mucormycosis* have

Disclosure Statement: S. Arif has nothing to disclose. J.R. Perfect: research grants, consulting services, honorariums, and advisory committees for Astellas, Pfizer, Merck, F2G, Vical, Viamet, Cidara, Scynexis, and TEVA.
Division of Infectious Diseases, Duke University Medical Center, 315 Trent Drive, PO Box 102359, Durham, NC 27710, USA
* Corresponding author.
E-mail address: sana.arif@duke.edu

Clin Chest Med 38 (2017) 555–573
http://dx.doi.org/10.1016/j.ccm.2017.04.014

been used somewhat interchangeably from a clinical standpoint. However, in this discussion the authors use the most recent designation of mucormycosis.

Epidemiology

The epidemiology of mucormycosis is very complex and not well understood. As Mucorales are a common part of the general environment, there can be differences in exposure, based on geographic location and seasonality.[4] A significant volume of the literature has focused on the development of mucormycosis in diabetic patients, and data on immunocompromised hosts are relatively limited but starting to increase.

A review of 929 cases of mucormycosis revealed that diabetes was the most commonly associated risk factor, affecting 36% of the reported cases.[5] In countries such as India, diabetes continues to remain the most common risk factor.[6,7] However, in more developed countries, the infection is encountered more frequently in patients with hematologic malignancies. A retrospective study from France identified 101 cases of mucormycosis, between 2003 and 2007, from the French hospital information system. It showed that the most common underlying condition was hematologic malignancies (50%), followed by diabetes (23%). Fifty-eight percent of the patients were men, and the mean patient age was 50.7 years. The median time from diagnosis of malignancy to the development of infection was 8.8 months. Twelve patients had received a hematopoietic SCT (HSCT), and the median time between HSCT and development of mucormycosis was 6.8 months.[8]

The Transplant Associated Infections Surveillance Network (TRANSNET) is a network of 24 transplant centers across the United States that collected data on invasive fungal infections (IFIs) in transplant recipients (SOT and HSCT) between 2001 and 2006. Eight percent of the cases in HSCT recipients were due to mucormycosis, with a 12-month cumulative incidence of 0.29%. The median time of onset of infection after transplantation was 135 days.[9] Among SOT recipients, the 12-month cumulative incidence was much lower at 0.07%. The highest incidence was seen in lung transplant (0.18%) and liver transplant (0.16%) recipients. Approximately 38% of the infections occurred within the first 6 months following transplantation. It was observed that the median time to infection after transplant was significantly shorter in liver transplant recipients (81 days), when compared with nonliver SOT recipients (533 days).[10]

There is concern that many studies might underestimate the true incidence of these infections as most studies only include patients with proven or probable infection, hence, missing many patients who do not meet the European Organization for Research and Treatment of Cancer/Mycoses Study Group's criteria.[10,11] At this time it is difficult to obtain robust histopathological confirmation of disease from many studies. However, it is largely thought that the number of cases have increased recently, though most of this is based on data from single centers.[12–14] The reasons for an increase in mucormycosis cases are unclear. It is likely multifactorial, including changes in immune suppressive regimens, stem cell sources, antimicrobial prophylaxis practices, and the ability to prolong life with aggressive chemotherapy and other adjunctive therapies.

Pathogenesis

The primary mode of acquiring mucormycosis is by inhalation of spores. The spores are typically 3 to 11 μm in size.[4] Hence, they can reach the alveolar spaces of the lung. Larger spores may get trapped in the nasal or sinus passages, leading to sinusitis. After inhalation, the spores tend to germinate into hyphae. Mononuclear and polymorphonuclear phagocytic cells are key in prevention of fungal proliferation at this stage. Factors such as corticosteroid use and uncontrolled diabetes can cause defective chemotaxis, impair phagocytosis, and impair the cell's intracellular killing mechanisms.[15]

The presence of burns or trauma can result in direct inoculation of the organism into the wound. Outbreaks have been dramatically associated with natural disasters, such as the tornado in Joplin, Missouri in 2011 and the Indian Ocean tsunami of 2004. It is also associated with the classic road rash resulting from motor cycle injuries. Health care–associated outbreaks have been linked to contaminated equipment, such as surgical dressings and tongue depressors, and from direct inoculation into tissue.[16]

The virulence factors of the various Mucorales species are not well understood. The fungus tends to attach to the extracellular protein matrix surrounding blood vessels. It is characterized as a vasotropic fungus. Animal model data suggest that the GRP78 receptor on the surface of endothelial cells facilitates invasion and damage of the cells by the mold.[17] The hyphae, thus, tend to be angioinvasive and cause significant tissue necrosis and thrombosis of vessels. This further impairs the ability of host immune mechanisms and antifungal agents to reach the site of infection, allowing the spread of infection.

Specific risk factors in solid organ transplantation

A case controlled study of 100 patients by Singh and colleagues[18] evaluated risk factors for the development of mucormycosis in SOT recipients. It was noted that the risk of infection was higher in patients with underlying renal failure and diabetes. Prior use of voriconazole was also linked to an increased risk of infection; even in animal models, exposure to voriconazole seems to accelerate the virulence of Mucorales. Exposing animals to voriconazole before infection selects for breakthrough mucormycosis in a mixed model of *Aspergillus fumigatus* and *Rhizopus oryzae* pulmonary infection.[19] Interestingly, the use of tacrolimus was found to be protective and led to a 4-fold decrease in the risk of zygomycosis. This protection might be related to antifungal properties associated with calcineurin inhibitors.[18] Similarly, statin exposure might reduce virulence of Mucorales and reduce the incidence of mucormycosis in diabetes.[20]

Liver transplant recipients are at a higher risk to develop infections earlier in their posttransplant period and are more likely to experience disseminated infection.[18,21] This risk is hypothesized to be related to iron overload. Iron is an essential growth factor for the Mucorales; they tend to use siderophores and iron permeases to acquire iron from the host. The presence of acidosis can decrease the ability of transferrin to bind iron, leading to more free iron in the bloodstream, which can, in turn, be acquired by the mold.[16] Overabundance of iron can also cripple vital host defense mechanisms, such as phagocytic activity, interferon-γ–mediated macrophage, and monocyte function, and alter T helper cell response.[18,22,23] Iron chelating agents, such as deferoxamine, are also a risk factor for infection, for these agents act to chelate iron from the human body; they paradoxically can serve as an external source of iron (xenosiderophore) for use by the members of the Mucorales family, thereby promoting their growth.[24]

Specific risk factors in hematopoietic stem cell transplant

A study from the Fred Hutchinson Cancer Center examined 29 HSCT recipients who were found to have mucormycosis. It was found that the onset of infection was usually greater than 90 days following transplantation. Furthermore, patients with an underlying diagnosis of myelodysplastic syndrome, male sex, and presence of severe graft-versus-host disease (GVHD) were considered at significant risk for infection.[12]

The role of voriconazole prophylaxis in the development of mucormycosis in this population remains controversial. As noted, experimental models indicate that exposure to voriconazole increases the virulence of certain Mucorales species.[10] However, a randomized double-blinded trial that compared the use of voriconazole with fluconazole as prophylaxis in HSCT recipients did not demonstrate a higher incidence of mucormycosis in the voriconazole arm.[25] On the other hand, a case controlled study showed that voriconazole prophylaxis was an independent risk factor to the development of zygomycosis in hematologic malignancy patients including HSCT recipients.[26] The authors think it is prudent to consider voriconazole exposure when evaluating the risk of mucormycosis in the HSCT population.

Clinical Presentation

The clinical presentation of mucormycosis can vary in accordance to the organ involved. Although mucormycosis can affect practically any organ in the body, the most common sites of involvement tend to be (1) sinuses, (2) pulmonary, (3) skin, (4) gastrointestinal (GI), and (5) others.

Sinusitis

The most common risk factor associated with sinus disease remains poorly controlled diabetes.[27] Most patients initially develop nasal congestion and purulent nasal discharge. The infection can involve one or all of the sinuses and has a tendency to spread into surrounding structures, such as the palate and orbit, or even develop intracranial extension. Patients often develop eschars on the palate and in the nasal cavity. Orbital involvement can present as orbital or preseptal cellulitis. Patients can have diplopia, ptosis, and complete vision loss. This is more commonly encountered when there is ethmoid sinus involvement, because from this sinus the infection can breach the lamina papyracea and invade the medial rectus muscle or even lead to cavernous sinus thrombosis, affecting cranial nerves III, IV, VI, and V (1, 2). Facial nerve palsies are commonly encountered as well. Intracranial infection can also present with epidural or subdural abscesses. Solitary meningitis is rarely encountered.[27]

Pulmonary

The lung tends to be the most common site of involvement in SOT recipients. The TRANSNET data showed that 53% of the patients had pulmonary involvement.[10] The pulmonary manifestations of mucormycosis are difficult to distinguish from those of invasive *Aspergillus*. Most patients present with a pneumonialike picture that does not respond to antibiotic therapy. Patients can have pleuritic chest pain and occasionally a pleural rub on examination. The infection is angioinvasive and can lead to necrosis of lung parenchyma. It can erode into blood vessels and lead to massive hemoptysis. Patients with pulmonary mucormycosis (PM) are more likely to succumb to disseminated infection rather than fulminate respiratory failure.[27] The mold can sometimes form fungal balls in pre-existing lung cavities. These balls can cause symptoms of a hypersensitivity pneumonitis or lead to an invasive infection over time.

Cutaneous

Primary cutaneous involvement is typically seen in immunocompromised patients with a disruption in the skin barrier. The lesion starts as local erythema and progresses to necrosis. If not treated promptly, it can progress to involve muscle and bone. Secondary involvement of the skin due to disseminated infection is uncommon, especially when compared with other molds, such as the *Fusarium* species. Mucorales are rarely cultured from blood cultures, and a positive blood culture from this organism is more likely to be due to contamination.

Gastrointestinal

Malnutrition in addition to direct immunosuppression is considered a risk factor for GI involvement. Patients can have various presentations from peptic ulceration to an ileal mass or neutropenic colitis. The stomach tends to be the most common site involved in the GI tract. Unfortunately, the diagnosis is missed in more than 50% of the cases and requires histopathology confirmation.

Diagnosis

Diagnosis of mucormycosis is challenging as signs and symptoms of the infection can vary. The current backbone of diagnostics is histopathology and culture. In the immunocompromised hosts, radiology may play a significant role in diagnosis. Conventional radiographs are frequently negative during the early stages of infection. Computed tomography (CT) radiography can provide early clues for diagnosis. However, the findings are often difficult to distinguish from those due to other IFIs. CT findings in PM can vary from nodules to consolidation and even cavitation. The halo signs, usually described for *Aspergillus* infections, can be seen in PM as well. The reverse halo sign or atoll sign is an area of ground-glass opacities surrounded by a ring of consolidation, which is more commonly associated with PM than with other IFIs. In a retrospective study, looking at acute leukemic patients who were diagnosed with PM, it was noted that 15 of 16 (94%) of them had the reverse halo sign on their imaging during the first

week of infection.[28] It is, therefore, thought to be a good indicator of possible PM in patients with hematologic malignancies. It should, however, be kept in mind that the reverse halo sign can also be seen in multiple other neoplastic and autoimmune conditions and is not diagnostically accurate.[29]

Sinus CT scans can give information regarding presence of invasive sinusitis. Sinusitis, especially in the presence of pulmonary infiltrates, is highly concerning for zygomycosis in the appropriate host.[30] An endoscopic sinus examination by an ear, nose, and throat physician can aid in diagnosis and provide tissue for culture and histopathology.

Classically, histopathology shows nonseptate, irregularly branching, thin-walled, broad hyphae in the tissue. However, if patients have been receiving a mold active antifungal agent at the time of sampling, the appearance of the hyphae may be altered. Additionally, even for an experienced pathologist, it can be difficult to differentiate septate from nonseptate hyphae in a tissue specimen.[31] Mucorales tend not to stain deeply with fungal stains like periodic acid-Schiff stain or Gomori methenamine silver stain. A hematoxylin and eosin stain can be helpful at times.[4]

Most of the species tend to grow better at 37°C than at 25°C.[32] Sabouraud media is commonly used, and the colonies tend to appear greyish in color. Care should be taken when setting up the culture to not overprocess the tissue specimen, as that may damage the hyphae and lead to a negative culture. Even with careful preparation of tissue, cultures can frequently be negative when the fungus is observed in the tissue sections. Microscopic examination of the sporangia and hyphae is used to identify specific genus and species from viable cultures. However, matrix-assisted laser desorption ionization time-of-flight mass spectroscopy (MALDI-TOF) is also an upcoming technology in mycology that will play a larger role in identifications of molds.[33] Overall the yield of tissue cultures tends to be low. These pathogens are a common part of the environment; thus, positive cultures need to be interpreted with caution to rule out contamination or commensals in certain situations. It is important to clinically correlate patients' risk factors and syndrome with the culture result.

Interestingly, even though the organisms are angioinvasive, blood cultures are typically negative, unless the lumen of a vascular catheter is involved.[34] As Mucorales do not typically release beta-D-glucan into the bloodstream, the 1,3 beta-D-glucan assay is typically negative. Galactomannan testing is classically negative as well, though rarely positives have been documented.[35] Various molecular tests, such as polymerase chain reaction (PCR) assays, which can be performed on fresh tissue samples and even paraffin wax–embedded tissue, are under development; but none are yet commercially available.[34] A new and potentially important step in diagnosis is the use of PCR directly on the specimen, such as bronchoalveolar lavage and blood. Impressively, in one study circulating Mucorales DNA was detected in 81% of cases; this positive result was detected early in infections and was potentially useful as a quantitative measurement for judging treatment success.[36]

Treatment

Antifungal therapy

Amphotericin B (AMB) is the mainstay of antifungal therapy against mucormycosis. It binds to ergosterol and damages the fungal cell membrane ultimately leading to cell death. The combination of AMB and surgery is known to have a mortality benefit.[37] Delay in the initiation of AMB at the time of diagnosis of infection is associated with a 2-fold increase in mortality.[38] In more recent years, the lipid formulations (liposomal and lipid complex) are preferred over amphotericin deoxycholate because of their better safety profiles.[39] Response rates (complete and partial) to lipid formulations are reported to vary from 32% to 100%, whereas those from AMB-deoxycholate are reported to vary from 0% to 60%.[24] Studies directly comparing response rates of different formulations are sparse. The typical recommended dose for liposomal AMB is 3 to 5 mg/kg. The Ambizygo multicenter trial evaluated the use of a higher dose of liposomal AMB (10 mg/kg) for initial treatment of mucormycosis. This study demonstrated a 45% response rate by week 12; however, 40% of the patients developed nephrotoxicity during that time.[40]

Posaconazole was the first azole to have consistent activity against the Mucorales and be studied for treatment. It is recommended for salvage therapy. A retrospective review of 91 patients with mucormycosis who were unable to tolerate polyene therapy showed that 60% of them had a positive response to posaconazole. The response rate did not differ according to site of infection.[41] Initially, it was only available as an oral solution that needed a low gastric pH for absorption; there were issues with attaining sufficient serum concentrations. However, recently, the new sustained-release tablet and the intravenous formulation have become available, which have overcome those limitations. As the drug can be safely given orally, it is often used to treat infections after initial induction therapy with AMB. Posaconazole is also used for antifungal prophylaxis in neutropenic patients. In a randomized clinical trial, posaconazole was found to be superior to fluconazole and itraconazole in preventing invasive fungal infections.[42] Because there are wide variations in posaconazole susceptibility between various species, it may be reasonable to check in vitro activity of the strain against the azole.

Isavuconazole is a newer azole that became available in 2015. It does have Food and Drug Administration (FDA) approval for treatment of mucormycosis. The VITAL study was an open-label multicenter study that showed that isavuconazole had activity against mucormycosis that was comparable with AMB. Among the 37 patients who were studied (16 salvage and 21 as primary treatment), 14% had a complete response and 17% had a partial response at the end of therapy.[43] The advantage of isavuconazole is that it can be used in patients with reduced renal function and less commonly causes QT prolongation unlike the other extended spectrum azoles. However, it can cause QT shortening in some patients; its use is contraindicated in individuals with familial short QT syndrome. It is available as an intravenous and oral formulation. Although drug levels for isavuconazole can be obtained, there is currently no standard interpretation.

Echinocandins by themselves do not have any direct activity in vitro against the Mucorales. However, certain species like R oryzae express the target enzyme for echinocandins. Additionally, murine data in mice with diabetic ketoacidosis or neutropenia showed improved survival when the combination therapy for an echinocandin and liposomal AMB was used. The mechanism for this synergy is not well understood,[44] but it may be related to altering the cell wall to allow a more robust immune response. A small retrospective study of patients with rhinocerebral mucormycosis showed improved 30-day success rate in patients given liposomal AMB and caspofungin in comparison with those given the lipid formulation of AMB therapy alone (100% vs 45%).[45] However, it should be noted that this study was conducted primarily on diabetic patients and did not involve many patients with malignancy or transplantation. Another study compared outcomes in 101 patients with mucormycosis before and after the era of combination therapy and did not find a significant difference in 90-day mortality.[46] Evidence behind the use of combination therapy is far from robust but given the high mortality of mucormycosis, combination therapy is frequently used as part of salvage therapy.

Murine model studies suggest that the combination of posaconazole and liposomal-AMB does not provide any additional benefit over use of liposomal AMB by itself.[47] No human trials have been performed evaluating the combination of posaconazole or isavuconazole with polyenes.[48]

Surgery

Mucormycosis tends to be angioinvasive, leading to significant thrombosis and tissue necrosis. This adversely affects the penetration of antifungals and immune mechanisms into the infected tissue. Removal of devitalized tissue plays a vital role in treatment. Surgical intervention is usually guided with the help of frozen sections to enable the acquisition of clean surgical margins. The combination of surgery with antifungal therapy has been shown to improve survival. One multicenter study that looked at 31 SOT recipients with PM noted improved 90-day survival in patients who underwent surgical debridement (14.0% vs 52.9%, $P<.05$).[24] Similarly, another study evaluating patients with cancer showed a correlation with surgical debridement and favorable outcomes.[49] It should be noted that there may be selection bias in these studies, because patients who are less sick and have fewer comorbid conditions are more likely to be selected for surgical intervention.

Granulocyte infusion

Granulocyte colony-stimulating factor (G-CSF) and granulocyte macrophage colony-stimulating factor (GM-CSF) have been shown to increase the oxidative burst and phagocytosis capabilities of polymorphonuclear cells.[50] One murine study also indicated that mice given a combination of liposomal AMB and GM-CSF had better outcomes than those who were given liposomal AMB alone.[51] This finding raises the possibility of using these agents as adjuvant therapy for mucormycosis. On the other hand, clinical data on this strategy are very limited and it should be kept in mind that these factors are very expensive and can have side effects, such as lung injury. Therefore, they should be used with caution on a case-by-case basis.

Hyperbaric oxygen

Granulocytes tend to kill fungi using an oxygen-dependent mechanism, such as generation of free radicals in an oxidative burst. The limiting factor for these mechanisms is usually the availability of oxygen. Hyperbaric oxygen (HBO) provides an increased supply, hence, amplifying the killing activity of these cells. HBO tends to reverse acidosis and, therefore, augment AMB activity. The use of HBO also decreases fungal proliferation and

accelerates tissue healing due to the release of growth factors.[52] The data documenting the benefit of HBO in the management of mucormycosis is largely based on case reports and small case series, but it is used an as an adjunctive therapy to surgery and antifungal therapy in cases of cutaneous and rhinocerebral infection.

Iron chelating agents

As previously discussed, iron plays an important role in the metabolism and growth of Mucorales. Newer iron chelating agents, such as deferiprone and deferasirox, can exert antifungal activity by effectively starving the fungus of iron. Unlike deferoxamine, they do not act as siderophores for the fungus. Animal data suggest that deferasirox was as effective as liposomal AMB and that the combination of liposomal AMB and deferasirox led to improved survival.[53] However, the DEFEAT *Mucor* study, which randomized 20 patients with mucormycosis to liposomal AMB plus deferasirox or liposomal AMB plus placebo, showed a higher 90-day mortality in the deferasirox arm (82% vs 22%, $P = .01$).[54] This small study needs to be interpreted with caution, as the number of patients was small and more patients with an underlying malignancy ended up in the deferasirox arm. Thus, adjunctive use of iron chelators is generally not recommended except on a case-by-case basis. In summary, treatment is a 3-part strategy for mucormycosis: control of underlying disease, surgical debridement of devitalized tissue, and primarily AMB therapy.

FUSARIUM

Fusarium is a ubiquitous mold, commonly found in the water supply and soil. The genus consists of more than 200 different species. These species are divided into 10 different phylogenetic complexes. Initially the anamorphs and teleomorphs both had individual names. However, this nomenclature was abolished in 2013, after the International Code of Nomenclature for algae, fungi, and plants advised against using dual nomenclature.[55] Most of the species are plant pathogens, but close to 70 different species have been associated with human infection. The bulk of human infections are due to members of the *Fusarium solani* complex, followed by those of the *Fusarium oxysporum* complex.[56]

Epidemiology and Risk Factors

Fusarium typically causes systemic infections in severely immunocompromised hosts. The TRANSNET data, which delineated all IFIs in SOT and HSCT recipients, showed that *Fusarium* accounted for 21.9% of the non-*Aspergillus* mold infections, hence, making it the most common cause of fungal infections in this population, following *Aspergillus* and Mucorales. *Fusarium* infection was more frequently seen in HSCT recipients compared with SOT recipients (31 vs 6 cases). Although *F solani* was the most commonly isolated species, responsible for 10% of all the cases, it should be noted that 22% of the *Fusarium* isolates could not be identified at a species level.[10]

In a multicenter study, including centers from Brazil and United States, which identified 61 cases, the estimated incidence of fusariosis was 5.97 cases per 1000 SCTs. The incidence was noted to be higher in allogeneic SCT recipients as compared with autologous SCT recipients. Among the allogeneic SCT recipients, the incidence was higher (20.19 per 1000 transplants) in recipients of an HLA mismatched related donor compared with those who received an HLA matched donor (5 per 1000 transplants). At the time of diagnosis, 46% of the patients were neutropenic. Disseminated fusariosis was most commonly seen within the first 100 days after transplant. The median time between transplantation and diagnosis of infection was 64 days.[57] Most studies suggest at least a bimodal distribution of cases: (1) an early peak before engraftment and (2) a late peak after engraftment.[57,58] It was observed that patients who developed infection early in the posttransplant period were more likely to be neutropenic, have received antithymocyte globulin, and to be on insulin for hyperglycemia. In comparison, those who developed the infection at later time points were usually not neutropenic but were more likely to have GVHD and to have received a nonmyeloablative preconditioning regimen.[57,59]

A study that evaluated 8 patients with AML, without an SCT who developed fusariosis, reported that the median time from start of chemotherapy to diagnosis of infection was 23.5 days. All patients had been neutropenic at the time of diagnosis, and the median duration of neutropenia was 22.5 days. Evaluation for risk factors in this study revealed that only active smoking was found to be significant (hazard ratio = 9.11, P = .004). Other factors, such as use of corticosteroids, cytarabine, or duration of neutropenia, were not found to be significantly associated with fusariosis.[59] The exact mechanism by which smoking predisposes to fusariosis is unclear, but it may be related to how smoking affects the immune system. *Fusarium* can be found as a contaminant in tobacco as well. Unfortunately, details of the smoking history were not evaluated in the study. Finally, this mold can reside in hospital water systems; therefore, attention should be paid to the hospital water from sinks, faucets, and showers in hospital outbreaks of fusariosis.[60]

Pathogenesis

The pathogenesis of fusariosis in humans is not well understood. *F solani* is thought to be the most virulent of the species. In a study whereby different species were inoculated in a murine model, all the mice injected with *F solani* died, whereas 100% of the ones given *Fusarium oxysporum*, *Fusarium verticillioides*, and *Fusarium proliferatum* survived.[61] How the virulence factors differ between the various species remains unclear.

Virulence factors

Mycotoxins are metabolites produced by fungi that can be harmful to other living things, including humans. *Fusarium* species are known to produce various mycotoxins. Grains infected with fusarial mycotoxins can lead to disease in humans, such as alimentary toxic aleukia. Some species tend to produce toxins, such as the T-2 toxin. Animal studies indicate that this toxin decreases chemotaxis of neutrophils and phagocytosis and protein synthesis by macrophages. Other toxins, such as deoxynivalenol, also impair the immune system by decreasing the number of lymphocytes and immunoglobulins. These toxins are also thought to cause dermal toxicity and, hence, can play a role in skin and soft tissue infections. Interestingly though, production of these toxins has not been confirmed in *Fusarium* species that cause invasive infections in humans.[62] Finally, the role of enzyme production in pathogenesis has not been documented. However, *Fusarium* species are able to attach themselves to foreign bodies, such as catheters and contact lenses.[62]

Host factors

As disseminated infections are more commonly encountered in immunocompromised hosts, the host immune system is thought to play a key role in prevention of infection. T-cell responses are thought to be important, because patients with HSCT, even after having recovered from neutropenia, are found to be at high risk for infection by *Fusarium* species.[57] Granulocytes also participate in host defense and are thought to decrease hyphal growth, whereas macrophages inhibit germination of conidia.[62]

Clinical Manifestations

Although in the immunocompetent hosts the most common manifestations of fusariosis tend to be keratitis and onychomycosis, the spectrum differs in the immunocompromised host.

Sinus infection

Inhalation of the spores and their subsequent germination in the sinuses can lead to the development of invasive sinusitis in the immunocompromised host. The features of fusarial sinusitis cannot be clinically distinguished from those of other fungal infections, such as *Aspergillus*.[63] It tends to present with nasal discharge, sinus pain, and obstruction. Patients can develop necrosis and eschar formation. Sinusitis can lead to lung involvement or even disseminated infection.

Skin infections

Localized single skin lesions are uncommon in the immunocompromised host; these are usually at the site of recent skin breakdown or preexisting fusarial onychomycosis. However, in a study that looked at 167 immunocompromised patients with invasive fusariosis, it was noted that greater than 50% of the patients presented with multiple skin lesions. Disseminated skin lesions were more common in neutropenic patients when compared with non-neutropenic immunocompromised hosts (94% vs 41%; *P*<.0001). In patients with disseminated disease, the most common skin finding was erythematous nodular lesions, which may or may not be associated with necrosis (87 vs 58 patients). The necrotic lesion seemed to be similar to ecthyma gangrenosum in 71 of the patients. Only 16 patients had a targetlike lesion (nodular lesion surrounded by ring of erythema). It was noted that the lesions seemed to be more commonly observed on the extremities but could occur anywhere on the body. Lesions can be appreciated in different stages of development on the same host. No particular pattern of skin lesions could be associated with any specific species of *Fusarium*.[64]

Pneumonia

Lung involvement is typically only seen in immunocompromised patients. It can be the primary source of infection or become secondarily involved due to hematogenous infection. A pneumonic process can be seen in approximately 54% of patients with fusariosis.[58] The signs and symptoms can be very nonspecific, and it can be difficult to differentiate from other causes of respiratory infection.

Fungemia and disseminated infection

Unlike other mold infections, *Fusarium* frequently yields a positive blood culture, which is thought to be due to its tendency to sporulate in vivo.[58,65] Although isolated fungemia is possible, it is usually associated with disseminated infection. In one study, 79% of the patients presented with disseminated infection, making it the most common presentation of *Fusarium* in patients with hematologic malignancies.[54] Patients usually present with fever, not responsive to standard antibiotic therapy, along with diffuse skin lesions and blood cultures positive for a mold. Other organ systems, such as sinuses, lungs, or eyes, can be secondarily involved as well. Patients are prone to hematogenous seeding of the eye leading to the development of endophtalmitis.[66]

Diagnosis

Isolation of *Fusarium* from a culture is the most effective way to reach a diagnosis. However, the clinical picture should be correlated with the positive culture, because there is widespread presence of the organism in the general environment and the culture could just represent contamination. Cultures can be taken from skin scrapings, corneal scrapings, bronchial lavage samples, and tissue cultures depending on the site of infection. Biopsy and culture of a skin lesion can be an important source of diagnostic information. According to one study, it can be the single source of diagnosis in 55% of the cases. Skin lesions can also precede fungemia by a median of 5 days in some patients.[64]

Unlike most other mold infections, disseminated fusariosis is more frequently associated with positive blood cultures. Studies have shown that approximately 50% of the patients tend to have positive blood cultures.[58,65] Although *Fusarium* can grow on standard blood culture medium, in cases whereby the inoculum is low, the organism tends to be detected earlier using specific fungal culture media.[67]

It should be kept in mind that patients can be infected with more than one species of *Fusarium* simultaneously.[68] *Fusarium* tends to grow readily on media that does not contain cycloheximide. Potato dextrose agar is one of the commonly used media for isolation. It should be incubated at 25°C. The colors of the colonies can vary markedly from lavender to gray.[69] The organism can have macroconidia (hyaline, multicellular, banana-like clusters with foot cells at the base of the macroconidium) and microconidia (hyaline, unicellular, ovoid to cylindrical in slimy beads or chains). The distinctive features of the conidia are used to identify the organism at a species level; however, this can be fairly tricky even for the experienced eye.[70] MALDI-TOF and PCR assays are being used more frequently to enable precise species identification.[71,72] These tests are not routine at this time, and such assays have not been standardized within most clinical laboratories.

In patients with skin or sinus involvement, a biopsy for pathology along with culture can be helpful. It can be difficult to identify the mold in tissue as the hyphae appear similar to those of *Scedosporium* and *Aspergillus*. They all have narrow, hyaline septate hyphae; although *Aspergillus* tends to show fixed 45° angle branching, the branching angle in *Fusarium* can vary between 45° and 90°.[73] The organism can also show adventitious sporulation, the presence of hyphae and yeastlike structures together, which is highly suggestive of fusariosis in the high-risk population. In situ hybridization in paraffin-embedded tissue specimens can be considered in cases whereby suspicion is high and cultures are negative.[69]

The radiographic findings of pulmonary fusariosis are largely similar to those of *Aspergillus*, and it is impossible to differentiate between the two based solely on imaging. A study that looked at radiographic findings in patients with pulmonary fusariosis showed that 25% of them had normal chest radiographs. Among 11 patients with known fusariosis who underwent CT scans, 82% of them were found to have either solitary or multiple nodules. No lobar predominance was observed, whereas 55% of the patients had a lung mass on imaging. Masses usually involved the segmental-subsegmental airways. Occasionally, ground-glass opacities or pleural effusions were seen; but no patients were found to have a halo sign or tree in bud opacities on imaging.[74]

Serum fungal markers, such as beta-D-glucan, can be positive in *Fusarium* infections; but this is very nonspecific. *Fusarium* can cross-react with the galactomannan assay.[75] In a study looking at 18 hematologic patients who had been screened regularly with galactomannan assay, it was found that 83% of them had at least one positive assay. The sensitivity and specificity was 83% and 67%, respectively. Galactomannan was positive before the diagnosis of invasive fusariosis in 11 of the 15 cases (73%).[76] Hence, *Fusarium* should be included in the differential in patients with a positive galactomannan assay.

Treatment

In cases of localized infection, such as sinus involvement or skin lesions, surgical debridement plays an essential role. However, in the case of systemic infection, antifungal agents are the mainstay of therapy. Unfortunately, no formal clinical trials have been performed regarding the treatment of fusariosis. Therefore, most of the recommendations have been gleamed from retrospective studies.[77] Animal studies have been attempted to evaluate various treatment regimens, but the results have largely been inconclusive.[78] The situation is further complicated by the lack of official break points, making it difficult to interpret minimum inhibitory concentration (MIC) data or appreciate its clinical relevance.

Many *Fusarium* species tend to have high MICs to nearly all available antifungal agents.[79–81] Susceptibility patterns for multiple species are also not available because of a lack of identification of the organism correctly at a species level.[56,80] However, the susceptibility patterns of various species in the genus are thought to differ appreciably,[82] with *F solani* being the most resistant.[83] Fluconazole, flucytosine, and the echinocandins do not have any activity against *Fusarium* species.[84,85]

Amphotericin B

Fusarium species tend to have a higher MIC to AMB compared with *Aspergillus*.[86] The efficacy of AMB has varied between various studies but was generally found to be low. Data from the Collaborative Exchange of Antifungal Research database, which evaluated treatment response to liposomal AMB in 26 patients with *Fusarium* infection, showed a 46% response rate, with an additional 3 (12%) patients remaining stable.[87] In another study, 42 patients with hematologic malignancies were treated with intravenous AMB; 32% of them responded to therapy, but only 21% of them were alive 90 days from diagnosis.[58]

Azoles

Older azoles, such as fluconazole and itraconazole, do not have good in vitro activity against *Fusarium* species. Although in vitro studies suggest that voriconazole does not have consistent in vitro activity against *Fusarium* species,[79,83] clinical outcomes are comparatively better. One study showed a 45% response rate among 11 patients with *Fusarium* infection.[88] Another investigation that studied 57 patients with invasive fusariosis, who had failed initial antifungal therapy, showed a 47% complete or partial response when placed on voriconazole as salvage therapy. It was seen that the presence of neutropenia at time of diagnosis adversely affected response rates (5% vs 33%). Patients with infection involving the lung/sinuses seemed to have a better response than those with central nervous system involvement, and the overall 90-day survival was only 42%.[89]

Clinical experience with using posaconazole is limited. A case series of 21 patients with fusariosis who were placed on posaconazole as salvage therapy showed a response rate of 48%. Efficacy was much lower in patients who were neutropenic or had recently undergone an HSCT.[90] The new extended-release tablet and intravenous formulation recently became available, increasing the likelihood of posaconazole being used as salvage therapy more frequently in the future.

Isavuconazole is a recently approved antifungal, which has some in vitro activity against *Fusarium* species; but clinical experience with it is limited.[91]

Combination therapy

The role of combination therapy remains controversial at this stage. There are case report data suggesting that combinations, such as AMB and voriconazole or an azole and terbinafine, may lead to better clinical responses.[92,93] On the other hand, there also remains the valid concern of antagonism between agents. Moreover, there might be differences in response between the various *Fusarium* species.[94] An in vitro study that evaluated interactions among various antifungal agents when used in combination to treat *Fusarium* species found that the combination of AMB and an azole was not synergistic, though additive in some cases. However, no cases of antagonism between the two drugs were documented. The combination of terbinafine and voriconazole was synergistic in 70% of the cases.[95] A study that looked at 73 cases of fusariosis, 18 of whom were treated with voriconazole in combination with another antifungal agent, did not demonstrate any additional survival benefit over patients who were treated with voriconazole alone.[89]

SCEDOSPORIUM

The genus *Scedosporium* primarily consists of 2 medically important species: *Scedosporium apiospermum* complex and *Scedosporium prolificans*. The teleomorph (sexual state) of *S apiospermum* is known as *Pseudallescheria apiosperma*. *Pseudallescheria boydii* was initially considered to be the teleomorph, but this was subsequently found to be a separate species.[96] *S prolificans* does not have a teleomorph and was subsequently found to be phylogenetically distinct in 2014 and renamed as *Lomentospora prolificans*.[97] In this article, the authors, however, discuss it in the *Scedosporium* section.

Epidemiology and Risk Factors

Scedosporium are ubiquitous in the environment. *S apiospermum* tends to be found more readily in areas with high organic pollution. They are able to survive in anaerobic conditions and in a high saline environment; hence, these fungi can be isolated from sewage, poultry manure, and swamps. Although their distribution is global, they are more commonly found in temperate climates. Geographically, *L prolificans* is typically seen in Australia, Spain, and in the southern United States. They tend to be associated more often with soil and animals. However, infections from both organisms can occur worldwide.[98] Nosocomial outbreaks have also been seen in hospitals where there was contamination of the ambient air.[99]

Infections are most frequently encountered in immunocompromised hosts. In a study that accumulated 162 cases of *L prolificans* from literature, it was observed that the median age of patients was 45 years, with 63.0% being men, 45.7% having an underlying malignancy, and 8.6% were SOT recipients. Seventy-two cases had disseminated infection, 81.9% of whom had a documented malignancy, usually hematological. The overall mortality was 46.9% and the mortality was 87.5% in patients with disseminated infection.[100] Similarly, another multicenter investigation that studied 80 transplant recipients (SOT and HSCT) demonstrated that 83% of the infections in the SOT population were due to *S apiospermum*. The median time for development of infection was 4.2 months after the transplant. However, in the HSCT recipients, *L prolificans* was more common and the median time to development of infection was 1.3 months. Most patients were receiving corticosteroids at the time of infection.[101]

Pathogenesis

Virulence factors

The fungus is most commonly acquired through the respiratory tract. If the conidia are not removed by the immune system, they are able to germinate. The hyphae grow and can lead to invasion of blood vessels and potentially disseminate hematogenously. We currently lack in-depth knowledge regarding the molecular mechanisms by which the fungus is able to invade host cells and propagate. The *Scedosporium* species tend to produce peptidases that may help them degrade human tissue.[102] Melanin is also thought to a play a role in fungal protection against host cell oxidative burst by acting as a scavenger of oxygen radicals. However, this phenomenon has not been specifically studied in *Scedosporium* species.[103] The organisms are also iron dependent and have siderophore activity.[98]

Host immune response

Alpha-glucan, a component of the cell wall of *P boydii*, is thought to play an important role in activating innate immunity. It is thought to play a key role in allowing engulfment of the organism by phagocytes. Alpha-glucan also acts as a stimulator for cytokine release.[104] Details of the cytokine responses during infection are not fully elucidated. However, one study did demonstrate that the release of interleukin 15 enhances polymorphonuclear cells-induced hyphae damage and oxidative burst in response to *S prolificans* but less so in response to *S apiospermum*.[105] Monocyte-derived macrophages are able to ingest and damage the *Scedosporium* hyphae. They also inhibit the germination of conidia.[103]

Clinical Manifestations

In the immunocompetent host, infection is usually acquired because of local trauma or after a near-drowning experience in polluted water.[106] In the immunocompromised hosts, more cases are due to inhalation of the fungus and subsequent hematogenous dissemination. However, trauma still remains a cause of infection in this population as well.

Pulmonary infection

The isolation of *Scedosporium* from a respiratory specimen does not always indicate invasive infection. It can also represent airway colonization. *Scedosporium* is very commonly isolated from the airways of patients with cystic fibrosis.[107] In immunocompetent hosts, this fungus is also associated with allergic bronchopulmonary symptoms and fungus ball formation in preexisting cavities. In transplant recipients, pulmonary infection tends to be the second most common site of invasive infection.[101] Patients usually present with fever, dyspnea, cough, pleuritic chest pain, and hemoptysis.

Disseminated infection

Disseminated infection is more commonly encountered in HSCT or SOT recipients compared with other immunosuppressed patients or normal hosts. In one study, it accounted for 46% of the *Scedosporium* cases in SOT and 69% of those in patients with an HSCT. SOT recipients with *L prolificans* were more likely to have fungemia, compared with those with *S apiospermum* (40.0% vs 4.7%).[101] Patients typically present with fever and varied symptoms. Skin lesions are frequently found in patients with disseminated infection. Sepsislike syndrome was only encountered in patients with an underlying hematologic malignancy.

Other infections

Scedosporium species also have a tropism for the central nervous system (CNS). The likelihood of CNS involvement was similar among transplant and nontransplant patients.[101] CNS involvement can present with headache, meningeal irritation, or altered mental status. CNS infection can also be part of a disseminated infection. Bone and joint infections can also occur and are usually associated with localized penetrating trauma. Ocular infections and sinus infections are well documented as well.

Diagnosis

The mainstay of diagnosis is isolation of the organism from culture and suggestive features on histopathology. The site of culture and biopsy would depend on the patients' symptoms. Histopathologically, *Scedosporium* can be difficult to distinguish from other fungi, such as *Aspergillus* and *Fusarium*, as it tends to produce hyaline septate hyphae. The branches occur at acute angles. Adventitious morphologic forms of *Scedosporium* can be seen in tissue, which help differentiate *Scedosporium* from *Aspergillus*. However, other fungi, such as *Fusarium* and *Acremonium*, can have similar features.[108]

The organisms grow readily on regular fungal media, such as Sabouraud agar. Special media with inhibitors can be considered when culturing respiratory specimens to hinder the growth of other fungi.[109] In cases of CNS involvement, cerebrospinal fluid (CSF) analysis tends to show pleocytosis, elevated protein, and at times decreased glucose. Growth from CSF specimens tends to be slow, and cultures can be negative in cases of walled off abscesses.[110] Blood cultures should be performed when disseminated infection is suspected as yield from blood cultures is higher with *Scedosporium* than with molds, such as *Aspergillus* and Mucorales. In one study, 70% of the blood cultures were found to be positive.[100]

Radiological findings in pulmonary *Scedosporium* infection can vary from diffuse lung infiltrates to a solitary lung nodule or presence of pleural effusion. The findings are nonspecific and can be similar to those seen in other invasive fungal infections.

Molecular tests, such as species-specific PCR assays, are still experimental and not routinely available.[111] Beta-D-glucan assay tends to be positive in *Scedosporium* infections, but this test result is nonspecific.[112]

Treatment

Although *Scedosporium* is an emerging fungus, it is still relatively rare; no clinical trials are available to guide the ideal duration of therapy. No standardized break points have been implemented either to guide therapy. The antifungal susceptibility pattern of the different species tends to vary.

A study looking at in vitro susceptibilities of clinical and environmental isolates revealed that *S apiospermum* tends to have lower MICs to voriconazole compared with other antifungal agents.

Fluconazole and flucytosine do not have activity against the *Scedosporium apiopermum* complex. The activity of terbinafine and echinocandins varies across isolates. It was also noted that most of the species did not have a normal MIC (minimum inhibitory concentration)/MEC (minimum effective concentration) distribution, thus, making predicting a susceptibility pattern difficult and increasing the importance of susceptibility testing on individual patient isolates. *L prolificans* isolates were resistant to AMB, itraconazole, posaconazole, and isavuconazole. Voriconazole was considered the most active, although its MIC was much higher than the MIC seen with other species, such as *S apiospermum*. Micafungin was found to have moderate in vitro activity against *L prolificans*.

Voriconazole is typically the preferred agent to treat *Scedosporium* infections.[113] One study evaluated the treatment response to voriconazole in 107 patients with *Scedosporium* infection. The success rate was highest in patients with skin and soft tissue infections and lower in those with CNS disease. The response was lower in patients with an underlying hematologic malignancy (45%) compared with SOT recipients (63%). Forty-five out of 70 patients with *S apiospermum* infection had a good response to therapy, but the response was lower at 44% in patients with *L prolificans* infection. Species and underlying disease were both significant prognostic factors for survival. Overall the mortality was 40%.[114]

Combination therapy is frequently attempted for *Scedosporium* infections, especially for *L prolificans*. It should be noted that there are no official guidelines by the Clinical and Laboratory Standards Institute for performing synergy studies. One in vitro study demonstrated that the combination of voriconazole with terbinafine showed synergy in nearly all isolates of *L prolificans* studied and decreased the MIC by 16 dilutions.[115] Other in vitro studies have shown synergy between AMB, voriconazole and micafungin, although with a low frequency. There are limited case report data showing correlation between in vitro and in vivo synergy.[116,117]

Surgical debridement can improve outcomes in patients, and it should be considered in all cases when possible.[100] Patients with hematologic malignancies and HSCT were noted to have worse outcomes. On the other hand, reversal of neutropenia was found to be an independent factor in reducing mortality.[100] This finding brings up the consideration of using immunotherapies, such as G-CSF, as adjuvants. Altough this is occasionally used, its efficacy remains unknown. Animal studies did not show any benefit or improved outcomes in combining the use of G-CSF with antifungal agents.[118]

DEMATIACEOUS MOLD

This group is heterogeneous and includes more than 70 different fungal genera. The unifying feature tends to be that most of these fungi produce melanin; hence, their cell walls appear pigmented. These mold infections are sometimes referred to as phaeohyphomycosis. The word literally means "condition of fungi with dark hyphae."[119] It should be noted that mycetoma and chromoblastomycosis are also sometimes included in this group of organisms but are not discussed in this review.

Most of the organisms in this group tend to be ubiquitous, saprophytic plant pathogens that can cause infections in humans. *Bipolaris spp*, *Cladophialophora bantania*, *Ochroconis gallopava*, *Alternaria spp*, *Wangiella dermatitidis*, *Phialophora spp*, and *Curvularia spp* are some of the organisms within this group.

Epidemiology

Recently, it has been proposed that the number of cases due to phaeohyphomycosis has been increasing. This increase could partially be due to an overall increase in the number of immunocompromised patients.[120,121] A review of the TRANSNET data revealed that 2.6% of the IFIs were due to phaeohyphomycosis. There was no significant difference in the number of cases in SOT versus HSCT recipients. The mean age of patients was 50.4 years, and 58% of them were male. The median time to onset of infection posttransplant was longer in SOT compared with HSCT recipients (685 days vs 100 days, $P<.001$). Among the HSCT recipients, 92.3% of the cases occurred in those who had received an allogeneic HSCT. In SOT recipients, 53% of all the phaeohyphomycosis cases occurred in lung transplants. Species from 14 different genera were isolated in the cases; but interestingly, 32% of the cases were due to *Alternaria* species.[122] Because of the rarity of cases, risk factors for these infections have not been well studied.

Pathogenesis

Humans usually acquire the fungi either by inhalation or percutaneous injury. Trauma can lead to direct inoculation of the pathogen at the site of skin disruption. After inhalation, the fungus can cause allergic or invasive disease involving the sinuses or the lung. We do not have a good understanding of host immune responses to these fungi. Based on the increasing frequency of these infections in immunocompromised hosts, it is thought that both cellular and cell-mediated immunity likely play an important role in host defense.

Our knowledge regarding the virulence factors of these organisms or how they invade the host tissue is limited. Melanin is thought to be a virulence factor in these fungi. Molecular studies in which the gene for melanin production was knocked out revealed that mutants without melanin were more likely to be killed by neutrophils.[123] Some data also suggest that the presence of melanin protects the fungus against host cell oxidative burst.[124]

Clinical Manifestations

The dematiaceous molds can cause a wide variety of clinical syndromes. They can cause superficial infections, such as onychomycosis, skin and soft tissue nodules, and keratitis, to deep infections, such as cerebral abscesses and disseminated infections. Review of TRANSNET data revealed that cutaneous infections were the most common site (53%) of involvement in SOT recipients, whereas in the HSCT recipients the lungs were most frequently affected (57%). Blood and CNS involvement was uncommon.[122]

Respiratory

In the respiratory tree, dematiaceous molds can cause allergic symptoms, such as allergic fungal rhino sinusitis (AFRS) and allergic bronchopulmonary mycosis (ABPM). Although it was initially thought that *Aspergillus* was the main fungus responsible for such syndromes, more recently members of the dematiaceous mold family are now thought to be responsible for a significant number of the cases. *Bipolaris, Curvularia, Exserohilum,* and *Drechslera* species are the most common pathogens associated with AFRS and ABPM.[125] The fungi cause an allergic response and are not invasive in these cases. However, it should be noted that these syndromes are predominantly seen in immunocompetent patients and ABPM is especially linked to those with asthma.

Immunocompromised individuals are more likely to present with invasive pneumonia. The signs and symptoms of pulmonary disease can be vague, such as dyspnea and cough. Hemoptysis can also be seen. Invasive sinusitis is also a relatively common manifestation. In a series of 39 cases, 36% went on to have sinus involvement. Of the 14 cases with sino-nasal disease, sinus pain, epistaxis, and nasal septum perforation were the most common presentations. Maxillary sinus was the most common site of involvement, followed by the ethmoid sinus. Interestingly, CT scan showed findings of sinusitis in 71% of the cases; but sinus wall invasion was appreciated in 20% of these patients, indicating that a high suspicion of invasion should be maintained despite a lack of changes on imaging.[121]

Disseminated infection

Disseminated infection is typically found in immunocompromised hosts. However, cases have also been identified in patients with no apparent risk factors.[126,127] In the TRANSNET data, 55% of the patients with phaeohyphomycosis developed disseminated infection and *Alternaria* was the genus most commonly present.[122] Another investigation that studied 39 patients, predominantly with hematologic malignancies, showed that 33% went on to develop disseminated infection; no predominant genus was observed.[121] Fungemia is usually seen in cases of disseminated *Scedosporium*, but it is relatively uncommon with other genera. In one series with 7 hematologic malignancy patients, who developed fungemia, it was observed that all of them had a central line, which was thought to be the source of infection.[121]

Diagnosis

Histopathology and culture are the cornerstone of diagnosis for this group of fungi. They can present with varied forms in tissue, from budding yeast and pseudohyphae to moniliform or true hyphae. Although most of the fungi will appear brown on staining, *Bipolaris, Alternaria* and *Curvularia* can appear to have hyaline hyphae in tissue. A Fontana-Masson stain can be used to detect the presence of melanin.

Most of these organisms can grow on a standard fungal culture media. However, positive cultures must be interpreted with caution as they can be colonizers in both respiratory and skin culture specimens. Microscopic features specific to each genus can be used to differentiate the fungi. The details of these features are beyond the scope of this review. The yield of blood cultures is only high in cases of disseminated infection due to *Scedosporium* species.

Radiographic features are similar to those of other fungal infections and can only be used as an adjuvant in diagnosis. No current serologic markers are available. PCR-based tests are currently under development and are being used in research studies, but they are not yet commercially available.[128]

Treatment

In addition to medical management, surgical debridement should be considered wherever possible to debulk the infection and increase the likelihood of a positive outcome. As there are no randomized clinical trials available, the optimal duration and choice of antifungal agents are not known; these have to be decided on a case-by-case basis.

Although in vitro susceptibility testing is being performed with increasing frequency, there are still no established clinical break points available. Among the azoles, itraconazole, voriconazole and posaconazole have good activity against most of the dematiaceous fungi; the MIC values typically tend to be less than 0.125 µg/mL. Fluconazole does not have reliable activity against this group of organisms.[129] In vitro data suggest that isavuconazole is an additional agent that can be used against these fungi.[130,131] Like the azoles, AMB has good activity against most genera except *Scedosporium*; however, it is typically not the first line of therapy. In one study, univariate analysis showed use of AMB for therapy as a risk factor for increased mortality.[121] Flucytosine has reasonably good activity against many members of the dematiaceous mold group, but not all. It is only used in combination therapy because solitary use can lead to rapid development of resistance.[132] The activity of echinocandins is variable among the multiple genera in this group of fungi; hence, they are not frequently used.[133] Data on the utility of combination therapy are very limited.

SUMMARY

IFIs with molds in immunocompromised patients can frequently complicate the complex management of these fragile patients. It is essential that accurate identification of the IFI occurs, and then a careful and committed management plan must be made using a variety of information and experience to allow successful management of both the infection and the underlying disease.

REFERENCES

1. Kwon-Chung KJ. Taxonomy of fungi causing mucormycosis and entomophthoramycosis (zygomycosis) and nomenclature of the disease: molecular mycologic perspectives. Clin Infect Dis 2012;54(Suppl 1):S8–15.
2. Hibbett DS, Binder M, Bischoff JF, et al. A higher-level phylogenetic classification of the Fungi. Mycol Res 2007;111(Pt 5):509–47.
3. Spellberg B, Walsh TJ, Kontoyiannis DP, et al. Recent advances in the management of mucormycosis: from bench to bedside. Clin Infect Dis 2009; 48(12):1743–51.
4. Farmakiotis D, Kontoyiannis DP. Mucormycosis. Infect Dis Clin North Am 2016;30(1):143–63.
5. Roden MM, Zaoutis TE, Buchanan WL, et al. Epidemiology and outcome of zygomycosis: a review of 929 reported cases. Clin Infect Dis 2005;41(5): 634–53.
6. Bala K, Chander J, Handa U, et al. A prospective study of mucormycosis in north India: experience from a tertiary care hospital. Med Mycol 2015; 53(3):248–57.
7. Chakrabarti A, Singh R. Mucormycosis in India: unique features. Mycoses 2014;57(Suppl 3):85–90.
8. Lanternier F, Dannaoui E, Morizot G, et al. A global analysis of mucormycosis in France: the RetroZygo Study (2005-2007). Clin Infect Dis 2012;54(Suppl 1):S35–43.
9. Kontoyiannis DP, Marr KA, Park BJ, et al. Prospective surveillance for invasive fungal infections in hematopoietic stem cell transplant recipients, 2001-2006: overview of the Transplant-Associated Infection Surveillance Network (TRANSNET) database. Clin Infect Dis 2010;50(8):1091–100.
10. Park BJ, Pappas PG, Wannemuehler KA, et al. Invasive non-Aspergillus mold infections in transplant recipients, United States, 2001-2006. Emerg Infect Dis 2011;17(10):1855–64.
11. Fox ML, Barba P, Heras I, et al. A registry-based study of non-Aspergillus mould infections in recipients of allogeneic haematopoietic cell transplantation. Clin Microbiol Infect 2015;21(1):e1–3.
12. Marr KA, Carter RA, Crippa F, et al. Epidemiology and outcome of mould infections in hematopoietic stem cell transplant recipients. Clin Infect Dis 2002;34(7):909–17.
13. Chamilos G, Luna M, Lewis RE, et al. Invasive fungal infections in patients with hematologic malignancies in a tertiary care cancer center: an autopsy study over a 15-year period (1989-2003). Haematologica 2006;91(7):986–9.
14. Lewis RE, Cahyame-Zuniga L, Leventakos K, et al. Epidemiology and sites of involvement of invasive fungal infections in patients with haematological malignancies: a 20-year autopsy study. Mycoses 2013;56(6):638–45.
15. Ibrahim AS, Spellberg B, Walsh TJ, et al. Pathogenesis of mucormycosis. Clin Infect Dis 2012; 54(Suppl 1):S16–22.
16. Benedict K, Park BJ. Invasive fungal infections after natural disasters. Emerg Infect Dis 2014;20(3): 349–55.
17. Liu M, Spellberg B, Phan QT, et al. The endothelial cell receptor GRP78 is required for mucormycosis pathogenesis in diabetic mice. J Clin Invest 2010; 120(6):1914–24.
18. Singh N, Aguado JM, Bonatti H, et al. Zygomycosis in solid organ transplant recipients: a prospective, matched case-control study to assess risks for disease and outcome. J Infect Dis 2009;200(6): 1002–11.

19. Lewis RE, Liao G, Wang W, et al. Voriconazole pre-exposure selects for breakthrough mucormycosis in a mixed model of Aspergillus fumigatus-Rhizopus oryzae pulmonary infection. Virulence 2011;2(4):348–55.

20. Bellanger AP, Tatara AM, Shirazi F, et al. Statin concentrations below the minimum inhibitory concentration attenuate the virulence of Rhizopus oryzae. J Infect Dis 2016;214(1):114–21.

21. Singh N, Sun HY. Iron overload and unique susceptibility of liver transplant recipients to disseminated disease due to opportunistic pathogens. Liver Transpl 2008;14(9):1249–55.

22. Cunningham-Rundles S, Giardina PJ, Grady RW, et al. Effect of transfusional iron overload on immune response. J Infect Dis 2000;182(Suppl 1): S115–21.

23. Omara FO, Blakley BR. The effects of iron deficiency and iron overload on cell-mediated immunity in the mouse. Br J Nutr 1994;72(06):899–909.

24. Sun HY, Singh N. Mucormycosis: its contemporary face and management strategies. Lancet Infect Dis 2011;11(4):301–11.

25. Wingard JR, Carter SL, Walsh TJ, et al. Randomized, double-blind trial of fluconazole versus voriconazole for prevention of invasive fungal infection after allogeneic hematopoietic cell transplantation. Blood 2010;116(24):5111–8.

26. Kontoyiannis DP, Lionakis MS, Lewis RE, et al. Zygomycosis in a tertiary-care cancer center in the era of Aspergillus-active antifungal therapy: a case-control observational study of 27 recent cases. J Infect Dis 2005;191(8):1350–60.

27. Kontoyiannis DP, Lewis RE. Invasive zygomycosis: update on pathogenesis, clinical manifestations, and management. Infect Dis Clin North Am 2006; 20(3):581–607, vi.

28. Legouge C, Caillot D, Chretien ML, et al. The reversed halo sign: pathognomonic pattern of pulmonary mucormycosis in leukemic patients with neutropenia? Clin Infect Dis 2014;58(5): 672–8.

29. Georgiadou SP, Sipsas NV, Marom EM, et al. The diagnostic value of halo and reversed halo signs for invasive mold infections in compromised hosts. Clin Infect Dis 2011;52(9):1144–55.

30. Chamilos G, Marom EM, Lewis RE, et al. Predictors of pulmonary zygomycosis versus invasive pulmonary aspergillosis in patients with cancer. Clin Infect Dis 2005;41(1):60–6.

31. Lanternier F, Sun HY, Ribaud P, et al. Mucormycosis in organ and stem cell transplant recipients. Clin Infect Dis 2012;54(11):1629–36.

32. Kontoyiannis DP, Chamilos G, Hassan SA, et al. Increased culture recovery of Zygomycetes under physiologic temperature conditions. Am J Clin Pathol 2007;127(2):208–12.

33. Sanguinetti M, Posteraro B. Identification of molds by MALDI-TOF mass spectrometry. J Clin Microbiol 2016;55(2):369–79.

34. Walsh TJ, Gamaletsou MN, McGinnis MR, et al. Early clinical and laboratory diagnosis of invasive pulmonary, extrapulmonary, and disseminated mucormycosis (zygomycosis). Clin Infect Dis 2012; 54(Suppl 1):S55–60.

35. Borras R, Rosello P, Chilet M, et al. Positive result of the Aspergillus galactomannan antigen assay using bronchoalveolar lavage fluid from a patient with an invasive infection due to Lichtheimia ramosa. J Clin Microbiol 2010;48(8):3035–6.

36. Millon L, Herbrecht R, Grenouillet F, et al. Early diagnosis and monitoring of mucormycosis by detection of circulating DNA in serum: retrospective analysis of 44 cases collected through the French Surveillance Network of Invasive Fungal Infections (RESSIF). Clin Microbiol Infect 2015;22(9):810.e1–8.

37. Tedder M, Spratt JA, Anstadt MP, et al. Pulmonary mucormycosis: results of medical and surgical therapy. Ann Thorac Surg 1994;57(4):1044–50.

38. Chamilos G, Lewis RE, Kontoyiannis DP. Delaying amphotericin B-based frontline therapy significantly increases mortality among patients with hematologic malignancy who have zygomycosis. Clin Infect Dis 2008;47(4):503–9.

39. Hamill RJ. Amphotericin B formulations: a comparative review of efficacy and toxicity. Drugs 2013; 73(9):919–34.

40. Lanternier F, Poiree S, Elie C, et al. Prospective pilot study of high-dose (10 mg/kg/day) liposomal amphotericin B (L-AMB) for the initial treatment of mucormycosis. J Antimicrob Chemother 2015; 70(11):3116–23.

41. van Burik JA, Hare RS, Solomon HF, et al. Posaconazole is effective as salvage therapy in zygomycosis: a retrospective summary of 91 cases. Clin Infect Dis 2006;42(7):e61–65.

42. Cornely OA, Maertens J, Winston DJ, et al. Posaconazole vs. fluconazole or itraconazole prophylaxis in patients with neutropenia. N Engl J Med 2007; 356(4):348–59.

43. Marty FM, Ostrosky-Zeichner L, Cornely OA, et al. Isavuconazole treatment for mucormycosis: a single-arm open-label trial and case-control analysis. Lancet Infect Dis 2016;16(7):828–37.

44. Ibrahim AS, Gebremariam T, Fu Y, et al. Combination echinocandin-polyene treatment of murine mucormycosis. Antimicrob Agents Chemother 2008; 52(4):1556–8.

45. Reed C, Bryant R, Ibrahim AS, et al. Combination polyene-caspofungin treatment of rhino-orbital-cerebral mucormycosis. Clin Infect Dis 2008; 47(3):364–71.

46. Abidi MZ, Sohail MR, Cummins N, et al. Stability in the cumulative incidence, severity and mortality of

101 cases of invasive mucormycosis in high-risk patients from 1995 to 2011: a comparison of eras immediately before and after the availability of voriconazole and echinocandin-amphotericin combination therapies. Mycoses 2014;57(11):687–98.

47. Ibrahim AS, Gebremariam T, Schwartz JA, et al. Posaconazole mono- or combination therapy for treatment of murine zygomycosis. Antimicrob Agents Chemother 2009;53(2):772–5.

48. Spellberg B, Ibrahim A, Roilides E, et al. Combination therapy for mucormycosis: why, what, and how? Clin Infect Dis 2012;54(suppl 1):S73–8.

49. Kontoyiannis DP, Wessel VC, Bodey GP, et al. Zygomycosis in the 1990s in a tertiary-care cancer center. Clin Infect Dis 2000;30(6):851–6.

50. Tragiannidis A, Groll AH. Hyperbaric oxygen therapy and other adjunctive treatments for zygomycosis. Clin Microbiol Infect 2009;15:82–6.

51. Rodriguez MM, Calvo E, Marine M, et al. Efficacy of liposomal amphotericin B combined with gamma interferon or granulocyte-macrophage colony-stimulating factor for treatment of systemic zygomycosis in mice. Antimicrob Agents Chemother 2009; 53(8):3569–71.

52. Kaide CG, Khandelwal S. Hyperbaric oxygen: applications in infectious disease. Emerg Med Clin North Am 2008;26(2):571–95, xi.

53. Ibrahim AS, Gebermariam T, Fu Y, et al. The iron chelator deferasirox protects mice from mucormycosis through iron starvation. J Clin Invest 2007; 117(9):2649–57.

54. Spellberg B, Ibrahim AS, Chin-Hong PV, et al. The Deferasirox–AmBisome Therapy for Mucormycosis (DEFEAT Mucor) study: a randomized, double-blinded, placebo-controlled trial. J Antimicrob Chemother 2012;67(3):715–22.

55. Hawksworth DL. A new dawn for the naming of fungi: impacts of decisions made in Melbourne in July 2011 on the future publication and regulation of fungal names. IMA Fungus 2011;2(2):155–62.

56. Guarro J. Fusariosis, a complex infection caused by a high diversity of fungal species refractory to treatment. Eur J Clin Microbiol Infect Dis 2013; 32(12):1491–500.

57. Nucci M, Marr KA, Queiroz-Telles F, et al. Fusarium infection in hematopoietic stem cell transplant recipients. Clin Infect Dis 2004;38(9):1237–42.

58. Nucci M, Anaissie EJ, Queiroz-Telles F, et al. Outcome predictors of 84 patients with hematologic malignancies and Fusarium infection. Cancer 2003;98(2):315–9.

59. Garnica M, da Cunha MO, Portugal R, et al. Risk factors for invasive fusariosis in patients with acute myeloid leukemia and in hematopoietic cell transplant recipients. Clin Infect Dis 2015;60(6):875–80.

60. Anaissie EJ, Kuchar RT, Rex JH, et al. Fusariosis associated with pathogenic fusarium species

colonization of a hospital water system: a new paradigm for the epidemiology of opportunistic mold infections. Clin Infect Dis 2001;33(11): 1871–8.

61. Mayayo E, Pujol I, Guarro J. Experimental pathogenicity of four opportunist Fusarium species in a murine model. J Med Microbiol 1999;48(4):363–6.

62. Nelson PE, Dignani MC, Anaissie EJ. Taxonomy, biology, and clinical aspects of Fusarium species. Clin Microbiol Rev 1994;7(4):479–504.

63. Davoudi S, Kumar VA, Jiang Y, et al. Invasive mould sinusitis in patients with haematological malignancies: a 10 year single-centre study. J Antimicrob Chemother 2015;70(10):2899–905.

64. Nucci M, Anaissie E. Cutaneous infection by Fusarium species in healthy and immunocompromised hosts: implications for diagnosis and management. Clin Infect Dis 2002;35(8):909–20.

65. Boutati EI, Anaissie EJ. A significant emerging pathogen in patients with hematologic malignancy: ten years' experience at a cancer center and implications for management. Blood 1997;90(3): 999–1008.

66. Rezai KA, Eliott D, Plous O, et al. Disseminated Fusarium infection presenting as bilateral endogenous endophthalmitis in a patient with acute myeloid leukemia. Arch Ophthalmol 2005;123(5): 702–3.

67. Hennequin C, Ranaivoarimalala C, Chouaki T, et al. Comparison of aerobic standard medium with specific fungal medium for detecting fusarium spp in blood cultures. Eur J Clin Microbiol Infect Dis 2002;21(10):748–50.

68. Guarro J, Nucci M, Akiti T, et al. Mixed infection caused by two species of Fusarium in a human immunodeficiency virus-positive patient. J Clin Microbiol 2000;38(9):3460–2.

69. Nucci M, Anaissie E. Fusarium infections in immunocompromised patients. Clin Microbiol Rev 2007;20(4):695–704.

70. Guarro J, Gene J. Fusarium infections. criteria for the identification of the responsible species. Mycoses 1992;35(5–6):109–14.

71. Marinach-Patrice C, Lethuillier A, Marly A, et al. Use of mass spectrometry to identify clinical Fusarium isolates. Clin Microbiol Infect 2009;15(7): 634–42.

72. Hennequin C, Abachin E, Symoens F, et al. Identification of fusarium species involved in human infections by 28S rRNA gene sequencing. J Clin Microbiol 1999;37(11):3586–9.

73. Liu K, Howell DN, Perfect JR, et al. Morphologic criteria for the preliminary identification of fusarium, paecilomyces, and acremonium species by histopathology. Am J Clin Pathol 1998;109(1):45–54.

74. Marom EM, Holmes AM, Bruzzi JF, et al. Imaging of pulmonary fusariosis in patients with hematologic

malignancies. Am J Roentgenol 2008;190(6): 1605–9.

75. Tortorano AM, Esposto MC, Prigitano A, et al. Cross-reactivity of Fusarium spp. in the Aspergillus galactomannan enzyme-linked immunosorbent assay. J Clin Microbiol 2012;50(3):1051–3.

76. Nucci M, Carlesse F, Cappellano P, et al. Earlier diagnosis of invasive fusariosis with Aspergillus serum galactomannan testing. PLoS One 2014; 9(1):e87784.

77. Cornely OA, Arikan-Akdagli S, Dannaoui E, et al. ESCMID and ECMM joint clinical guidelines for the diagnosis and management of mucormycosis 2013. Clin Microbiol Infect 2014;20(Suppl 3):5–26.

78. Guarro J. Lessons from animal studies for the treatment of invasive human infections due to uncommon fungi. J Antimicrob Chemother 2011;66(7): 1447–66.

79. Azor M, Gené J, Cano J, et al. In vitro antifungal susceptibility and molecular characterization of clinical isolates of Fusarium verticillioides (F. moniliforme) and Fusarium thapsinum. Antimicrob Agents Chemother 2008;52(6):2228–31.

80. Azor M, Cano J, Gené J, et al. High genetic diversity and poor in vitro response to antifungals of clinical strains of Fusarium oxysporum. J Antimicrob Chemother 2009;63(6):1152–5.

81. Alastruey-Izquierdo A, Cuenca-Estrella M, Monzon A, et al. Antifungal susceptibility profile of clinical Fusarium spp. isolates identified by molecular methods. J Antimicrob Chemother 2008;61(4): 805–9.

82. Tortorano AM, Prigitano A, Dho G, et al. Species distribution and in vitro antifungal susceptibility patterns of 75 clinical isolates of Fusarium spp. from Northern Italy. Antimicrob Agents Chemother 2008;52(7):2683–5.

83. Azor M, Gené J, Cano J, et al. Universal in vitro antifungal resistance of genetic clades of the Fusarium solani species complex. Antimicrob Agents Chemother 2007;51(4):1500–3.

84. Cornely OA, Schmitz K, Aisenbrey S. The first echinocandin: caspofungin. Mycoses 2002;45(Suppl 3):56–60.

85. Pujol I, Guarro J, Gene J, et al. In-vitro antifungal susceptibility of clinical and environmental Fusarium spp. strains. J Antimicrob Chemother 1997; 39(2):163–7.

86. Arikan S, Lozano-Chiu M, Paetznick V, et al. Microdilution susceptibility testing of amphotericin b, itraconazole, and voriconazole against clinical isolates of Aspergillus and Fusarium species. J Clin Microbiol 1999;37(12):3946–51.

87. Perfect JR. Treatment of non-Aspergillus moulds in immunocompromised patients, with amphotericin B lipid complex. Clin Infect Dis 2005;40(Suppl 6): S401–8.

88. Perfect JR, Marr KA, Walsh TJ, et al. Voriconazole treatment for less-common, emerging, or refractory fungal infections. Clin Infect Dis 2003;36(9): 1122–31.

89. Lortholary O, Obenga G, Biswas P, et al. International retrospective analysis of 73 cases of invasive fusariosis treated with voriconazole. Antimicrob Agents Chemother 2010;54(10):4446–50.

90. Raad II, Hachem RY, Herbrecht R, et al. Posaconazole as salvage treatment for invasive fusariosis in patients with underlying hematologic malignancy and other conditions. Clin Infect Dis 2006;42(10): 1398–403.

91. Thompson GR 3rd, Wiederhold NP. Isavuconazole: a comprehensive review of spectrum of activity of a new triazole. Mycopathologia 2010;170(5):291–313.

92. Durand-Joly I, Alfandari S, Benchikh Z, et al. Successful outcome of disseminated fusarium infection with skin localization treated with voriconazole and amphotericin B-lipid complex in a patient with acute leukemia. J Clin Microbiol 2003;41(10): 4898–900.

93. Inano S, Kimura M, Iida J, et al. Combination therapy of voriconazole and terbinafine for disseminated fusariosis: case report and literature review. J Infect Chemother 2013;19(6):1173–80.

94. Cordoba S, Rodero L, Vivot W, et al. In vitro interactions of antifungal agents against clinical isolates of Fusarium spp. Int J Antimicrob Agents 2008;31(2): 171–4.

95. Ortoneda M, Capilla J, Javier Pastor F, et al. In vitro interactions of licensed and novel antifungal drugs against Fusarium spp. Diagn Microbiol Infect Dis 2004;48(1):69–71.

96. Chen M, Zeng J, De Hoog GS, et al. The 'species complex' issue in clinically relevant fungi: a case study in Scedosporium apiospermum. Fungal Biol 2016;120(2):137–46.

97. Lackner M, de Hoog GS, Yang L, et al. Proposed nomenclature for Pseudallescheria, Scedosporium and related genera. Fungal Diversity 2014;67(1): 1–10.

98. Cortez KJ, Roilides E, Quiroz-Telles F, et al. Infections caused by Scedosporium spp. Clin Microbiol Rev 2008;21(1):157–97.

99. Guerrero A, Torres P, Duran MT, et al. Airborne outbreak of nosocomial Scedosporium prolificans infection. Lancet 2001;357(9264):1267–8.

100. Rodriguez-Tudela JL, Berenguer J, Guarro J, et al. Epidemiology and outcome of Scedosporium prolificans infection, a review of 162 cases. Med Mycol 2009;47(4):359–70.

101. Husain S, Muñoz P, Forrest G, et al. Infections due to Scedosporium apiospermum and Scedosporium prolificans in transplant recipients: clinical characteristics and impact of antifungal agent therapy on outcome. Clin Infect Dis 2005;40(1):89–99.

102. Larcher G, Cimon B, Symoens F, et al. A 33 kDa serine proteinase from Scedosporium apiospermum. Biochem J 1996;315(Pt 1):119–26.

103. Roilides E, Simitsopoulou M, Katragkou A, et al. Host immune response against Scedosporium species. Med Mycol 2009;47(4):433–40.

104. Bittencourt VC, Figueiredo RT, da Silva RB, et al. An alpha-glucan of Pseudallescheria boydii is involved in fungal phagocytosis and Toll-like receptor activation. J Biol Chem 2006;281(32):22614–23.

105. Winn RM, Gil-Lamaignere C, Roilides E, et al. Effects of interleukin-15 on antifungal responses of human polymorphonuclear leukocytes against Fusarium spp. and Scedosporium spp. Cytokine 2005;31(1):1–8.

106. Katragkou A, Dotis J, Kotsiou M, et al. Scedosporium apiospermum infection after near-drowning. Mycoses 2007;50(5):412–21.

107. Cimon B, Carrere J, Vinatier JF, et al. Clinical significance of Scedosporium apiospermum in patients with cystic fibrosis. Eur J Clin Microbiol Infect Dis 2000;19(1):53–6.

108. Schell WA. New aspects of emerging fungal pathogens. A multifaceted challenge. Clin Lab Med 1995;15(2):365–87.

109. Blyth CC, Harun A, Middleton PG, et al. Detection of occult Scedosporium species in respiratory tract specimens from patients with cystic fibrosis by use of selective media. J Clin Microbiol 2010;48(1):314–6.

110. Berenguer J, Diaz-Mediavilla J, Urra D, et al. Central nervous system infection caused by Pseudallescheria boydii: case report and review. Rev Infect Dis 1989;11(6):890–6.

111. Harun A, Blyth CC, Gilgado F, et al. Development and validation of a multiplex PCR for detection of Scedosporium spp. in respiratory tract specimens from patients with cystic fibrosis. J Clin Microbiol 2011;49(4):1508–12.

112. Odabasi Z, Paetznick VL, Rodriguez JR, et al. Differences in beta-glucan levels in culture supernatants of a variety of fungi. Med Mycol 2006;44(3):267–72.

113. Lackner M, de Hoog GS, Verweij PE, et al. Species-specific antifungal susceptibility patterns of Scedosporium and Pseudallescheria species. Antimicrob Agents Chemother 2012;56(5):2635–42.

114. Troke P, Aguirrebengoa K, Arteaga C, et al. Treatment of scedosporiosis with voriconazole: clinical experience with 107 patients. Antimicrob Agents Chemother 2008;52(5):1743–50.

115. Meletiadis J, Mouton JW, Meis JF, et al. In vitro drug interaction modeling of combinations of azoles with terbinafine against clinical Scedosporium prolificans isolates. Antimicrob Agents Chemother 2003;47(1):106–17.

116. Bhat SV, Paterson DL, Rinaldi MG, et al. Scedosporium prolificans brain abscess in a patient with chronic granulomatous disease: successful combination therapy with voriconazole and terbinafine. Scand J Infect Dis 2007;39(1):87–90.

117. Gosbell IB, Toumasatos V, Yong J, et al. Cure of orthopaedic infection with Scedosporium prolificans, using voriconazole plus terbinafine, without the need for radical surgery. Mycoses 2003;46(5–6):233–6.

118. Ortoneda M, Capilla J, Pastor FJ, et al. Interaction of granulocyte colony-stimulating factor and high doses of liposomal amphotericin B in the treatment of systemic murine scedosporiosis. Diagn Microbiol Infect Dis 2004;50(4):247–51.

119. Fothergill AW. Identification of dematiaceous fungi and their role in human disease. Clin Infect Dis 1996;22(Suppl 2):S179–84.

120. Schieffelin JS, Garcia-Diaz JB, Loss GE Jr, et al. Phaeohyphomycosis fungal infections in solid organ transplant recipients: clinical presentation, pathology, and treatment. Transpl Infect Dis 2014;16(2):270–8.

121. Ben-Ami R, Lewis RE, Raad II, et al. Phaeohyphomycosis in a tertiary care cancer center. Clin Infect Dis 2009;48(8):1033–41.

122. McCarty TP, Baddley JW, Walsh TJ, et al. Phaeohyphomycosis in transplant recipients: results from the transplant associated infection surveillance network (TRANSNET). Med Mycol 2015;53(5):440–6.

123. Feng B, Wang X, Hauser M, et al. Molecular cloning and characterization of WdPKS1, a gene involved in dihydroxynaphthalene melanin biosynthesis and virulence in Wangiella(Exophiala) dermatitidis. Infect Immun 2001;69(3):1781–94.

124. Schnitzler N, Peltroche-Llacsahuanga H, Bestier N, et al. Effect of melanin and carotenoids of Exophiala (Wangiella) dermatitidis on phagocytosis, oxidative burst, and killing by human neutrophils. Infect Immun 1999;67(1):94–101.

125. Manning SC, Schaefer SD, Close LG, et al. Culture-positive allergic fungal sinusitis. Arch Otolaryngol Head Neck Surg 1991;117(2):174–8.

126. Flanagan KL, Bryceson AD. Disseminated infection due to Bipolaris australiensis in a young immunocompetent man: case report and review. Clin Infect Dis 1997;25(2):311–3.

127. Khan JA, Hussain ST, Hasan S, et al. Disseminated Bipolaris infection in an immunocompetent host: an atypical presentation. J Pak Med Assoc 2000;50(2):68–71.

128. Schoch CL, Seifert KA, Huhndorf S, et al. Nuclear ribosomal internal transcribed spacer (ITS) region as a universal DNA barcode marker for Fungi. Proc Natl Acad Sci 2012;109(16):6241–6.

129. Brandt ME, Warnock DW. Epidemiology, clinical manifestations, and therapy of infections caused by dematiaceous fungi. J Chemother 2003;15(Suppl 2):36–47.

130. Badali H, de Hoog GS, Curfs-Breuker I, et al. Use of amplified fragment length polymorphism to identify 42 Cladophialophora strains related to cerebral phaeohyphomycosis with in vitro antifungal susceptibility. J Clin Microbiol 2010;48(7):2350–6.

131. Chowdhary A, Hagen F, Curfs-Breuker I, et al. In vitro activities of eight antifungal drugs against a global collection of genotyped Exserohilum isolates. Antimicrob Agents Chemother 2015;59(10): 6642–5.

132. Vermes A, Guchelaar HJ, Dankert J. Flucytosine: a review of its pharmacology, clinical indications, pharmacokinetics, toxicity and drug interactions. J Antimicrob Chemother 2000;46(2):171–9.

133. Espinel-Ingroff A. In vitro antifungal activities of anidulafungin and micafungin, licensed agents and the investigational triazole posaconazole as determined by NCCLS methods for 12,052 fungal isolates: review of the literature. Rev Iberoam Micol 2003;20(4):121–36.

Moving?

Printed and bound by CPI Group (UK) Ltd, Croydon, CR0 4YY

08/05/2025

01864701-0008